Cell Biology, Genetics, and Biochemistry for Pre-Clinical Students

Cell Biology, Genetics, and Biochemistry for Pre-Clinical Students

RENÉE J. LECLAIR

PDF AND EPUB FREE ONLINE AT: HTTPS://DOI.ORG/10.21061/CELLBIO

VIRGINIA TECH CARILION SCHOOL OF MEDICINE IN ASSOCIATION WITH VIRGINIA TECH PUBLISHING
BLACKSBURG, VA

Suggested citation: LeClair, Renée (2021). *Cell Biology, Genetics, and Biochemistry for Pre-Clinical Students.* Roanoke: Virginia Tech Carilion School of Medicine. https://doi.org/10.21061/cellbio. Licensed with CC BY-NC-SA 4.0 https://creativecommons.org/licenses/by-nc-sa/4.0.

Publisher: This work is published by the Virginia Tech Carilion School of Medicine in association with Virginia Tech Publishing, a division of the University Libraries at Virginia Tech.

Virginia Tech Carilion School of Medicine 2 Riverside Circle Roanoke, VA 24016 USA

Virginia Tech Publishing University Libraries at Virginia Tech 560 Drillfield Drive Blacksburg, VA 24061 USA https://publishing.vt.edu publishing@vt.edu

This work is also distributed by LibreTexts, Davis, CA USA info@libretexts.org. Note: The LibreTexts version of this work at https://med.libretexts.org/@go/page/37584 may differ from this version.

Peer review: This book has undergone single-blind peer review by five external reviewers.

Accessibility statement: Virginia Tech Publishing is committed to making its publications accessible in accordance with the Americans with Disabilities Act of 1990. The Pressbooks (HTML) and ePub versions of this text are tagged structurally and include alternative text, which allows for machine readability.

Publication cataloging information:
LeClair, Renée, author
Cell Biology, Genetics, and Biochemistry for Pre-Clinical Students / Renée LeClair
Pages cm
ISBN 978-1-949373-42-4 (PDF)
ISBN 978-1-949373-43-1 (ePub)
ISBN 978-1-957213-05-7 (Pressbooks) https://pressbooks.lib.vt.edu/cellbio
ISBN 978-1-949373-41-7 (Print)
URI (Universal Resource Identifier) http://hdl.handle.net/10919/102308
DOI https://doi.org/10.21061/cellbio

1. Biochemistry -- Textbooks
2. Cytology -- Textbooks
3. Cytogenetics -- Textbooks

   Title QH581.2 B613

Disclaimer: The information in this textbook is intended for educational purposes only and is not meant to take the place of medical care, diagnoses, or services. Please see your healthcare provider about any health concerns.

Cover art: Adapted from DNA double helix grooves by Biochemlife. CC BY SA 4.0.
Illustration and cover design: Kindred Grey

Contents

Introduction

Cell Biology, Genetics, and Biochemistry for Pre-Clinical Students is intended to address both necessary content and align with the preclerkship curricular needs. The utility of a flexible text can positively impact the learning environment and increase student engagement and performance. This text is made to be adaptable by using pieces and parts to suit students and inspire the addition of elements to this living resource. Features of this resource include:

- Detailed learning objectives are provided at the beginning of each subsection:
- High resolution, color contrasting figures illustrate concepts, relationships, and processes throughout
- Summary tables display detailed information
- Selected chapters provide additional sources of information
- Accessibility features including structured heads and alternative-text provide access for readers accessing the work via a screen-reader

This resource was designed to fill a gap in undergraduate medical education (UME) and support preclerkship education in the content area of basic science for medical education. Its content is aligned to USMLE(R) (United States Medical Licensing Examination) providing coverage of topics including: cell biology, genetics and biochemistry. Unlike traditional textbooks, the organization of this resource is driven by curricular structure, rather than subject area. As the format and design of UME differs across many programs, this resource is purposefully brief and flexible, allowing for rapid adaptation across programs. The resource is organized into small chapters that can be used to support student preparation in any arrangement. The sections are not intended to be all-inclusive, but rather primers for applied content delivery. Similarly, clinical context is only briefly discussed allowing the user to apply the basic content (delivered here) in the clinical context used by their specific curricular structure. In our curriculum, these topic areas are interwoven into problem-based learning cases. The cases and clinical correlates change regularly and having the flexibility of these short resources that can be applied to many scenarios across the first and second years of our curriculum is beneficial.

Over the past twenty years, medical education has undergone a rapid curricular restructuring. This is in part due to recommendations of the Flexner report,[1] coupled with the changes observed in millennial[2] and iGen learners. To accommodate the integration of additional core competencies, the majority of medical programs have moved away from discipline-based delivery and currently use some form of integrated curricular format.[3] This allows material to be presented in a more clinically realistic and pertinent format without the constraints of artificial discipline silos. This movement has had positive impacts on programmatic outcomes and student performance, but it has presented some challenges for curricular design, student engagement and educational resources.

The creation of this resource was intended to address three predominant challenges in medical education: need, student engagement and cost of textbooks. Although contemporary medical curricula have moved to a cohesive, integrated format, the required textbooks for undergraduate medical education remain traditional and discipline-based. In the absence of an integrated resource, students are requested to purchase and juggle preparation materials between many different discipline-based textbooks. Traditional textbooks are often designed to support subject-based courses, rather than a clinically centered education. (Medical schools are educating future physicians, not future biochemists, physiologists, etc.) A high volume of content, some of it lacking alignment with class sessions coupled with restrictions on student contact time imposed by accrediting bodies, means that faculty across the country are having to rethink preparation materials to facilitate efficient, focused learning experiences.

This resource is intended to provide learners with a high-level view of relevant topical areas that will be further elaborated on within the classroom setting. Unlike other traditional textbooks, it is not intended to include all content a learner would need about the relevant subject area but to function as a stepping stone towards mastery of the content.

As programs embrace the philosophy of student-directed learning embedded in adult learning theory, more simplified readily available resources will be essential to support this fast-paced learning of health professional educational programs. The short-divided nature of the resource makes it flexible and adaptable to many different curricular settings as topic areas can be quickly divided or separated for ideal use. While there are many factors that can contribute to a student's lack of preparation, lengthy textbook resources for a single integrated classroom session have a significant negative impact. So while an integrated curricular model enhances many aspects of learning, it makes using traditional textbooks cumbersome and disjointed for students. This resource hopes to address this concern.

Finally, there is a wealth of "medical" content freely accessible online, and students can find themselves spending a significant amount of time trying to identify alternative resources that may—or may not—be appropriate. Faculty taking ownership to identify and adapt realistic materials for each session reduces the concern that students are finding misinformation through internet sources, and this project allows faculty to create a resource that harnesses the best attributes of many different formats into a product that best supports the learning environment. Otherwise, external online resources are also likely to contain extraneous content that is not aligned with the classroom learning objectives (akin to subject-based textbook chapters), so it can also reduce the perceived worth of preparation. If the integrated resource is generated correctly, concisely and accurately by the faculty, the students will gain trust, rely on the vetted resources and prepare for the active classroom.

— Renée LeClair

Notes

1. Cooke M, Irby DM, Ph D, et al. American Medical Education 100 Years after the Flexner Report. 2006:1339-1344.
2. Roberts DH, Newman LR, Schwartzstein RM. Twelve tips for facilitating Millennials' learning. *Medical Teacher*. 2012;34:274-278.
3. VanTassel-Baska J, Wood S. The integrated curriculum model (ICM). *Learning and Individual Differences*. 2010;20(4):345-357.

Acknowledgments

Funding and In-Kind Support
Publication of this work is made possible in part through the support of VIVA (Virtual Library of Virginia), LibreTexts, the Open Education Initiative of the University Libraries at Virginia Tech, and Virginia Tech Publishing.

Peer Reviewers
Llanie Nobile, Marquette University
Jan Pitcairn, University of New England College of Osteopathic Medicine
Anamika Sengupta, University of the Incarnate Word School of Osteopathic Medicine
Douglas Spicer, University of New England College of Osteopathic Medicine
Kathryn Thompson, University of New England College of Osteopathic Medicine

Editorial Team
Managing Editor: Anita Walz
Graphic Design and Editorial Assistance: Kindred Grey
Alternative Text: Sophia DeSimone

Special Thanks
Henry Jakubowski, Emeritus, College of Saint Benedict and Saint John's University
Delmar Larson, Founder, LibreTexts
Christa Miller, Accessible Technologies, Virginia Tech

About the Author

Renée J. LeClair is an Associate Professor in the Department of Basic Science Education at the Virginia Tech Carilion School of Medicine, where her role is to engage activities that support the departmental mission of developing an integrated medical experience using evidence-based delivery grounded in the science of learning. She received a Ph.D. at Rice University and completed a postdoctoral fellowship at the Maine Medical Center Research Institute in vascular biology. She became involved in medical education, curricular renovation, and implementation of innovative teaching methods during her first faculty appointment, at the University of New England, College of Osteopathic Medicine. In 2013, she moved to a new medical school, University of South Carolina, School of Medicine, Greenville. The opportunities afforded by joining a new program and serving as the Chair of the Curriculum committee provided a blank slate for creative curricular development and close involvement with the accreditation process. During her tenure she developed and directed a team-taught student-centered undergraduate medical course that integrated the scientific and clinical sciences to assess all six-core competencies of medical education.

Instructor Resources

How to Adopt This Book

This is an open textbook. That means that this book is freely available and you are welcome to use, adapt, and share this book with attribution according to the Creative Commons NonCommercial ShareAlike 4.0 (CC BY-NC-SA 4.0) license https://creativecommons.org/licenses/by-nc-sa/4.0. (Many, but not all images, illustrations, etc in this book are licensed under CC BY 4.0.)

Instructors reviewing, adopting, or adapting this textbook are encouraged to register at https://bit.ly/interest-preclinical. This assists the Open Education Initiative at Virginia Tech in assessing the impact of the book and allows us to more easily alert instructors of additional resources, features and opportunities.

Finding Additional Resources for Your Course

The main landing page for the book is https://doi.org/10.21061/cellbio.

This page includes:

- Links to multiple electronic versions of the textbook (PDF, ePub, HTML)
- Links to the instructor resource-sharing portal
- Link to errata document
- Links to other books within this series

Sharing Resources You've Created

Have you created any supplementary materials for use with Cell Biology, Genetics, and Biochemistry for Pre-Clinical Students such as presentation slides, activities, test items, or a question bank? If so, please consider sharing your materials related to this open textbook. Please tell us about resources you wish to share by using this form: https://bit.ly/interest-preclinical or by directly sharing resources under an open license to the public-facing instructor sharing portal https://www.oercommons.org/groups/pre-clinical-resources/10133.

Customizing This Book

The Creative Commons Attribution NonCommercial-ShareAlike 4.0 license https://creativecommons.org/licenses/by-nc-sa/4.0/legalcode on this book allows customization and redistribution which is NonCommercial, that is "not primarily intended for or directed towards commercial advantage or monetary compensation."

Best practices for attribution are provided at https://wiki.creativecommons.org/wiki/ Best_practices_for_attribution.

This book is hosted in PDF and ePub in VTechWorks, in HTML in Pressbooks and via the LibreTexts platform. Pressbooks and LibreTexts platforms both offer customization/remixing.

Feedback

To report an error or omission, please use https://bit.ly/feedback-preclinical.

We welcome additional feedback at publishing@vt.edu.

1. Biochemistry Basics

Learning Objectives

- Review basic amino acid structure and determine the functional capabilities of amino acids based on their R-groups.
- Review how enzymes catalyze specific reactions essential to a cell and how these reactions have specific chemistry based on the K_m and V_{max} of the enzyme.
- Determine how the kinetics of an enzyme can be altered by cofactors, coenzymes, inhibitors, and activators.

About this Chapter

This chapter is for reference only and contains basic information on amino acid structure and enzyme regulation. The fundamental building blocks of proteins and enzymes are amino acids. Their unique structures and functional groups allow for specific interactions that can enhance enzyme activity, facilitate folding of individual motifs, and provide stability for the protein structure as a whole. The ability to regulate enzyme activity is an essential component to cellular homeostasis. Enzymes can be regulated by many extrinsic factors that will increase or decrease product production, change enzyme concentration, or change substrate availability. Regardless of the mechanisms of regulation, pathway control will be a recurring component to all biochemistry. It should be noted that the mechanisms discussed here are not fully inclusive but highlight the most commonly used mechanisms of regulation in the biochemical reactions presented in the rest of the content.

1.1 Amino Acids

There are twenty commonly occurring amino acids in mammalian proteins (nine essential and eleven nonessential). Each amino acid has a carboxyl group, a primary amino group, and a unique side chain (R-group) bonded to the α-carbon atom. At physiologic pH (approximately 7.4), amino acids are present as zwitter ions with the carboxyl group forming the negatively charged carboxylate ion (COO^-), and the amino group is protonated (NH_3^+) (figure 1.1).

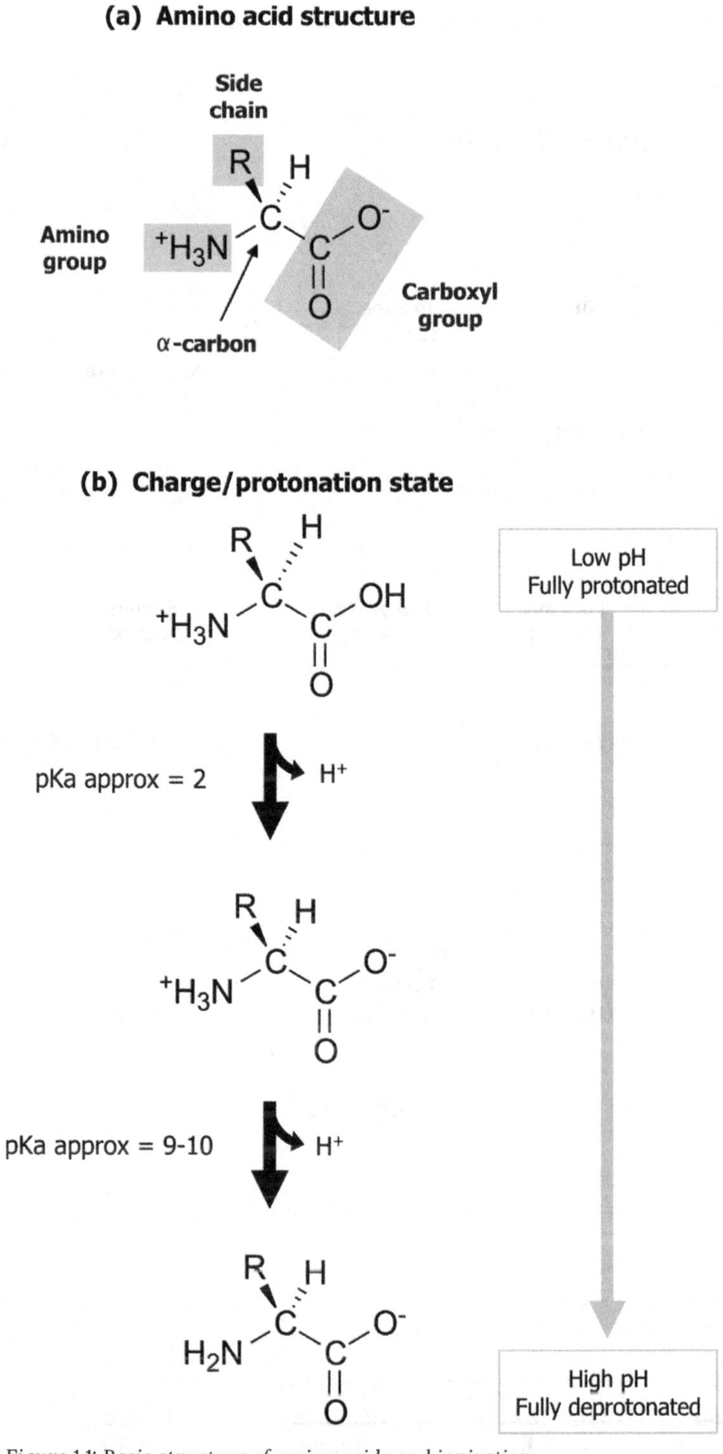

Figure 1.1: Basic structure of amino acids and ionization.

Amino acids can be grouped largely by the functionality of their R-group (figure 1.2).

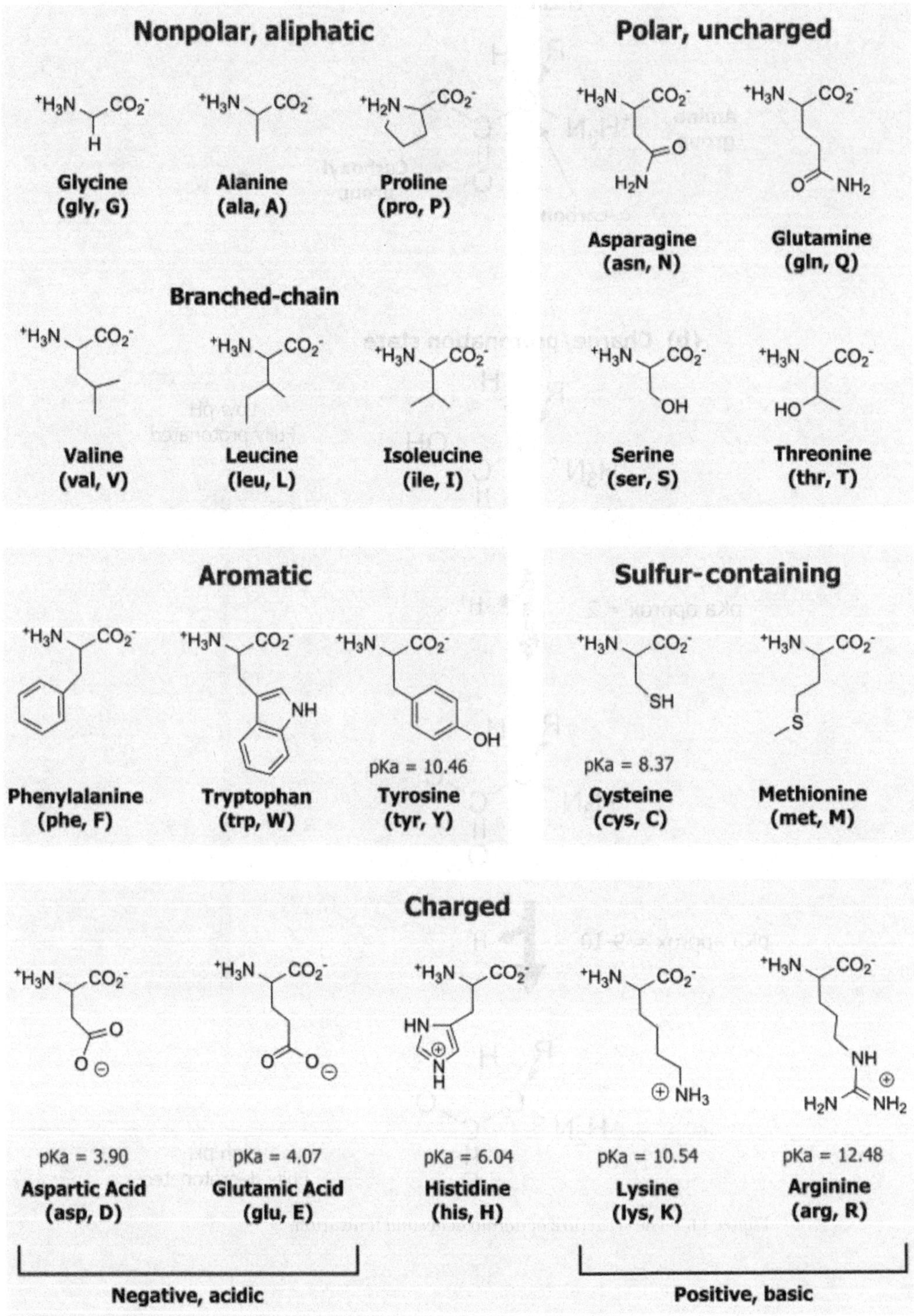

Figure 1.2: Chart of amino acids.

Although it is not essential to memorize the structures of the amino acids, a strong understanding of their general characteristics will be very helpful.

Amino acid functional groups

The primary sequence of a protein is determined by the amino acids in the chain and how these individual units function as a group. More generally, amino acids can be characterized as polar or nonpolar. These fundamental characteristics will determine where the residue resides within the protein (surface or core, within a transmembrane domain or part of the active site) and how the amino acid contributes to folding and catalysis.

Nonpolar residues

Nonpolar amino acids can be further divided into: uncharged (aromatic and nonpolar aliphatic) and sulfur-containing groups. Nonpolar uncharged side chains do not gain or lose protons or participate in hydrogen or ionic bonding. These amino acids typically cluster in the internal regions of a protein, away from the aqueous interface. The exception to this is if these amino acids are present as part of a membrane-bound protein, and in this case, the amino acids may be exposed in the transmembrane region. Proline is also of note, as it forms an unconventional peptide bond and will add a kink in the primary structure of a protein. Sulfur-containing amino acids can participate in disulfide linkages, which are used to stabilize interactions between peptide chains or tertiary structures.

Polar residues

Amino acids with uncharged polar R-groups may participate in hydrogen bonding and undergo modifications such as phosphorylation. Tyrosine, serine, and threonine all have a hydroxyl group within the R-group, and they can also be readily modified by kinase-mediated phosphorylation.

Some amino acids are charged at a physiological pH and can be acidic or basic. These side chains may donate or accept protons, respectively, and the most notable charged amino acid is histidine, which can function as a buffer at a physiological pH.

1.1 References and resources

Text

Ferrier, D. R., ed. *Lippincott Illustrated Reviews: Biochemistry*, 7th ed. Philadelphia: Wolters Kluwer Health/ Lippincott Williams & Wilkins, 2017, Chapter 1: Amino Acids, Chapter 2: Protein Structure.

Lieberman, M., and A. Peet, eds. *Marks' Basic Medical Biochemistry: A Clinical Approach*, 5th ed. Philadelphia: Wolters Kluwer Health/Lippincott Williams & Wilkins, 2018, Chapter 6: Amino Acids in Proteins, Chapter 8: Enzymes as Catalysts, Chapter 9: Regulation of Enzymes.

Figures

Grey, Kindred, Figure 1.1 Basic structure of amino acids and ionization. 2021. Chemical structure by Henry Jakubowski. https://archive.org/details/1.1_20210924. CC BY 4.0.

Grey, Kindred, Figure 1.2 Chart of amino acids. 2021. Chemical structure by Henry Jakubowski. https://archive.org/details/1.2_20210924. CC BY 4.0.

1.2 Enzyme Kinetics

Many translated proteins are also enzymes with a specific metabolic function within the cell. Enzymes help reduce the amount of transition state energy required for a reaction to move forward through several mechanisms:

1. Stabilizing the substrate within the active site,
2. Excluding water from the reaction site,
3. Stabilizing the transition state, and
4. Using cofactors or coenzymes to help with group transfer.

The kinetics of enzyme-catalyzed reactions is mainly determined by the properties of the catalyst. Like all catalysts, the enzyme [E] creates a new reaction pathway. Initially, the substrate [S] is bound to the free enzyme [ES] (figure 1.3).

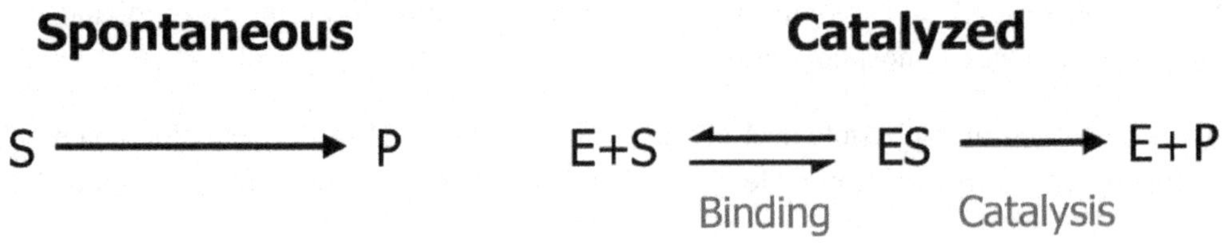

Figure 1.3: Basics of enzyme kinetics.

The rate of this enzyme reaction can be described by the Michaelis-Menten equation, which relates the the initial velocity (v_i) to the concentration of substrate [S] and the two parameters K_m and V_{max}. The V_{max} is defined as the maximal velocity that can be achieved at an infinite substrate concentration, while the K_m is defined as the substrate concentration needed to reach 1/2 V_{max}. The Michaelis constant (K_m) characterizes the affinity of the enzyme for a substrate. A high affinity of the enzyme for a substrate therefore leads to a low K_m value, and vice versa (figure 1.4).

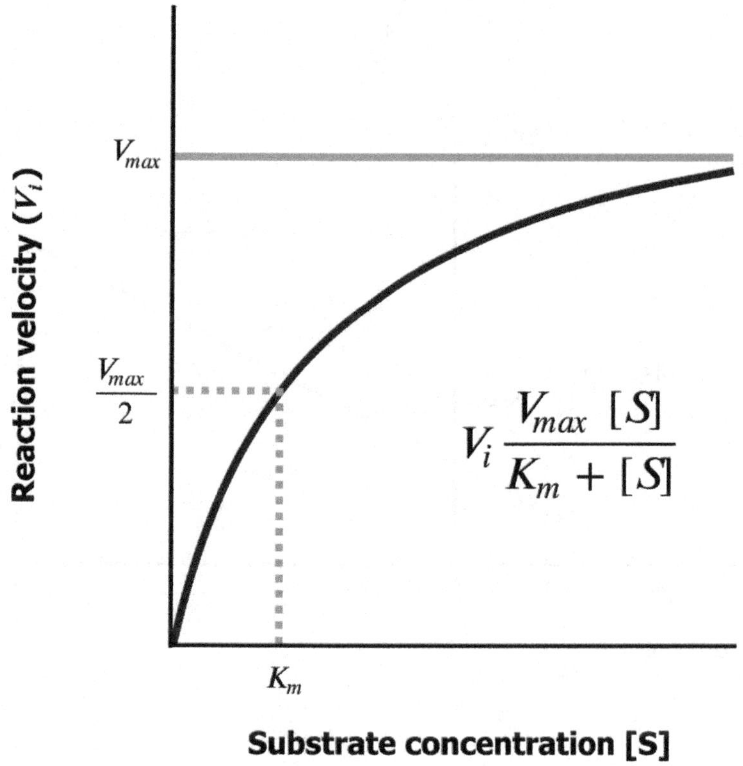

Figure 1.4: Graphical representation of the Michaelis–Menten equation.

Note

The Michaelis-Menten model contains simplifying assumptions (substrate binding is in equilibrium, formation of [P] is irreversible, [E] and [ES] are the only enzyme forms).

Since v_i approaches V_{max} asymptotically, it is difficult to read off reliable values for V_{max} or K_m from diagrams plotting v against [S] (figure 1.4). To alleviate this issue, the Michaelis-Menten equation can be arranged in such a way that the measured points lie on a straight line. In the Lineweaver Burk plot, 1/v is plotted against 1/[S]. The intersections of the line of best fit with the axes then produce $1/V_{max}$ and $-1/K_m$ (figure 1.5).

$$\frac{1}{V} = \frac{K_m}{V_{max}} \left(\frac{1}{[S]}\right) + \frac{1}{V_{max}}$$

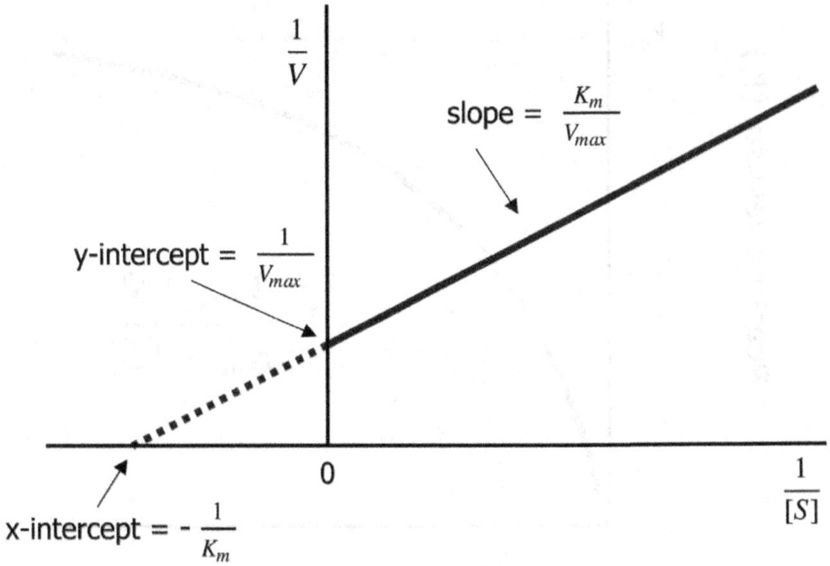

Figure 1.5: Lineweaver–Burk plot to illustrate Km and Vmax.

Factors influencing enzyme kinetics

The catalytic properties of enzymes, and consequently their activity, are influenced by numerous factors, which all must be optimized and controlled if activity measurements are to be performed in a useful and reproducible fashion. These factors include physical quantities (temperature or pressure), the chemical properties of the solution (pH or ionic strength), and the concentrations of all relevant substrates, cofactors, coenzymes, and inhibitors. The role of cofactors (inorganic) or coenzymes (organic) is often to accept or donate electrons in a reaction or to temporarily stabilize the substrate in the course of the reaction. Depending on the type of interaction with the enzyme, a distinction is made between soluble coenzymes and prosthetic groups.

1. **Soluble coenzymes** are bound to the enzyme during a reaction, undergo a chemical change, and are then released again. The original form of the coenzyme is regenerated by a second, independent reaction.
2. **Prosthetic groups** are coenzymes that are tightly bound to the enzyme (sometimes covalently), and remain associated with the enzyme during the reaction. The part of the substrate bound by the coenzyme after release of the first product is then transferred in a second reaction to another substrate or coenzyme of the same enzyme. Many coenzymes are aromatic compounds that cannot be synthesized de novo in animal cells.
3. **Metal ions** can also serve as cofactors. Their functions are variable; some stabilize the native conformation of an enzyme active site, while others are involved in oxidation–reduction reactions or facilitate catalysis by polarizing chemical bonds within the substrate.

Enzyme regulation

Competitive and noncompetitive inhibition

Enzymes can be inhibited or activated by interference from other compounds. These will influence the reaction by changing the K_m or V_{max} of the reaction. Most enzyme inhibitors act reversibly and do not cause permanent changes in the enzyme. However, there are also irreversible inhibitors that modify the target enzyme covalently and permanently. These are termed suicide inhibitors.

Inhibitors can be categorized as competitive or noncompetitive, and this can be determined by comparing the kinetics of the normal versus inhibited reactions.

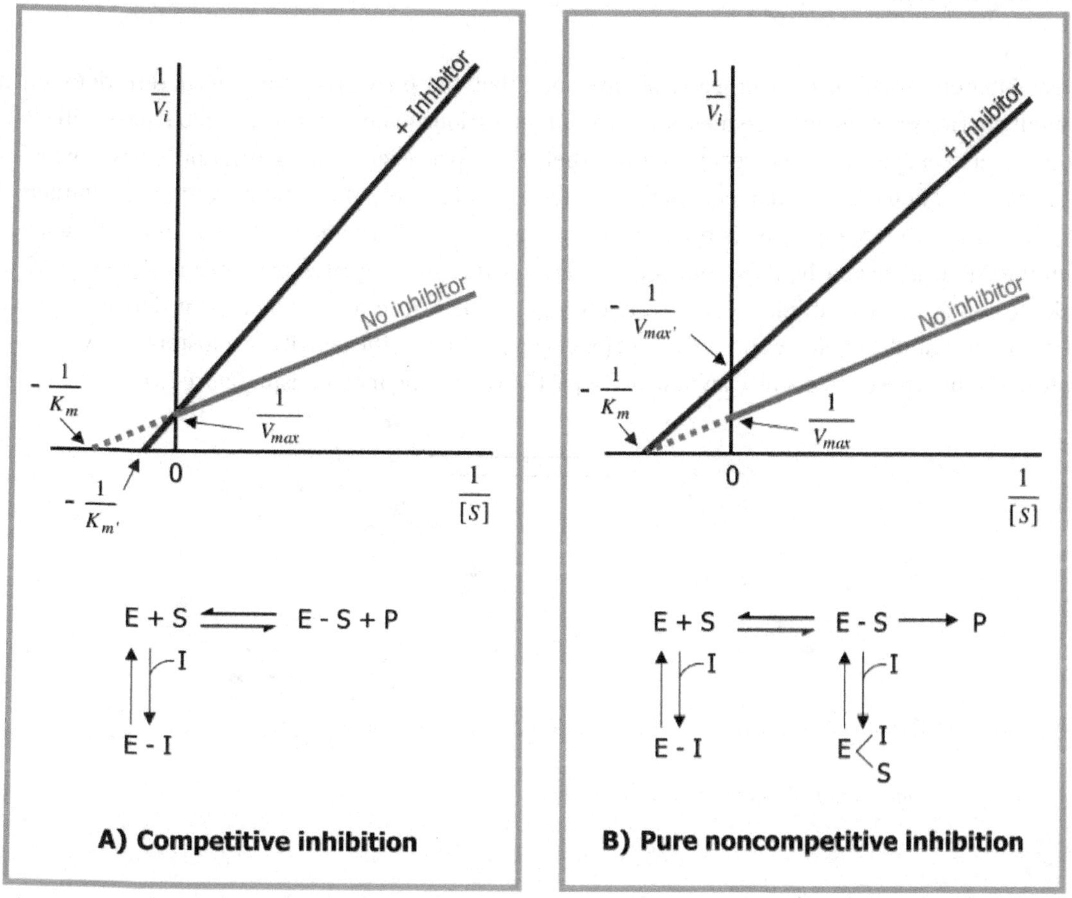

Figure 1.6: Competitive vs. noncompetitive inhibition.

Competitive inhibitors bind the enzyme at the active site and compete with the substrate for binding. Many function as substrate analogs. In the presence of the inhibitor, a higher substrate concentration is therefore needed to achieve a half-maximum rate; the Michaelis constant K_m increases. When substrate concentrations are elevated, this will ultimately displace the inhibitor, and V_{max} will be reached. The maximum rate, V_{max}, is therefore not influenced by competitive inhibitors. In this case, there is no change on V_{max} as competition can be overcome by increasing the concentration of substrate, but there is an increase in the apparent K_m, as a greater substrate concentration is needed to reach V_{max} (figure 1.6(a)).

In contrast, noncompetitive inhibitors bind the enzyme on a site alternative to the substrate binding site, and therefore its effects cannot be overcome by increasing the substrate. In this case, K_m remains unchanged, but k_{cat} (the rate of product formation), and thus V_{max}, decreases. Irreversible inhibitors usually result in a noncompetitive type of inhibition because the concentration of active enzyme [E] decreases (figure 1.6(b)).

The action of inhibitors can be illustrated clearly in the Lineweaver-Burk plot. In this type of plot, the intercept of the approximation lines with the y-axis corresponds to $1/V_{max}$, while the x-axis intercept gives the value of $-1/K_m$. This is why the straight lines obtained in the absence (blue) and presence of a competitive inhibitor (A, red) intersect on the y-axis ($1/V_{max}$), unchanged), while noncompetitive inhibitors (B, red) result in a straight line with a higher y-intercept but unchanged x-intercept ($1/V_{max}$) increased, K_m) unchanged) (figure 1.6).

Allosteric regulation

The Michaelis-Menten model of enzyme catalysis assumes that the enzyme's spatial structure does not alter with substrate binding. However, many enzymes are present in various conformations, which have different catalytic properties. Allosteric enzymes can be recognized by their S-shaped (sigmoidal) saturation curves, which cannot be described using the Michaelis-Menten equation. In allosteric enzymes, the binding efficiency initially rises with increasing [S], because the free enzyme is present in a low-affinity conformation, which is gradually converted into a higher-affinity form. It is only at high [S] values that a lack of free binding sites becomes noticeable and the binding efficiency decreases again. The affinity of allosteric enzymes is therefore not constant, but depends on the type and concentration of the ligand. Inhibitors and activators (effectors) influence the activity of allosteric enzymes by stabilizing certain conformations. These effects play an important part in regulating metabolism (figure 1.7).

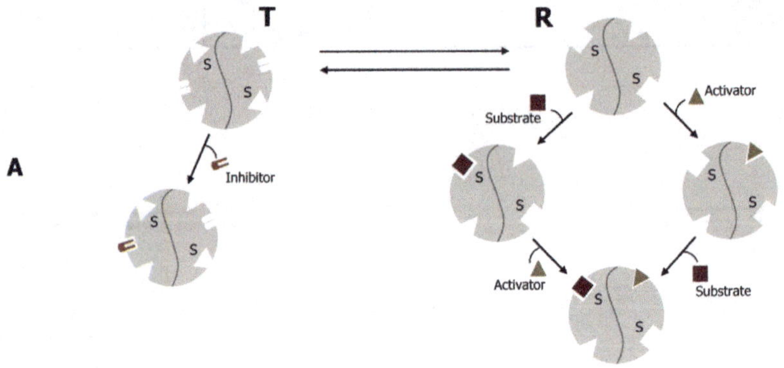

Figure 1.7(a): Allosteric enzyme regulation.

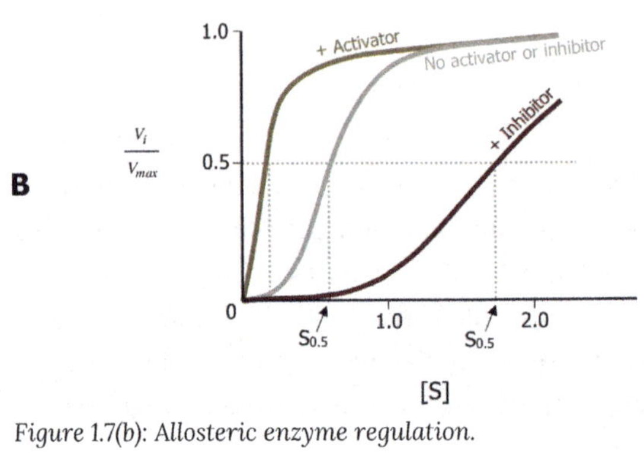

Figure 1.7(b): Allosteric enzyme regulation.

Similar to noncompetitive inhibitors, allosteric effectors will bind sites alternative to the active site. Allosteric activators typically stabilize the relaxed conformation of an enzyme (R), and increase the rate of substrate binding of the subsequent subunits. This is called cooperativity. In contrast, allosteric inhibitors will stabilize the tense (T) conformation of a protein and will increase substrate off (release) rate. The best example of this is with oxygen binding to hemoglobin, which has a quaternary structure with four binding sites for oxygen.

Enzyme regulation through covalent modification

Enzyme function can also be modified through covalent modification such as phosphorylation. These are typically post-translational modifications that can take place in the golgi or through kinase-mediated interactions. For example, glycogen phosphorylase requires phosphorylation for activation. Phosphorylation will be an integral means of regulation of enzymes during metabolic pathways.

1.2 References and resources

Text

Ferrier, D. R., ed. *Lippincott Illustrated Reviews: Biochemistry*, 7th ed. Philadelphia: Wolters Kluwer Health/ Lippincott Williams & Wilkins, 2017, Chapter 1: Amino Acids, Chapter 2: Protein Structure.

Lieberman, M., and A. Peet, eds. *Marks' Basic Medical Biochemistry: A Clinical Approach*, 5th ed. Philadelphia: Wolters Kluwer Health/Lippincott Williams & Wilkins, 2018, Chapter 6: Amino Acids in Proteins, Chapter 8: Enzymes as Catalysts, Chapter 9: Regulation of Enzymes.

Figures

Grey, Kindred, Figure 1.3 Basics of enzyme kinetics. 2021. https://archive.org/details/1.3_20210924. CC BY 4.0.

Lieberman M, Peet A. Figure 1.4 Graphical representation of the Michaelis-Menten equation. Adapted under Fair Use from Marks' Basic Medical Biochemistry. 5th Ed. pp 152. Figure 9.2 A graph of the Michaelis-Menten equation. 2017.

Lieberman M, Peet A. Figure 1.5 Lineweaver-Burk plot to illustrate Km and Vmax. Adapted under Fair Use from Marks' Basic Medical Biochemistry. 5th Ed. pp 153. Figure 9.3 The Lineweaver-Burk transformation for the Michaelis-Menten equation. 2017.

Lieberman M, Peet A. Figure 1.6 Competitive vs. noncompetitive inhibition. Adapted under Fair Use from Marks' Basic Medical Biochemistry. 5th Ed. pp 156. Figure 9.6 Lineweaver-Burk plots of competitive and purenoncompetitive inhibition. 2017.

Lieberman M, Peet A. Figure 1.7 Allosteric enzyme regulation. Adapted under Fair Use from Marks' Basic Medical Biochemistry. 5th Ed. pp 157. Figure 9.8 Activators and inhibitors of an allosteric enzyme (simplified model). 2017.

2. Basic Laboratory Measurements

Learning Objectives

- Evaluate clinical data to determine pathways involved in metabolic homeostasis.
- Recognize the utility of values for blood lactate, urinalysis, ALT/AST, and lipid profiles in clinical decision making.
- Determine how enzymes are regulated by comparing the role of inhibitors and activators, with examples, including: transition state inhibitors, irreversible inhibitors, and competitive and noncompetitive inhibitors/activators (see section 1.2).
- Identify vitamins as cofactors and necessary components of biological systems and begin to associate common symptoms with nutritional deficiencies.

About this Chapter

The cell is the most fundamental unit of all eukaryotic organisms. Its components and their cellular interactions are essential to the inner workings of the human body. Cells are primarily influenced by:

- the surrounding environment,
- through cell-cell interactions, and
- through circulating signals or hormones.

As a clinician, your first indication of changes to these cellular components will be illustrated by the signs and symptoms of your patient. Following this generalized assessment, you will begin to dissect out a clinical diagnosis by interpreting basic lab values. Each of these elements are indicative of molecular changes ultimately leading to the presentation you are challenged with.

2.1 Laboratory Values and Biochemical Correlates

A comprehensive metabolic panel (CMP) is a blood test that measures a variety of compounds (such as blood glucose and electrolytes), and it can be used to determine fluid balance, kidney function, and liver function, as well as other key metabolic functions. It is often used to determine health status (or metabolic dysfunction) and gives you insight into changes in biochemical reactions. Other diagnostics such as a complete blood count (CBC) may also be used but will not be discussed here.

How to read a CMP both clinically and biochemically will help hone the skills of diagnosis and maintenance of health status in patients. Additional laboratory tests such as a lipid profile, blood lactate, or urinalysis may also be ordered to supplement information from the CMP.

Deviations in any of these values can help determine changes in substrate availability, cofactors, and vitamin or enzymatic deficiencies. It will also help you better understand how biochemical pathways can influence clinical signs and symptoms.

Comprehensive metabolic panel

A CMP is often administered as part of a routine physical exam or for monitoring of specific conditions that impact kidney and liver functions. The results include the following tests (table 2.1):

Analyte	**Normal range**
Chemistries	
Glucose	70–100 mg/dL
Calcium	8.4–10.5 mg/dL
Protein	
Total protein	6.1–8.0 g/dL
Albumin	3.2–4.6 g/dL
Electrolytes	
Sodium	135-144 mmol/L
Potassium	3.6–5.0 mmol/L
Chloride	101–111 mmol/L
CO2	21–35 mmol/L
Kidney tests	
Blood urea nitrogen (BUN)	5–20 mg/dL
Creatinine	0.44–1.00 mg/dL
Liver tests	
Alkaline phosphatase (ALP)	38–126 IU/L
Aspartate amino transferase (AST)	14.9–39.9 IU/L
Alanine amino transferase (ALT)	11–43 IU/L
Bilirubin, total	0.0–1.2 mg/dL
Globulin	1.5–3.5 g/dL
Direct bilirubin	<0.3 mg/dL

Table 2.1: Normal values for a typical comprehensive metabolic panel. These values will be given to you when evaluating information.

Glucose – This energy source for the body is maintained in a very narrow range. Metabolic pathways are in place to balance both glucose uptake and glucose output to keep this value constant. Glucose homeostasis is regulated hormonally, and deviations from normal values could suggest metabolic or hormonal deficiencies (chapter 4 and chapter 5).

Calcium – This is one of the most important minerals in the body; it is essential for the proper functioning of muscles, nerves, and cardiac tissue. It is a cofactor in processes such as blood clotting and bone formation. Other vitamins also play key roles in these pathways (vitamin K in clotting and vitamin D in bone formation), so understanding this value may give insights into other potential deficiencies.

Proteins

Albumin – Albumin is a major serum protein produced in the liver and is a nonspecific carrier of many lipid soluble vitamins and other hydrophobic compounds. It is also essential for maintaining oncotic pressure. Decreases in serum albumin may be suggestive of nutritional deficiencies or changes in plasma volume as well as poor liver function. Therefore accessibility of lipid soluble vitamins, minerals, and hormones may be diminished secondarily to a decrease in albumin.

Total protein – Like serum albumin, a measure of total serum protein is useful to evaluate malnutrition or more chronic disorders such as inflammatory bowel disease. Increased production of immunoglobulins could also be detected here and would be indicative of chronic illness.

Electrolytes

Sodium – Sodium is vital to normal body processes, including nerve and muscle function. Hyponatremia can be suggestive of illness, diarrhea, or malnutrition, while hypernatremia is most often caused by an increased loss of water (dehydration) potentially due to endocrine disorders such as Cushing syndrome or diabetes insipidus.

Potassium – Potassium is critical for cardiac function, and although hypo or hyperkalemia can be indicative of a variety of disorders, it can be a critical indicator of maintenance of diabetes. Unmanaged diabetic individuals may present with hyperkalemia, however, inappropriate insulin administration will increase potassium uptake. Therefore poor management can cause a sudden drop in potassium (hypokalemia) leading to cardiac dysfunction.

CO_2 (carbon dioxide, bicarbonate) – CO_2 is produced from several oxidative pathways and is removed in the form of bicarbonate or through hemoglobin transport. Elevation of CO_2 could suggest a renal, respiratory, and/or metabolic concern, and additional laboratory values would need to be assessed to determine the root cause. These may include blood lactate, blood urea nitrogen (BUN), as well as arteriole blood gasses (ABG).

Chloride – Chloride is a negatively charged ion that works with other electrolytes (potassium, sodium, and bicarbonate) to help regulate both fluid and acid-base (pH) balance in the body. Chloride and electrolyte tests may help diagnose the cause of signs and symptoms such as prolonged vomiting, diarrhea, weakness, and difficulty breathing (respiratory distress).

Kidney tests

Blood urea nitrogen (BUN) – Urea is a waste product of amino acid metabolism filtered out of the blood by the kidneys. It is a primary means of nitrogen disposal, and conditions that affect the kidneys have the potential to affect the amount of urea in the blood. This value is also indicative of deficiencies in amino acid metabolism, or changes in urea cycle activity or protein catabolism (section 5.3).

Creatinine – This waste product is produced in the muscles and filtered out by the kidneys. Urinary levels of creatinine are a good indicator of how the kidneys are working.

Liver tests

Alkaline phosphatase (ALP) – ALP is an enzyme found in the liver and other tissues such as bone. Elevated levels of ALP are most commonly caused by liver disease or other pathologies that increase cell damage leading to the release of ALP in the blood. Other disorders that impact bone growth may also increase ALP.

Alanine amino transferase (ALT) – ALT is an enzyme found predominantly in the liver and kidney. It is important in movement of ammonia (through the process of transamination) in tissues, and an elevation of ALT in circulation suggests liver damage (or potentially muscle damage) (section 5.3).

Aspartate amino transferase (AST) – AST is also a transferase needed in nitrogen metabolism found especially within the heart and liver. It is also a useful test for detecting liver damage. The ratio of ALT/AST can be used to distinguish between disorders such as alcoholic versus nonalcoholic fatty liver disease (section 5.3).

Bilirubin – Bilirubin is a waste product produced by the degradation of heme. Heme degradation within the liver is a normal part of red blood cell turnover, but elevated bilirubin could also be indicative of excessive hemolysis (due to deficiencies in NAPDH or increased oxidative stress) or biliary obstructions. Bilirubin values can be reported as direct (conjugated) or indirect (unconjugated) bilirubin. As conjugation takes place in the liver, decreased conjugated bilirubin or increased unconjugated bilirubin would suggest liver dysfunction (figure 2.1).

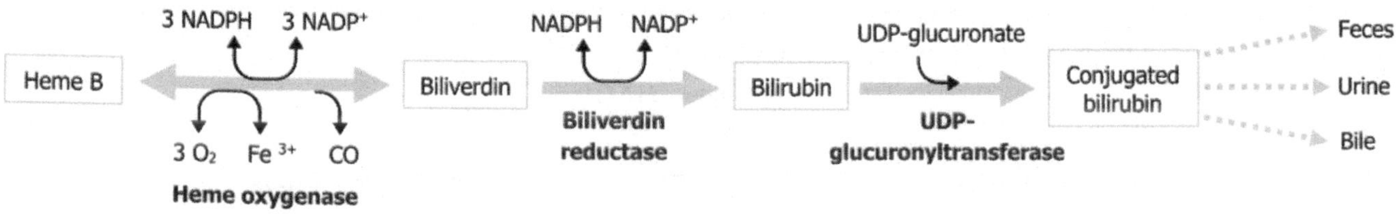

Figure 2.1: Heme degradation.

Lipid profile

A lipid profile (table 2.2) is often used to assess risk of developing cardiovascular disease (CVD) or to monitor the effectiveness of a dietary or pharmacological intervention.

Serum measurement	Desirable levels
Total cholesterol	<200 mg/dL
Low-density lipoprotein cholesterol (LDL-C)	<100 mg/dL
High-density lipoprotein cholesterol (HDL-C)	over 40 mg/dL for females; over 60 mg/dL for males
Triglycerides (TGs)	<150 mg/dL
TG to HDL ratio (calculated)	<5

Table 2.2: Desirable (optimal) values for lipids. Ranges of intermediate and high can also be found for these values.

Total cholesterol – This measurement takes in to account various forms of cholesterol in circulation. It is the total of high-density lipoprotein (HDL), low-density lipoprotein (LDL), and 20 percent of the triglyceride measurement. This is key to determining your cholesterol ratio (total/HDL), which should be below 5 with an ideal ratio being 3.5.

High-density lipoprotein cholesterol (HDL-C) – HDL is predominantly involved in reverse cholesterol transport because it removes excess cholesterol from peripheral tissues and carries it to the liver for removal or use. It has several key interactions with very low-density lipid (VLDL) particles in circulation that assist in lipid metabolism.

Low-density lipoprotein cholesterol (LDL-C) – LDL is often called "bad cholesterol" because it can deposit excess cholesterol in walls of blood vessels, which can contribute to atherosclerosis.

Triglycerides – This is a measurement of circulating triacylglycerols (TAG), which are primarily transported by VLDL particles. TAG levels should be less than 150 mg/dL, and increased TAG may suggest endocrine deficiencies or metabolic defects.

Variations of normal in a lipid profile could be suggestive of heritable disorders, poor diet, or lipid uptake, decreased lipid storage, or excessive synthesis. The combination of these values will help determine what aspect of lipid metabolism is altered (chapter 6).

Lactate

Serum lactate levels may also be measured in conjunction with a complete metabolic panel. Serum lactate should be negligible under normal conditions, however, elevated lactate could be suggestive of excessive anaerobic metabolism, such as is the case in intense exercise or deficiency in oxygen transport caused by ischemic injury. This could also be caused by inappropriate diversion of substrate such as is the case in some enzymatic deficiencies (pyruvate dehydrogenase deficiency) or changes in NADH levels (figure 2.2).

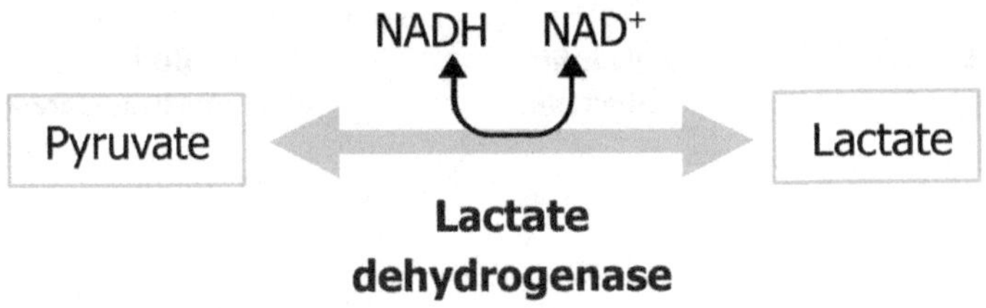

Figure 2.2: Reaction catalyzed by lactate dehydrogenase.

Urinalysis (includes a visual, chemical, and microscopic exam)

Visual exam and the microscopic exam

Although both the visual and microscopic exam are very essential components to this analysis, these will not be focused on here. The color of urine can vary, most often shades of yellow, from very pale or colorless to very dark or amber. Red-colored urine can also occur when blood is present; yellow-brown or greenish-brown urine may be a sign of bilirubin in the urine. Urine clarity refers to how clear the urine is. This could be defined as: clear, slightly cloudy, cloudy, or turbid. "Normal" urine can be clear or cloudy.

A microscopic examination will typically be done when there are abnormal findings on the physical or chemical examination. Cells and other substances that may be seen include the following: red blood cells (RBCs), white blood cells (WBCs), epithelial cells, bacteria, yeast and parasites, trichomonas, casts, and crystals. If the crystals are from substances that are not normally in the urine, they are considered "abnormal." Abnormal crystals may indicate an abnormal metabolic process. Some of these include: calcium carbonate, cystine, tyrosine, and leucine. Urinary presence of some amino acids can be suggestive of amino acid metabolic disorders (chapter 8).

Chemical exam

Much like the CMP, the chemical analysis of a urine sample can be very indicative of biochemical derangement. A review of the following components is helpful in making a clinical diagnosis.

Specific gravity (SG) – Specific gravity is a measure of urine concentration. This test simply indicates how concentrated the urine is.

pH – Urine is typically slightly acidic, about pH 6, but can range from 4.5 to 8. The kidneys play an important role in maintaining the acid-base balance of the body. Therefore, any condition that produces acids or bases in the body, such as acidosis or alkalosis, or the ingestion of acidic or basic foods, can directly affect urine pH.

Protein – The protein test provides an estimate of the amount of albumin in the urine. Normally, there should be no protein (or a small amount of protein) in the urine. When urine protein is elevated, a person has a condition called proteinuria; this could be caused by a variety of health conditions. Healthy people can have temporary or persistent proteinuria due to stress, exercise, fever, aspirin therapy, or exposure to cold, for example.

Glucose – Glucose is normally not present in urine. When glucose is present, the condition is called glucosuria. This condition can result from either an excessively high glucose level in the blood, such as may be seen in individuals with uncontrolled diabetes. Other reducing sugars, galactose or fructose, may also be present in the urine if a metabolic deficiency occurs (section 9.1).

Some other conditions that can cause glucosuria include hormonal disorders, liver disease, medications, and pregnancy. When glucosuria occurs, other tests such as a fasting blood glucose test are usually performed to further identify the specific cause.

Ketones – Ketones are also not normally found in the urine. They are intermediate products of fat metabolism and can be produced when an individual does not eat enough carbohydrates such as in fasting conditions or high-protein diets. When carbohydrates are not available, the body metabolizes fat to generate ATP for baseline metabolic function. Strenuous exercise, exposure to cold, frequent, prolonged vomiting, and several digestive system diseases can also increase fat metabolism, resulting in ketonuria (section 5.2).

In a person who has diabetes, ketones in urine may be an early indication of insufficient insulin. Insufficient insulin response can result in impaired glucose oxidation and consequently results in aberrant fat metabolism. Oxidation of fatty acids provides substrate for ketogenesis, which can cause ketosis and potentially progress to ketoacidosis, a form of metabolic acidosis. Excess ketones and glucose are dumped into the urine by the kidneys in an effort to flush them from the body.

Hemoglobin and myoglobin – The presence of hemoglobin in urine indicates blood in the urine (known as hematuria).

A small number of RBCs are normally present in urine, however, as these numbers elevate, this will result in a positive test result. These results are interpreted with the microscopic exam. For example, a positive test result here with no visible RBCs in the urine would suggest the presence of myoglobin only, which could be due to strenuous exercise or muscle damage.

Leukocyte esterase – Leukocyte esterase is an enzyme present in most white blood cells (WBCs). A few white blood cells are normally present in urine, however, when the number of WBCs in urine increases significantly, this screening test will become positive. When this test is positive and/or the WBC count in urine is high, it may indicate that there is inflammation in the urinary tract or kidneys.

Nitrite – Many normal bacteria can convert nitrate (normally present in urine) to nitrite (not normally present in urine). When bacteria are present in the urinary tract, they can cause a urinary tract infection, which could be diagnosed by a positive nitrite test result.

Bilirubin – Bilirubin is not present in the urine of healthy individuals (figure 2.1). The presence of bilirubin in urine is an early indicator of liver disease and can occur before clinical symptoms such as jaundice develop. Only conjugated bilirubin is present in the urine.

Urobilinogen – Urobilinogen is normally present in urine in low concentrations. It is formed in the intestine from bilirubin, and a portion of it is absorbed back into the blood. Positive test results may indicate liver diseases such as viral hepatitis, cirrhosis, liver damage due to drugs or toxic substances, or conditions associated with increased RBC destruction (hemolytic anemia).

2.1 References and resources

Text

Ferrier, D. R., ed. *Lippincott Illustrated Reviews: Biochemistry*, 7th ed. Philadelphia: Wolters Kluwer Health/ Lippincott Williams & Wilkins, 2017, Chapter 27: Nutrition: Overview, Chapter 28: Micronutrients: Vitamins, Chapter 29: Micronutrients: Minerals.

Le, T., and V. Bhushan. *First Aid for the USMLE Step 1*, 29th ed. New York: McGraw Hill Education, 2018, 65–71.

Figures

Grey, Kindred, Figure 2.1 Heme degradation. 2021. https://archive.org/details/2.2_20210924. CC BY 4.0.

Grey, Kindred, Figure 2.2 Reaction catalyzed by lactate dehydrogenase. 2021. https://archive.org/details/2.4_20210924. CC BY 4.0.

2.2 Vitamins as Coenzymes

Nutritional basics

Many of the metabolic enzymes discussed in this course require essential coenzymes for optimal activity. An individual's nutritional status has the potential to greatly influence their ability to efficiently oxidize fuels, and this can lead to deviations from clinical norms or illness, which would be illustrated on an individual's CMP.

It is important to be aware of the presentation of these nutritional deficiencies as they can manifest as hypoglycemia, different types of anemia, or physiological symptoms.

Overview

Vitamins are organic compounds that, for the most part, we cannot synthesize through endogenous metabolism in adequate quantities (with the exceptions of vitamins B_3, D, and K). To address these nutritional needs, we must consume vitamins as part of a balanced diet or supplement through a variety of mechanisms. Below are some key aspects of the roles vitamins play within metabolism and common symptoms associated with deficiencies (table 2.3).

Note

Water-soluble vitamins

- Water-soluble vitamins include: ascorbic acid (vitamin C), thiamin (vitamin B_1), riboflavin (vitamin B_2), niacin (vitamin B_3), pantothenic acid (vitamin B_5), pyridoxine, pyridoxal, and pyridoxamine (vitamin B_6), biotin (vitamin B_7), and cobalamin (vitamin B_{12}).
- Readily excreted in the urine, toxicity is rare.
- Deficiencies can occur quickly.
- Water-soluble vitamins are precursors of coenzymes for the enzymes of intermediary metabolism.

Fat-soluble vitamins

- Fat-soluble vitamins include: vitamins A, D, K, and E.
- They are released, absorbed, and transported (in chylomicrons) with dietary fat.
- They are not readily excreted, and significant quantities are stored in the liver and adipose tissue.
- Most function as transcriptional regulators.
- Only one fat-soluble vitamin (vitamin K) has a coenzyme function.
- Consumption of vitamins A and D in excess of the dietary reference intakes can lead to accumulation of toxic quantities of these compounds.

Folic acid

Folic acid deficiency is a relatively common vitamin deficiency in the United States, presenting routinely as macrocytic anemia.

- Tetrahydrofolate (THF), the reduced coenzyme form of folate, receives one-carbon fragments from amino acid donors such as serine, glycine, and histidine, and transfers them to intermediates in the synthesis of amino acids, purines, and thymidine monophosphate (TMP, a pyrimidine nucleotide found in DNA).
- Inadequate serum levels of folate can be caused by increased demand (such as the case in pregnancy and lactation), inadequate dietary intake, poor absorption (caused by pathology of the small intestine), alcoholism, or treatment with drugs (for example, methotrexate).
- Folic acid supplementation before conception and during the first trimester has been shown to significantly reduce neural tube defects.

Cobalamin (vitamin B_{12})

Vitamin B_{12} is required in humans for two essential enzymatic reactions.

- One of the reactions is the remethylation of homocysteine to methionine, and the other involves the isomerization of methylmalonyl coenzyme A (CoA), which is produced during the degradation of some amino acids (isoleucine, valine, threonine, and methionine) and odd-chain fatty acids (FAs).
- Folic acid (as N5-methyl THF) is also required for one of the reactions needed for remethylation of homocysteine.
- Deficiency of B_{12} or folate results in elevated Hcy levels (chapter 8), however, only a deficiency of B_{12} will result in elevated levels of methylmalonic acid.
- Pernicious anemia is a type of vitamin B_{12} anemia caused by a lack of intrinsic factor. Intrinsic factor (IF) is released from the parietal cells and binds vitamin B_{12} so that it can be absorbed in the intestines.
- B_{12} is also important in the synthesis of S-adenosylmethionine (SAM), which plays an integral role in cellular methylation reactions and neurotransmitter synthesis.

Ascorbic acid (vitamin C)

The active form of vitamin C is ascorbic acid.

- Vitamin C is used as a coenzyme in hydroxylation reactions, such as in the hydroxylation of prolyl and lysyl residues of collagen.
- It is required for the maintenance of normal connective tissue as well as for wound healing.
- Vitamin C assists in the absorption of dietary iron by reducing ferric iron to the ferrous form.

Pyridoxine (vitamin B_6)

Vitamin B_6 is a term that encompasses all derivatives of pyridine including: pyridoxine, pyridoxal, and pyridoxamine.

- Pyridoxine serves as a precursor of the biologically active coenzyme, pyridoxal phosphate (PLP).
- PLP functions as a coenzyme for activation transfer reactions, particularly those that catalyze reactions involving amino acids (section 5.3).
- Isoniazid, a drug commonly used to treat tuberculosis, can induce a vitamin B_6 deficiency by forming an inactive derivative with PLP.
- Pyridoxine is the only water-soluble vitamin with significant toxicity. Sensory neuropathies can occur at intakes exceeding five times the Tolerable Upper Limit (UL). This is defined as the maximum amount of daily vitamins and minerals that you can safely take without risk of an overdose or serious side effects.

Thiamine (vitamin B_1)

Thiamine pyrophosphate (TPP) is the biologically active form of thiamine and is generated by the transfer of a pyrophosphate group from adenosine triphosphate (ATP) to thiamine.

- TPP is a coenzyme in the formation or degradation of α-ketols by transketolase (section 7.1) and in the oxidative decarboxylation of α-keto acids.
- The activity of both the pyruvate dehydrogenase complex and α-ketoglutarate dehydrogenase can be impaired if thiamine is deficient. This can lead to impaired production of ATP, impaired cellular function, and lactic acidosis.
- TPP is also required by branched-chain α-keto acid dehydrogenase of muscle.
- Activity of erythrocyte transketolase is used to diagnosis a thiamine deficiency.
- Beriberi is a severe thiamine-deficiency syndrome found in geographic areas with poor and restricted diets.
- Wernicke-Korsakoff syndrome can present in individuals with alcohol abuse disorder. Common symptoms include confusion, ataxia, and nystagmus.

Niacin (vitamin B_3)

Niacin, or nicotinic acid, is a substituted pyridine derivative. The biologically active coenzyme forms are nicotinamide adenine dinucleotide (NAD^+) and its phosphorylated derivative, nicotinamide adenine dinucleotide phosphate ($NADP^+$).

- Nicotinamide is readily deaminated in the body and, therefore, is nutritionally equivalent to nicotinic acid.
- NAD^+ and $NADP^+$ serve as coenzymes in oxidation-reduction reactions in which the coenzyme undergoes reduction of the pyridine ring by accepting a hydride ion.
- A deficiency of niacin causes pellagra, which encompasses the three Ds: dermatitis, diarrhea, and dementia.
- Hartnup disorder, characterized by defective absorption of tryptophan, can result in pellagra-like symptoms.

Riboflavin (vitamin B_2)

The two biologically active forms of B_2 are flavin mononucleotide (FMN) and flavin adenine dinucleotide (FAD), formed by the transfer of an adenosine monophosphate moiety from ATP to FMN.

- FMN and FAD are each capable of reversibly accepting two hydrogen atoms, forming $FMNH_2$ or $FADH_2$. FMN and FAD are bound tightly, or covalently, to flavoenzymes that catalyze the oxidation or reduction of a substrate.

- Riboflavin deficiency is not associated with a major human disease, although it frequently accompanies other vitamin deficiencies.

Biotin (vitamin B_7)

Biotin is a coenzyme in carboxylation reactions, in which it serves as a carrier of activated carbon dioxide (coenzyme for acetylCoA carboxylase and pyruvate carboxylase).

- Biotin is covalently bound to the ε-amino group of lysine residues in biotin-dependent enzymes.
- Biotin deficiency does not occur naturally because the vitamin is widely distributed in food.
- Excessive consumption of raw egg white as a source of protein can cause symptoms of biotin deficiency. Symptoms may include: dermatitis, glossitis, loss of appetite, and nausea. Raw egg white contains avidin, which is a glycoprotein that tightly binds biotin and prevents its absorption from the intestine.

Pantothenic acid

Pantothenic acid is a component of CoA, which functions in the transfer of acyl groups.

- CoA contains a thiol group that carries acyl compounds as activated thiol esters. Examples of such structures are succinyl-CoA, fatty acyl-CoA, and acetyl-CoA.
- Pantothenic acid is also a component of the acyl carrier protein domain of fatty acid synthase (section 4.4).
- The vitamin is widely distributed in a variety of foods, and deficiency is not well characterized in humans.

Vitamin A

The retinoids are a family of molecules that are related to dietary retinol (vitamin A).

- Vitamin A (and its metabolites) are important for vision, reproduction, growth, immune function, and maintenance of epithelial tissues.
- Retinoic acid is derived from the oxidation of retinol and mediates most of the actions of the retinoids.
- Retinol is oxidized to retinoic acid. Retinoic acid binds specifically to a family of nuclear receptors (retinoic acid receptors, RAR) and modulates gene expression in target tissues, such as epithelial cells. The activated retinoic acid-RAR complex binds to response elements on DNA and recruits activators or repressors to regulate retinoid-specific mRNA synthesis (figure 2.3).

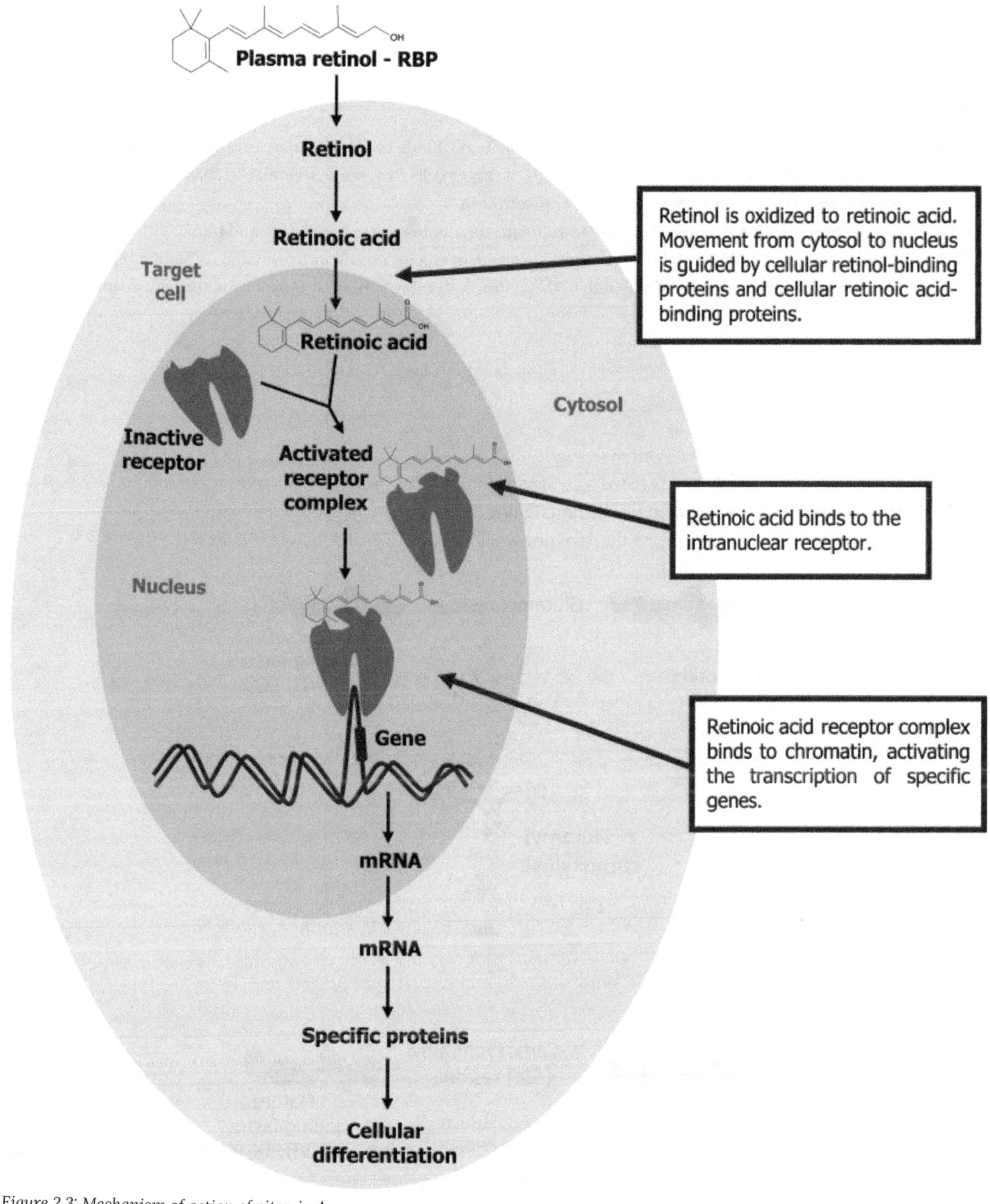

Figure 2.3: Mechanism of action of vitamin A.

Vitamin D

The D vitamins are a group of sterols that have a hormone-like function.

- The active molecule, 1,25-dihydroxycholecalciferol (calcitriol), binds to intracellular receptor proteins. The receptor complex interacts with DNA in the nucleus of target cells in a manner similar to that of vitamin A and either selectively stimulates or represses gene transcription.
- The most prominent actions of calcitriol are to regulate the plasma levels of calcium and phosphorus. Within the gastrointestinal tract, calcitriol increases the transcription of calcium transport proteins, calbindin-D proteins, which results in increased uptake of calcium. It also increases reabsorption of phosphorus through a similar mechanism.

Vitamin K

- The primary role of vitamin K is to serve as a coenzyme in the carboxylation of glutamic acid residues; this post-translational modification is required for the functioning of many proteins required for blood clotting.
- Vitamin K is required in the hepatic synthesis of prothrombin (factor II) and factors VII, IX, and X (figure 2.4).

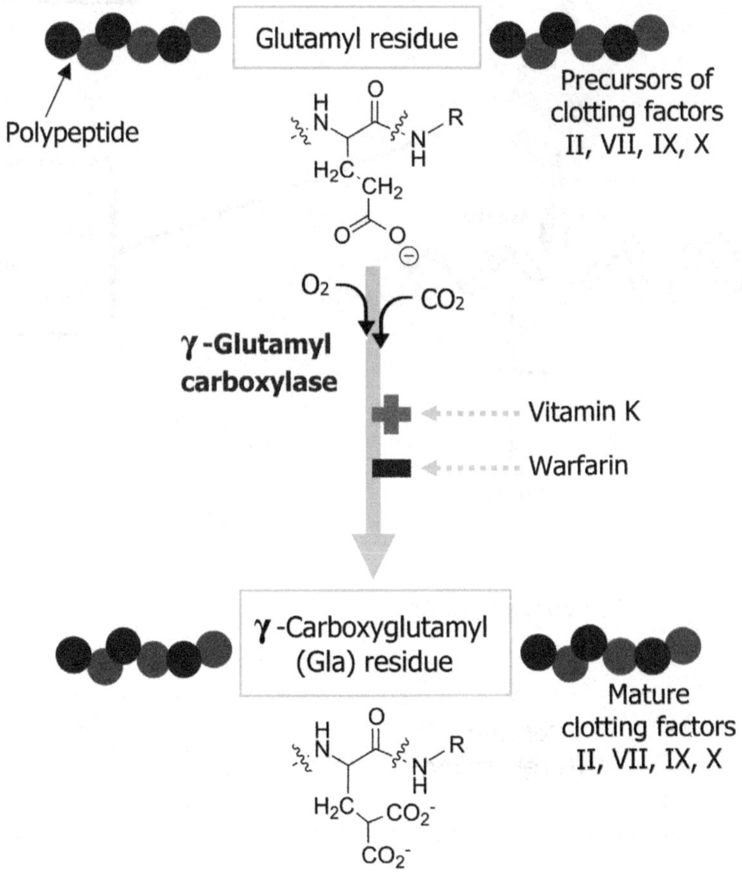

Figure 2.4: Vitamin K stimulates the maturation of clotting factors.

- The formation of carboxy-glutamyl (Gla) residues is sensitive to inhibition by warfarin, an analog of vitamin K that inhibits vitamin K epoxide reductase (VKOR), the enzyme required to regenerate the functional hydroquinone form of vitamin K.

Vitamin E

The E vitamins consist of eight naturally occurring tocopherols, of which α-tocopherol is the most active.

- The primary function of vitamin E is as an antioxidant in prevention of the nonenzymatic oxidation of cell components.
- Vitamin E deficiency in adults is usually associated with defective lipid absorption or transport.

Vitamin	Other names	Active form	Function	Deficiency	Signs and symptoms	Toxicity	Notes
Water soluble							
Vitamin B_9	Folic acid	Tetrahydrofolic acid	Transfer one-carbon units; synthesis of methionine, purines, and thymidine monophosphate	Megaloblastic anemia Neural tube defects	Anemia Birth defects	None	Administration of high levels of folate can mask vitamin B_{12} deficiency
Vitamin B_{12}	Cobalamin	Methylcobalamin Deoxyadenosyl cobalamin	Coenzyme for reactions: • homocysteine → methionine • methylmalonyl-CoA → succinyl-CoA	Pernicious anemia Dementia Spinal degeneration	Megaloblastic anemia Neuropsychiatric symptoms	None	Pernicious anemia is treated with intramuscular or high-dose oral vitamin B_{12}
Vitamin C	Ascorbic acid	Ascorbic acid	Antioxidant Coenzyme for hydroxylation reactions, for example: In procollagen: • proline → hydroxyproline • lysine → hydroxylysine	Scurvy	Sore, spongy gums Loose teeth Poor wound healing	None	Benefits of supplementation not established in controlled trials
Vitamin B_6	Pridoxine Pyridoxamine Pyridoxal	Pyridoxal phosphate	Coenzyme for enzymes, particularly in amino acid metabolism	Rare	Glossitis Neuropathy	Yes	Deficiency can be introduced by isoniazid Sensory neuropathy occurs at high doses
Vitamin B_1	Thiamine	Thiamine pyrophosphate	Coenzyme of enzymes catalyzing: • pyruvate → acetyl-CoA • α-ketoglutarate → succinyl-CoA • ribose 5-P + xylulose 5-P → sedoheptulose 7-P + glyceraldehyde 3-P • branched-chain α-keto acid oxidation	Beriberi Wernicke-Korsakoff syndrome (most common in alcoholics)	Tachycardia, vomiting, convulsions Apathy, loss of memory, dysregulated eye movements	None	
Niacin	Nicotinic acid Nicotinamide	NAD^+ $NADP^+$	Electron transfer	Pellagra	Dermatitis Diarrhea Dementia	None	High doses of niacin used to treat hyperlipidemia
Vitamin B_2	Riboflavin	FMN FAD	Electron transfer	Rare	Dermatitis Angular stomatitis	None	
Biotin		Enzyme-bound biotin	Carboxylation reactions	Rare		None	Consumption of large amounts of raw egg whites (which contain a protein, avidin, that binds biotin) can induce a biotin deficiency

Vitamin	Other names	Active form	Function	Deficiency	Signs and symptoms	Toxicity	Notes
Pantothenic acid		Coenzyme A	Acyl carrier	Rare		None	
Fat soluble							
Vitamin A	Retinol Retinal Retinoic acid β-Carotene	Retinol Retinal Retinoic acid	Maintenance of reproduction Vision Promotion of growth Differentiation and maintenance of epithelial tissues Gene expression	Infertility Night blindness Retardation of growth Xerophthalmia	Increased visual threshold Dryness of cornea	Yes	B-Carotene not acutely toxic, but supplementation is not recommended Excess vitamin A can increase incidence of fractures
Vitamin D	Cholecalciferol Ergocalciferol	1,25-dihydroxy-cholecalciferol	Calcium uptake Gene expression	Rickets (in children) Osteomalacia (in adults)	Soft, pliable bones	Yes	Vitamin D is not a true vitamin because it can be synthesized in skin; application of sunscreen lotions or presence of dark skin color decreases this synthesis
Vitamin K	Menadione Menaquinone Phylloquinone	Menadione Menaquinone Phylloquinone	γ-Carboxylation of glutamate residues in clotting and other proteins	Newborn Rare in adults	Bleeding	Rare	Vitamin K produced by intestinal bacteria Vitamin K deficiency common in newborns Intramuscular treatment with vitamin K is recommended at birth
Vitamin E	α-Tocopherol	Any of several tocopherol derivatives	Antioxidant	Rare	Red blood cell fragility leads to hemolytic anemia	None	Benefits of supplementation not established in controlled trials

Table 2.3: Summary table of vitamins.

2.2 References and resources

Text

Ferrier, D. R., ed. *Lippincott Illustrated Reviews: Biochemistry*, 7th ed. Philadelphia: Wolters Kluwer Health/ Lippincott Williams & Wilkins, 2017, Chapter 27: Nutrition: Overview, Chapter 28: Micronutrients: Vitamins, Chapter 29: Micronutrients: Minerals.

Le, T., and V. Bhushan. *First Aid for the USMLE Step* 1, 29th ed. New York: McGraw Hill Education, 2018, 65–71.

Figures

Ferrier D. Figure 2.3 Mechanism of action of Vitamin A. Adapted under Fair Use from Figure 28.20 Action of the retinoids. Lippincott Illustrated Reviews Biochemistry. 7th Ed. pp388. 2017. Chemical structure by Henry Jakubowski.

Grey, Kindred, Figure 2.4 Vitamin K stimulates the maturation of clotting factors. 2021. Chemical structure by Henry Jakubowski. https://archive.org/details/2.6_20210924. CC BY 4.0.

Tables

Table 2.3 adapted from Ferrier, D. R., ed. *Lippincott Illustrated Reviews: Biochemistry*, 7th ed. Philadelphia: Wolters Kluwer Health/Lippincott Williams & Wilkins, 2017.

3. Fed and Fasted State

Learning Objectives

- Describe the effect of insulin, glucagon, epinephrine, and cortisol on metabolic processes in the liver, adipose, and skeletal muscle and how these hormones function to regulate blood glucose homeostasis.
- Determine the fuels utilized by the liver, red blood cells, adipose, skeletal muscle in the fed and fasted states and determine the pathway(s) providing this substrate.
- Differentiate between insulin sensitive and insulin insensitive tissues; identify the GLUT transporters common to specific tissues and their clinical relevance.
- Review the signaling mechanisms used by insulin, glucagon, cortisol, and epinephrine.

About this Chapter

One of the fundamental homeostatic responses is the regulation of blood glucose by alterations in flux through metabolic pathways. This regulation includes both dietary intake of fuels, tissue uptake and oxidation of fuels, and storage and release of fuels under necessary conditions. Most of these processes are controlled hormonally by insulin, glucagon, cortisol, and epinephrine. Ultimately, these pathways ensure that both ATP levels are sufficient for an organism to sustain cellular activities and that blood glucose is maintained in a narrow window. Both processes are balanced without exhausting either fuel and energy resources.

3.1 Fed and Fasted States

Glucose homeostasis is fundamental to the human body and regulated primarily by the levels of four major hormones:

1. Insulin,
2. Glucagon,
3. Cortisol, and
4. Epinephrine.

The ratios of these hormones in circulation will dictate the activity of specific metabolic pathways that control glucose homeostasis in a range of 80 mg/dL to 120 mg/dL. There are many other hormones (thyroid hormone, growth hormone, etc.) and adipokines (adiponectin, leptin, etc.) that can influence glucose homeostasis, as well as neural mechanisms that control higher level functions such as hunger and satiety. These will not be the focus of this section.

Fed state metabolism

In the fed state, or postprandial, elevated glucose levels trigger the release of insulin from the pancreas. As insulin levels rise, there is an increase in glucose uptake, oxidation, and storage in peripheral tissues as well as increases in other anabolic pathways.

Under these conditions, most tissues (liver, skeletal muscle, adipose, brain, and red blood cells) will increase glucose uptake and oxidation (table 3.1 and figure 3.1).

Each tissue will take up glucose in the fed state using one of the glucose transporters (GLUT) known to facilitate glucose transport across the plasma membrane. This family of proteins can be broadly categorized as insulin-independent and insulin-dependent transporters.

Tissue type	**Fuel utilized in fed state**	**Primary glucose transporter**
Liver	Glucose	GLUT2 (insulin-independent)
Red blood cells	Glucose	GLUT1 (insulin-independent)
Brain	Glucose	GLUT1 and GLUT3 (insulin-independent)
Skeletal muscle	Glucose	GLUT4 (insulin-dependent)
Adipose	Glucose	GLUT4 (insulin-dependent)

Table 3.1: Summary table of fuels used in the fed state and uptake methods for important tissues.

Insulin-independent glucose uptake

The brain and red blood cells will always preferentially oxidize glucose regardless of hormone levels. Consequently, both tissues have a prevalence of GLUT1 transporters on the cell membrane. GLUT1 is present on the blood brain barrier, while GLUT3 is predominant on the brain. GLUT1 has a lower K_m (higher affinity) for glucose, ensuring glucose transport to these important tissues. Likewise, glucose uptake in the liver is also insulin-independent and is facilitated by GLUT2 transporters. The pancreas also predominantly expresses GLUT1 and is able to take up glucose in this manner.

Red blood cell metabolism

The red blood cell lacks mitochondria, therefore it oxidizes glucose under both fed and fasted conditions. Glucose can be oxidized by:

1. **Glycolysis**. Glucose is oxidized to pyruvate and converted to lactate, which will enter the Cori Cycle (section 4.1). (Lactate is returned to the liver and used as a substrate for gluconeogenesis.)
2. **Pentose phosphate pathway**. Glucose is initially oxidized to ribulose 5-phosphate. In addition to the production of this 5-C sugar, more importantly NADPH is produced, which is needed as a reducing agent in the red blood cell (section 7.1).

Brain metabolism

The brain will preferentially oxidize glucose under most conditions with the exception of starvation states.

Liver metabolism

In the liver, glucose is taken up in an insulin-independent manner, and the activity of the following processes increased in the fed state are summarized in figure 3.1 and tables 3.1 and 3.2.

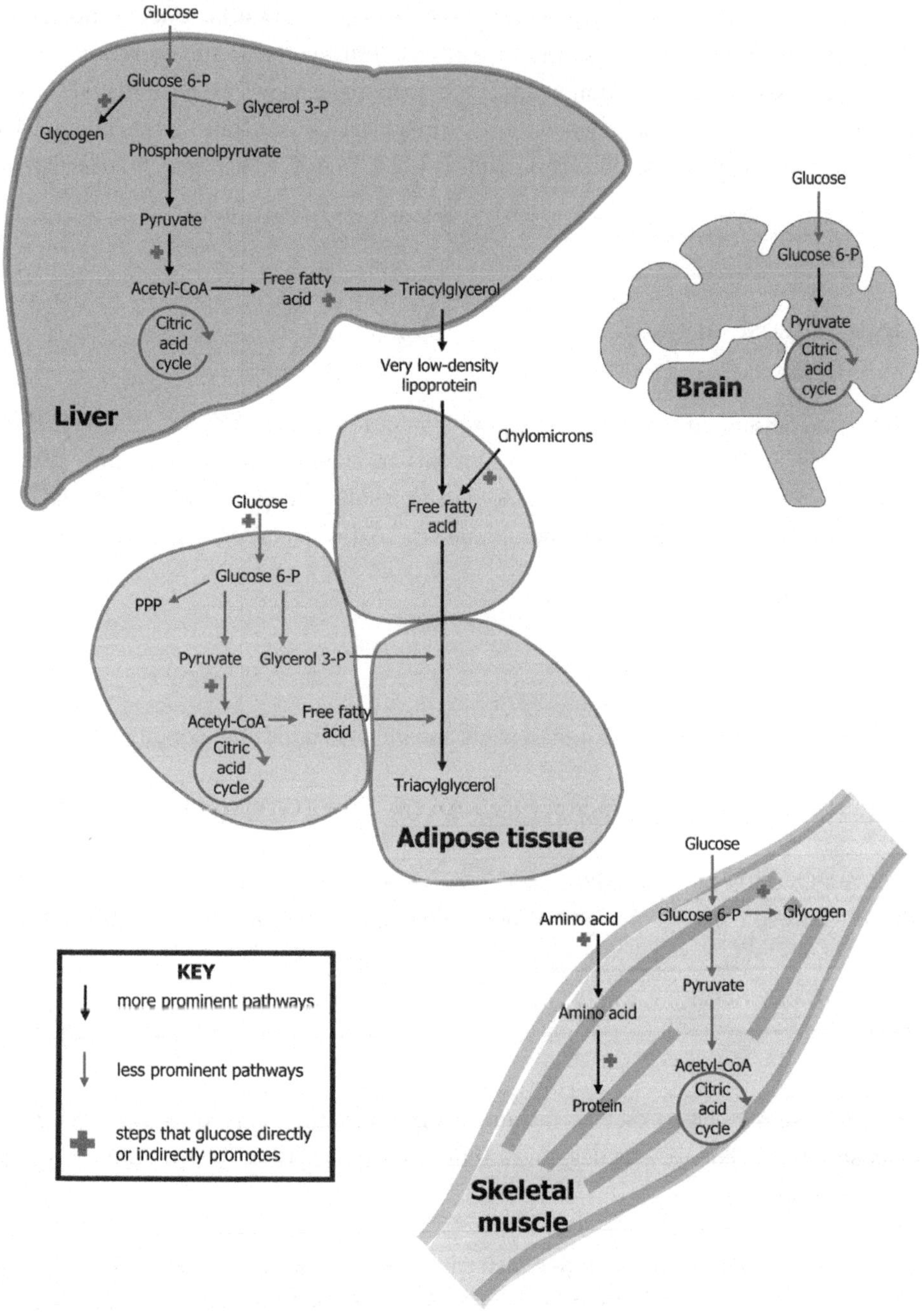

Figure 3.1: Overview of the fed state.

1. **Glycolysis**. Glucose will be oxidized to pyruvate, which can enter the TCA cycle after conversion to acetyl-CoA (section 4.1).
2. **Glycogen synthesis**. Glucose 6-phosphate is used to synthesize glycogen (section 4.5).
3. **Pentose phosphate pathway**. Glucose 6-phosphate can be used to generate five-carbon sugars and NADPH (section 7.1).
4. **Tricarboxylic acid cycle**. The TCA cycle will oxidize acetyl-CoA to generate NADH, $FADH_2$, and GTP. The acetyl-CoA that enters the cycle is fully oxidized and released as CO_2 (section 4.2).
5. **Cholesterol synthesis**. Acetyl-CoA transported to the cytosol is used to synthesize cholesterol, which can be used for many cellular processes (section 6.1).
6. **Fatty acid synthesis**. Excess citrate from the TCA cycle is shuttled out of the mitochondria and cleaved into oxaloacetate (OAA) and acetyl-CoA. The cytosolic acetyl-CoA can be used for fatty acid synthesis or cholesterol synthesis (section 4.4). Ultimately fatty acid synthesis leads to VLDL synthesis and secretion.
7. **Urea cycle**. Depending on diet and translation needs, excess amino acids will be deaminated through transamination reactions, and the nitrogen will enter the urea cycle as aspartate or free ammonia. Excess amino acids are not stored, rather the deaminated carbon skeletons can be stored as glycogen or triacylglycerol (section 5.3).

Insulin-dependent glucose uptake

In contrast, the skeletal muscle and adipose tissues require insulin for glucose uptake. GLUT4 is the primary glucose transporter on these tissues, and in the absence of insulin this transporter is predominantly bound to intracellular vesicles. When the cell receives a signal (via insulin binding the insulin receptor), this cell signaling event allows the GLUT4 containing vesicles to fuse with the plasma membrane where it will facilitate glucose uptake.

Skeletal muscle metabolism

The skeletal muscle will increase uptake of both amino acids and glucose under fed conditions.

1. **Glycolysis**. Glucose will be oxidized to pyruvate, which can enter the TCA cycle after conversion to acetyl-CoA (section 4.1).
2. **Protein synthesis**. Amino acids will be used for protein synthesis (anabolic metabolism).
3. **Glycogen synthesis**. Glucose 1-phosphate can be converted to UDP-glucose and stored as glycogen (section 4.5).

Adipose metabolism

In the adipose tissue, glucose as well as dietary fat and cholesterol (transported as chylomicrons; section 6.2) are taken up by the adipose tissue. Glucose has several potential fates described below, while dietary fat is stored as triacylglycerol.

1. **Glycolysis**. Glucose can be oxidized to pyruvate which can enter the TCA cycle after conversion to acetyl-CoA (section 4.1).
2. **Pentose phosphate pathway.** Glucose will be oxidized to generate NADPH needed for fatty acid synthesis (section 7.1).

3. **TAG synthesis**. Oxidation of glucose to glycerol 3-phosphate is needed for the synthesis of triacylglycerols (TAGs).

Pathway	Summary	Regulatory enzyme
Glycolysis	Glucose oxidation to pyruvate	Glucokinase/hexokinase Phosphofructokinase-1 Pyruvate kinase
Glycogen synthesis	Fuel storage	Glycogen synthase
Pentose pathway	NADPH and 5-C sugars production	Glucose 6-phosphate dehydrogenase
Tricarboxylic acid cycle	Oxidizes pyruvate to generate NADH and FADH2	Pyruvate dehydrogenase complex α-ketoglutarate dehydrogenase Isocitrate dehydrogenase
Cholesterol synthesis	Produces steroid hormone precursor	HMG-CoA reductase
Fatty acid synthesis	Produces free fatty acids and transported as VLDL for fuel storage in peripheral tissues	Acetyl-CoA carboxylase
Urea cycle	Nitrogen disposal	Carbamoyl phosphate synthetase I

Table 3.2: Summary of metabolism during the fed state.

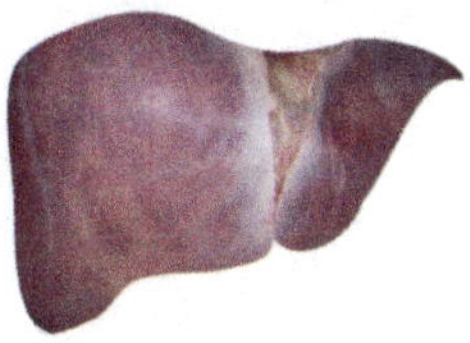
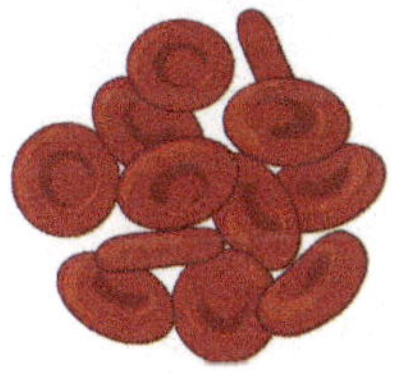
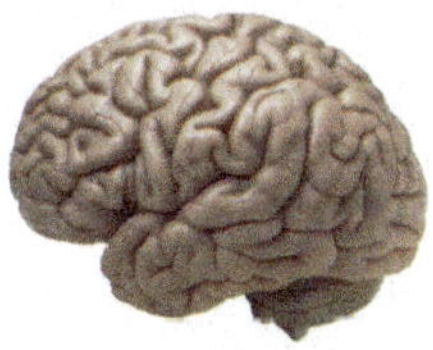
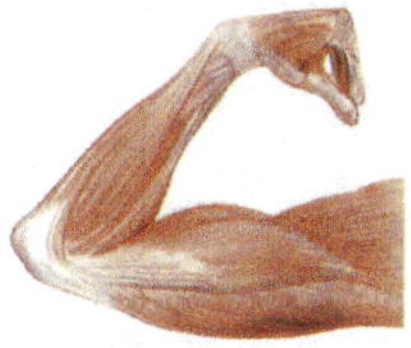
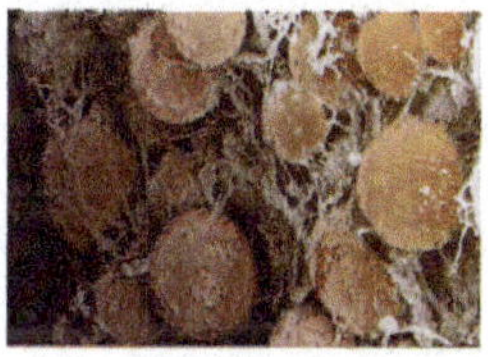

Fasted state metabolism

Approximately two hours after a meal, the decrease in serum glucose levels will lead to decreased insulin production in the pancreas. At this point in fasted state metabolism, the insulin to glucagon ratio becomes less than 1 (insulin low; glucagon high) with an additional increase of cortisol and epinephrine. Under these conditions tissues will transition to utilizing alternative fuels for energy as a means of maintaining glucose homeostasis. Fasted state metabolism will have limited impact on the oxidation of glucose by the brain and red blood cells, but it will lead to an increase in fatty acid oxidation by both the skeletal muscle and the liver (figure 3.6). The fatty acids oxidized by these tissues are released through the process of epinephrine-mediated lipolysis from the adipose. In the fasted state, the liver will primarily release glucose using both gluconeogenesis and glycogenolysis for the maintenance of blood glucose.

Tissue type	Fuel utilized in the fasted state	Pathway providing the fuel
Liver	Fatty acids	Lipolysis in the adipose
Red blood cells	Glucose	Hepatic glycogenolysis and gluconeogenesis
Brain	Glucose	Hepatic glycogenolysis and gluconeogenesis
Skeletal muscle	Fatty acids	Lipolysis in the adipose

Table 3.3: Summary table of fuels used in the fasted state and the pathways providing the fuel source.

Liver metabolism

The primary role of the liver in the fasted state is to synthesize and release glucose. To facilitate this task, the liver will use circulating free fatty acids as the primary fuel source to generate energy (ATP) for these homeostatic processes. (These processes are summarized in figure 3.2 and tables 3.3 and 3.4)

1. **Glycogenolysis.** Hepatic glycogenolysis provides glucose that is released into the bloodstream to maintain blood glucose and provide an oxidizable substrate for the brain and RBCs (section 4.5).
2. **Gluconeogenesis.** This is an anabolic process that synthesizes glucose from lactate, amino acids, or glycerol. This process is heavily reliant on the ATP generated from β-oxidation. The glucose produced is released into the bloodstream to maintain blood glucose and provide an oxidizable substrate for the brain and RBCs (section 5.1).
3. **Fatty acid β-oxidation.** This is the process by which free fatty acids are oxidized to produce acetyl-CoA, NADH, and $FADH_2$. It is a high energy yielding process and is required to generate ATP in the fasted state (section 5.2).
4. **Ketogenesis.** This process utilizes the acetyl-CoA produced through β-oxidation to produce β-hydroxybutyrate and acetoacetate. These ketone bodies can be oxidized by peripheral tissues; the liver cannot oxidize ketone bodies (section 5.2).
5. **Urea cycle.** Cortisol initiated protein catabolism provides amino acids needed as a substrate for gluconeogenesis. In order to use the carbon skeletons (keto-acids), the amino acids must be deaminated and the ammonia is disposed of through the synthesis of urea; nitrogen will enter the urea cycle as aspartate or free ammonia (section 5.3).

Red blood cell metabolism

The red blood cell lacks mitochondria, therefore it oxidizes glucose under both fed and fasted conditions. The metabolism of this tissue remains largely unchanged.

Brain metabolism

The brain will oxidize glucose under most conditions with the exception of starvation states. Under normal fasting conditions, although ketones will be synthesized, the brain will not transition to utilizing them as a predominant source of fuel until extended fasting has occurred (days).

Skeletal muscle metabolism

The skeletal muscle will increase uptake of fatty acids and ketones.

1. **Fatty acid β-oxidation.** This is the process by which free fatty acids are oxidized to produce acetyl-CoA, NADH, and $FADH_2$ (section 5.2).
2. **Oxidation of ketones.** Ketone bodies taken up by the skeletal muscle can be reconverted to acetyl-CoA and oxidized in the TCA cycle (section 5.2).
3. **Protein catabolism.** Cortisol-mediated protein catabolism is also active and supplies amino acids for gluconeogenesis in the liver.

Adipose metabolism

The most important process in the adipose tissue during the fasted state is lipolysis.

1. **Lipolysis**. This process will release fatty acids from stored triacylglycerols and provides an oxidizable substrate for the skeletal muscle and liver (section 5.2).

Pathway	Summary	Regulatory enzyme
Glycogenolysis	Provides glucose for maintenance of blood glucose	Glycogen phosphorylase
Gluconeogenesis	Provides glucose for maintenance of blood glucose	Glucose 6-phosphatase Fructose 1,6-biphosphatase PEPCK/pyruvate carboxylase
Lipolysis	Releases free fatty acids from adipose	Hormone sensitive lipase
Fatty acid β-oxidation	Generates ATP in the fasted state	Carnitine palmitoyltransferase
Ketogenesis	Generates ketone bodies	Driven by substrate availability HMG-CoA synthase
Urea cycle	Nitrogen disposal	Carbamoyl phosphate synthetase I

Table 3.4: Summary of metabolism during the fasted state.

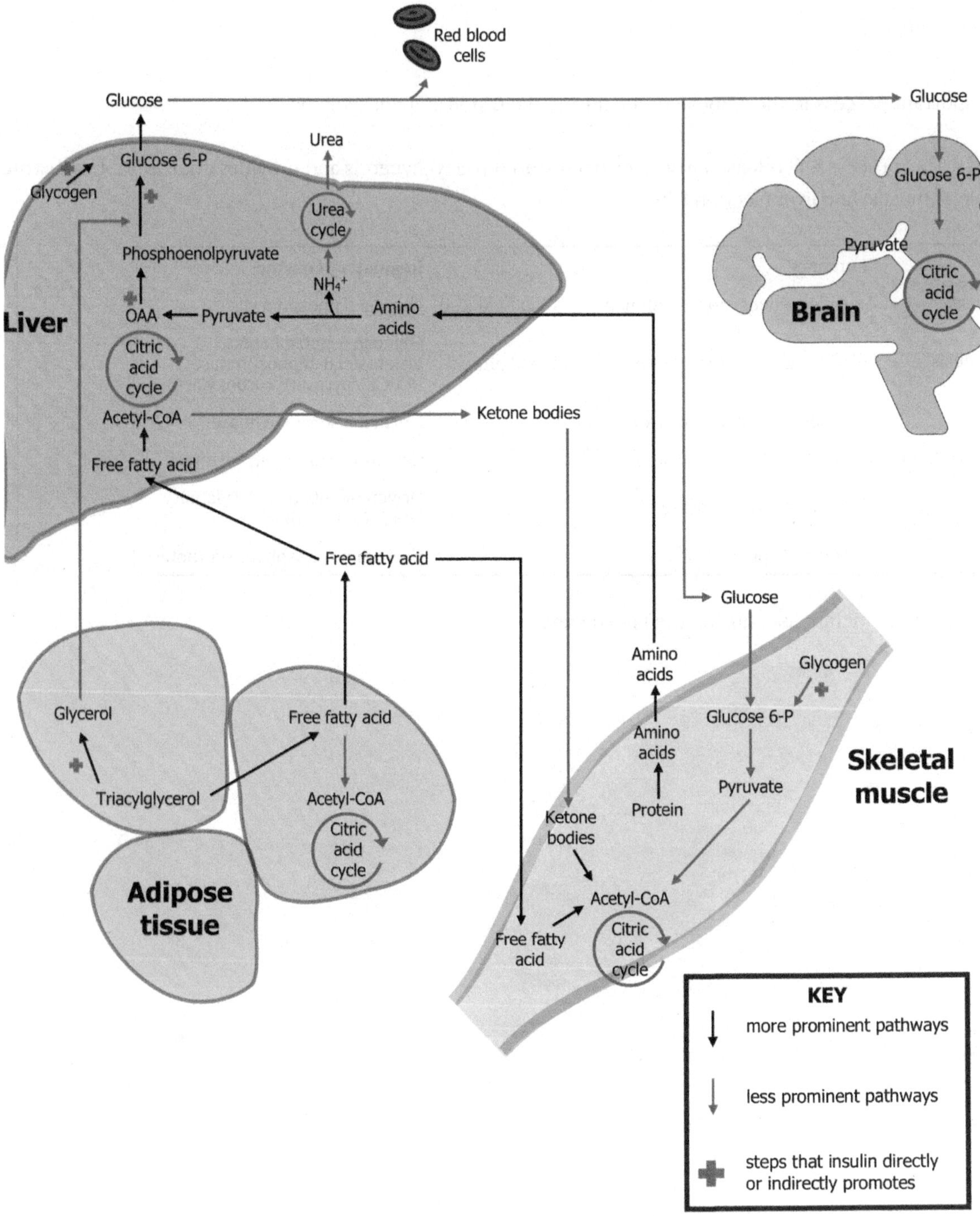

Figure 3.2: Overview of fasted state metabolism.

3.1 References and resources

Text

Ferrier, D. R., ed. *Lippincott Illustrated Reviews: Biochemistry*, 7th ed. Philadelphia: Wolters Kluwer Health/ Lippincott Williams & Wilkins, 2017, Chapter 24: Fed Fast Cycle.

Le, T., and V. Bhushan. *First Aid for the USMLE Step* 1, 29th ed. New York: McGraw Hill Education, 2018, 91, 324–325

.

Lieberman, M., A. and Peet, eds. *Marks' Basic Medical Biochemistry: A Clinical Approach*, 5th ed. Philadelphia: Wolters Kluwer Health/Lippincott Williams & Wilkins, 2018, Chapter 2: The Fed or Absorptive State, Chapter 3: The Fasted State.

Figures

Arm muscles anatomical. Public domain. From wpclipart.

Gregory D, Marshall D, Fat cells. CC BY 4.0. From Welcome Collection.

Grey, Kindred, Figure 3.1: Overview of fed state metabolism. 2021. CC BY 4.0. Added Liver by Liam Mitchell from the Noun Project, Brain by Maxicons from the Noun Project, and Muscle by Laymik from the Noun Project.

Grey, Kindred, Figure 3.2: Overview of fasted state metabolism. 2021. CC BY 4.0. Added Liver by Liam Mitchell from Noun Project, Brain by Maxicons from Noun Project, Muscle by Laymik from Noun Project, red blood cells by Lucas Helle from Noun Project.

Häggström M, Liver (transparent). Public domain. From Wikimedia Commons.

LadyofHats, Osmotic pressure on blood cells diagram. Public domain. From Wikimedia Commons.

_DJ_, Human brain on white background. 2005. CC BY-SA 2.0. From Flickr.

4. Fuel for Now

Learning Objectives

Glycolysis and the pyruvate dehydrogenase complex

- Compare the K_ms of glucokinase and hexokinase and relate this activity to their tissue specific activity.
- Determine flux through glycolysis based on the regulation of phosphofructokinase 1 and 2 (PFK1 / PFK2), pyruvate kinase (PK), and the pyruvate dehydrogenase complex.
- Describe the regulation and necessary cofactors of the pyruvate dehydrogenase complex (PDC).

Tricarboxylic acid cycle (TCA) and electron transport chain (ETC)

- Describe the impact of the ratio of $NADH/NAD^+$ and ATP/ADP on flux through the tricarboxylic acid cycle (isocitratedehydrogenase and α-ketoglutarate) and the ETC.
- Determine the relevance of the TCA cycle for providing key intermediates to other synthetic pathways (i.e. heme synthesis) and the need to replenish TCA cycle intermediates.
- Evaluate the role of the malate-aspartate shuttle and the glycerol 3-phosphate shuttle in transferring NADH across the mitochondrial membrane.
- Determine the impact of inhibitors and uncouplers on the ETC.

Fatty acid synthesis

- Describe fatty acid synthesis, including the location of the pathway, substrate, and regulation of acetyl-CoA carboxylase.

Glycogen synthesis

- Determine how glycogen synthesis is regulated in the liver and skeletal muscle (key enzyme: glycogen synthase).

About this Chapter

This chapter will focus on the pathways involved fuel usage in the fed state. Under these conditions, insulin is elevated and glucose uptake by most tissues is increased. The increase in fuel availability enhances both ATP production and fuel storage. Whether fuel is oxidized or stored depends on the regulation of various hepatic pathways (glycolysis, tricarboxyilc acid cycle (TCA), electron transport chain (ETC), fatty acid synthesis, and glycogen synthesis), and they all act in concert to maintain metabolic efficiency. The most important part of each of these pathways will be understanding the key regulatory enzymes and how flux can be altered through these regulatory mechanisms.

4.1 Glycolysis and the Pyruvate Dehydrogenase Complex (PDC)

Glycolysis can be divided into two parts, the preparative phase, which requires two ATP, and the energy producing phase, which produces NADH and ATP. The net result of glucose oxidation through glycolysis is two ATP, two NADH and two pyruvate. Briefly, the process of glycolysis starts with the phosphorylation of a glucose molecule (six-carbon sugar). The addition of a phosphate group traps the glucose in the cell where it will undergo isomerization to fructose 6-phosphate and further phosphorylation to fructose 1,6-bisphosphate. From here, fructose 1,6-bisphosphate is cleaved by aldolase B into two three-carbon compounds, which will ultimately produce two pyruvate. Under aerobic conditions, the pyruvate will enter the mitochondria and be oxidized to acetyl-CoA, which will enter the TCA cycle. When oxygen is limited or energy demands exceed oxygen delivery for ATP, the cell will rely on anaerobic glycolysis. In this case, lactate dehydrogenase will oxidize the NADH generated from glycolysis by reducing cytosolic pyruvate to lactate. Under these conditions oxygen is not required to reoxidize NADH, and therefore the process is referred to as anaerobic. The energy produced through this process is much less than through aerobic oxidation and therefore less favorable (figure 4.1).

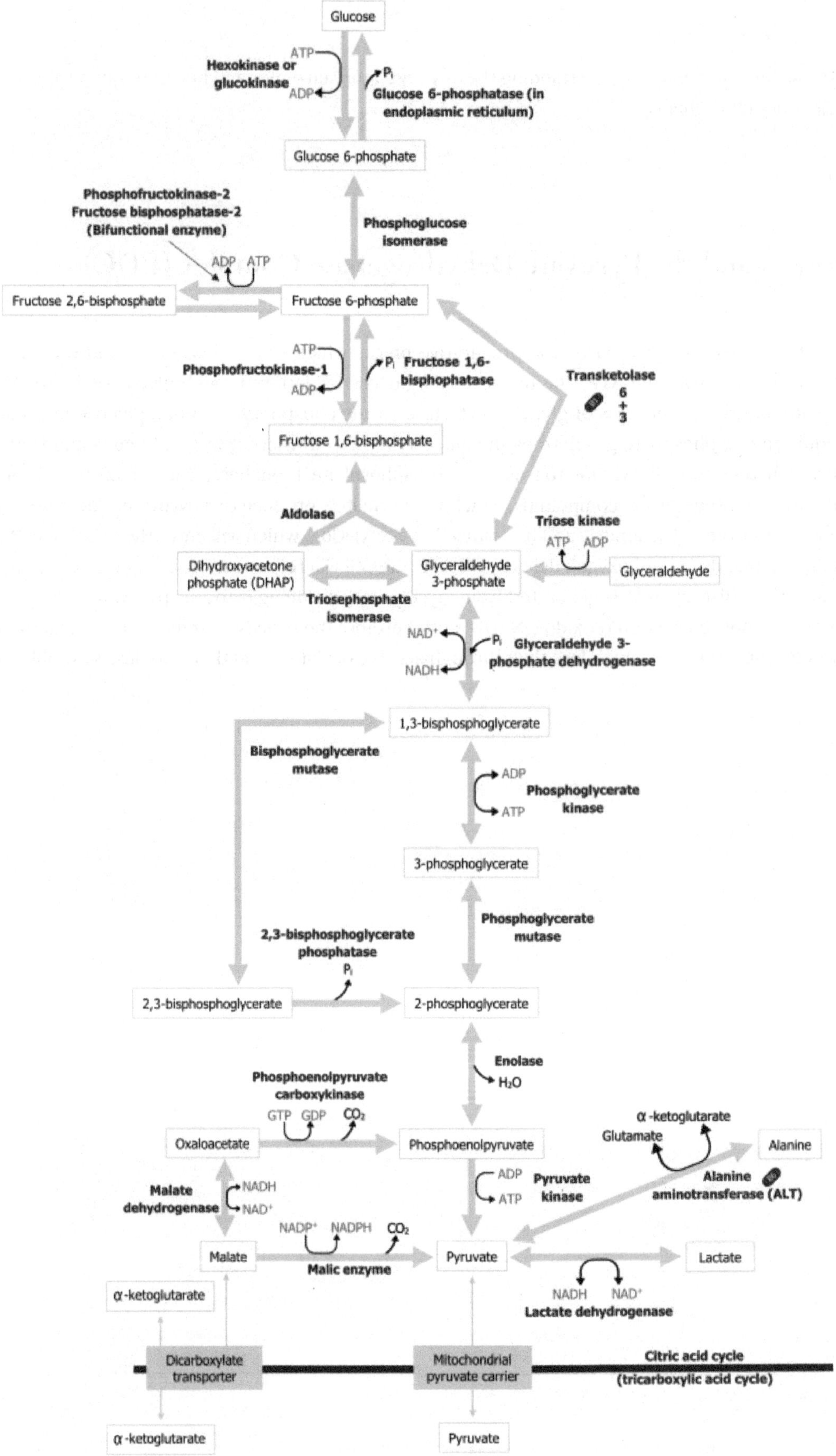
Glucose
ATP
Hexokinase or glucokinase
ADP
P_i
Glucose 6-phosphatase (in endoplasmic reticulum)
Glucose 6-phosphate
Phosphofructokinase-2
Fructose bisphosphatase-2
(Bifunctional enzyme)
Phosphoglucose isomerase
ADP ATP
Fructose 2,6-bisphosphate
Fructose 6-phosphate
ATP
Phosphofructokinase-1
ADP
P_i
Fructose 1,6-bisphophatase
Transketolase
6
+
3
Fructose 1,6-bisphosphate
Aldolase
Triose kinase
ATP ADP
Dihydroxyacetone phosphate (DHAP)
Glyceraldehyde 3-phosphate
Glyceraldehyde
Triosephosphate isomerase
NAD^+
P_i
Glyceraldehyde 3-phosphate dehydrogenase
NADH
1,3-bisphosphoglycerate
Bisphosphoglycerate mutase
ADP
Phosphoglycerate kinase
ATP
3-phosphoglycerate
Phosphoglycerate mutase
2,3-bisphosphoglycerate phosphatase
P_i
2,3-bisphosphoglycerate
2-phosphoglycerate
Enolase
H_2O
Phosphoenolpyruvate carboxykinase
GTP GDP CO_2
α-ketoglutarate
Glutamate
Oxaloacetate
Phosphoenolpyruvate
Alanine
ADP
Pyruvate kinase
ATP
Alanine aminotransferase (ALT)
Malate dehydrogenase
NADH
NAD^+
$NADP^+$ NADPH CO_2
Malate
Malic enzyme
Pyruvate
Lactate
α-ketoglutarate
NADH NAD^+
Lactate dehydrogenase
Dicarboxylate transporter
Mitochondrial pyruvate carrier
Citric acid cycle
(tricarboxylic acid cycle)
α-ketoglutarate
Pyruvate

Figure 4.1: Summary of glycolysis. The three regulated steps of the process will be the focus, and those are catalyzed by the enzymes glucokinase/hexokinase, phosphofructokinase 1 (PFK1), and pyruvate kinase. All other steps in glycolysis are reversible (as indicated by the arrows) and are also used in gluconeogenesis.

Regulation of glycolysis

Glycolysis in the liver has three primary regulated and irreversible steps (figure 4.1).

Glucokinase: Glucose to glucose 6-phosphate

In the liver, glucose is taken up through an insulin-independent process mediated by GLUT2 transporters. Following this, glucose must be phosphorylated to be trapped in the cell. The phosphorylation of glucose to glucose 6-phosphate is catalyzed by glucokinase (figure 4.2) in the liver.

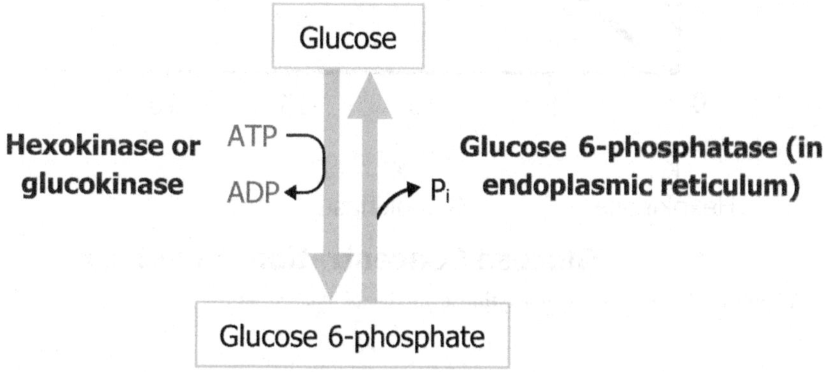

Figure 4.2: Regulatory step committed by hexo or glucokinase. The first regulatory step in glycolysis is the phosphorylation of glucose by hexo or glucokinase. The reverse reaction, which is part of gluconeogensis, is catalyzed by glucose 6-phosphatase.

In skeletal muscle, and most other peripheral tissues, glucose is phosphorylated by hexokinase.

Glucokinase and hexokinase perform the same reaction but have very different enzyme kinetics. Glucokinase (in the liver) has a higher K_m (lower affinity for glucose) when compared to hexokinase. In the liver, this enzyme will phosphorylate glucose only when glucose concentrations are high such as in the fed state. Glucokinase also has a high V_{max} and is therefore not rapidly saturated. This allows for continuous glucose uptake when glucose levels are high allowing for glucose storage and the rapid removal of glucose from circulation, minimizing the likelihood of hyperglycemia. In contrast, hexokinase has a lower K_m and a high affinity for glucose (figure 4.3). This enzyme becomes rapidly saturated over a very small range of glucose concentrations.

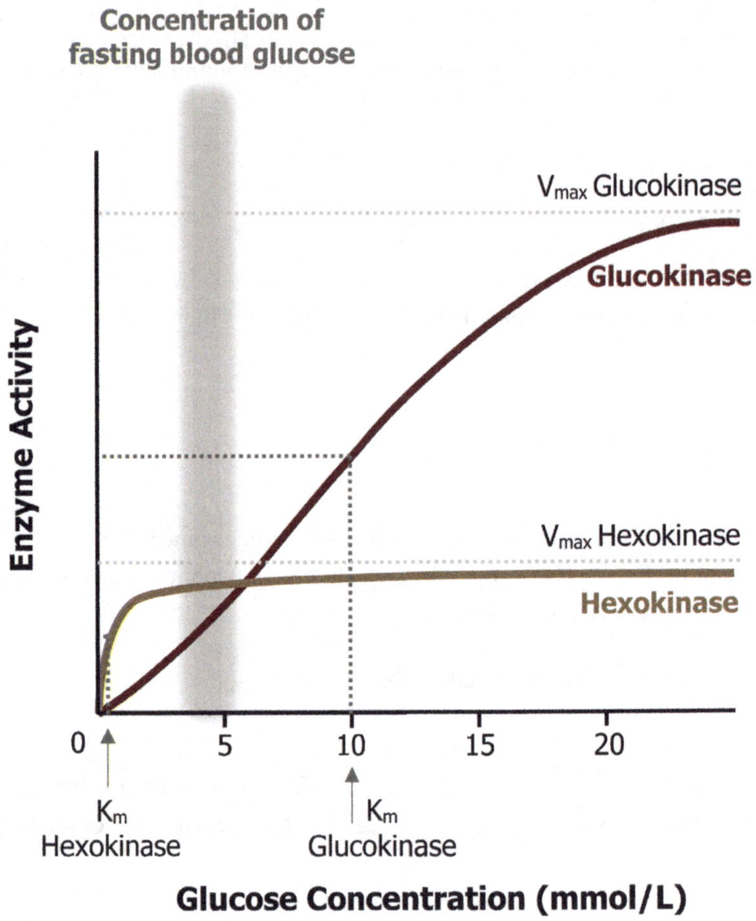

Figure 4.3: Comparison of glucokinase and hexokinase kinetics.

Regulation of glucokinase and hexokinase

Hexokinase is regulated through feedback inhibition where glucose 6-phosphate will compete with glucose for substrate binding. On the other hand, glucokinase is regulated through an alternative mechanism involving the glucokinase regulatory binding protein (GKRP). This protein will bind glucokinase and trap it in the nucleus. When glucose is high, glucokinase is released into the cytosol to phosphorylate glucose. As fructose 6-phosphate levels increase, this will inhibit the glucokinase reaction by enhancing the rebinding of glucokinase to GKRP, trapping it in the nucleus (figure 4.4).

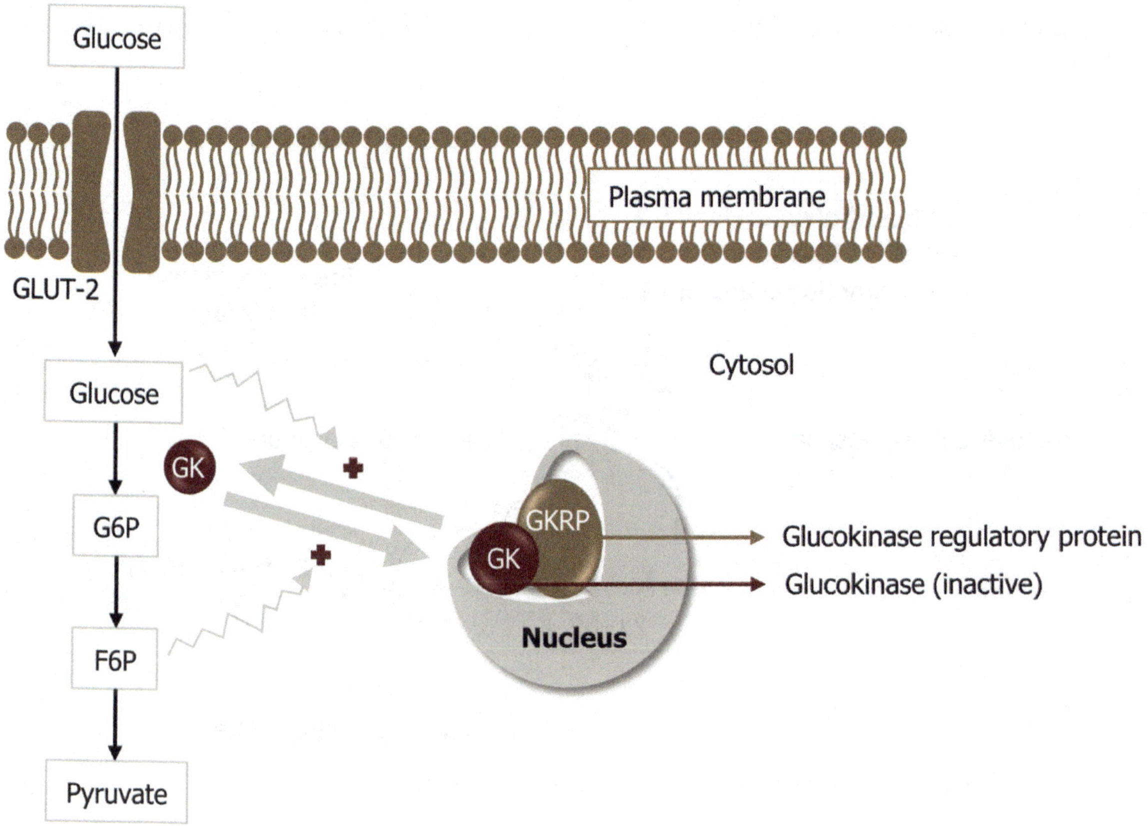

Figure 4.4: Regulation of glucokinase by glucokinase regulatory protein.

Phosphofructokinase 1 (PFK1): Fructose 6-phosphate to fructose 1,6-bisphosphate

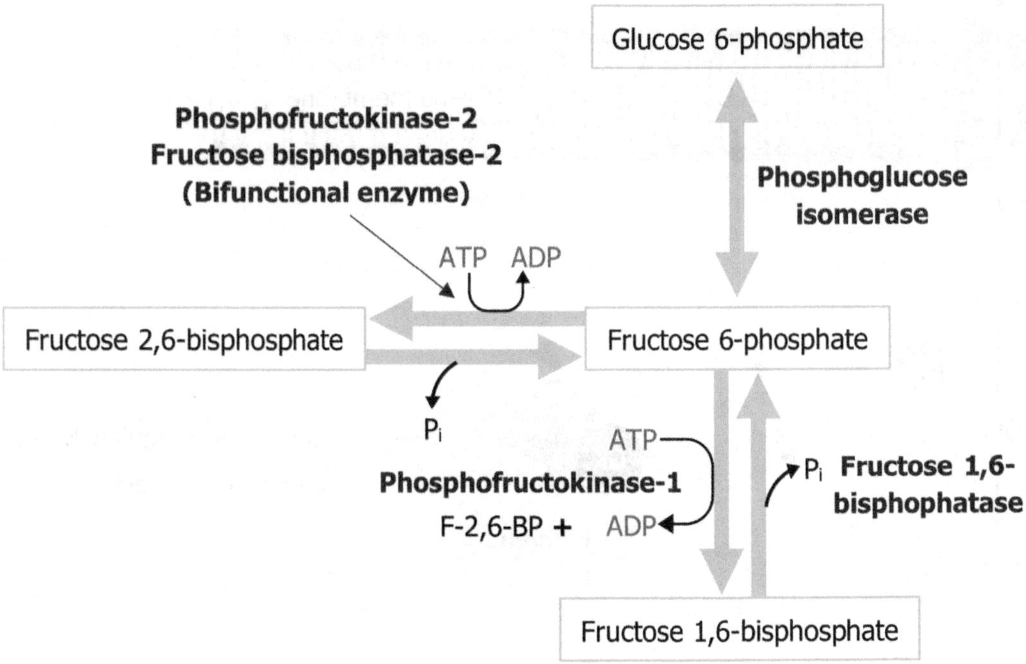

Figure 4.5: Regulation of PFK1 by fructose 2,6-bisphosphate generated by PFK2.

Following glucose phosphorylation to glucose 6-phosphate, the glucose 6-phosphate can be used for glycogen synthesis or the pentose phosphate pathway. Substrate that continues through glycolysis is isomerized to fructose 6-phosphate, which is the substrate for the reaction catalyzed by phosphofructokinase 1 (PFK1).

Regulation of phosphofructokinase 1 (PFK1)

Regulation of phosphofructokinase 1 is primarily through allosteric activation by AMP and fructose 2,6-bisphosphate. High AMP levels would indicate a lack of energy within the cell, and this would increase flux through glycolysis by enhancing the activity of PFK1. PFK1 is also inhibited by citrate and ATP; levels of these compounds are indicative of a high energy state, suggesting there are sufficient oxidation productions and glucose is diverted to storage pathways.

Fructose 2,6-bisphosphate is an important regulator of glycolysis, formed by a shunt in the glycolytic pathway. When there is an excess of fructose 6-phosphate in the cell, this substrate is accepted by phosphofructokinase 2 (PFK2) and converted to fructose 2,6-bisphosphate. This compound, fructose 2,6-bisphosphate, functions as an allosteric activator of PFK1. Additionally, PFK2 can be regulated by covalent modification such as phosphorylation. PFK2 is a bifunctional enzyme and only functions as a kinase when insulin is high and it is dephosphorylated. Under fasted conditions, when glucagon is high, this leads to the phosphorylation and inactivation of PFK2; when the enzyme is phosphorylated, it functions as a phosphatase and is referred to as fructose 2,6-bisphosphatase (FBP2) (figure 4.5).

Pyruvate kinase: Phosphoenol pyruvate to pyruvate

Following the synthesis of fructose 1,6-phosphate, aldolase will cleave this substrate into dihydroxyacetone and glyceraldehyde 3-phosphate. These three carbon compounds will be used to synthesize pyruvate in the final regulatory step of the pathway catalyzed by pyruvate kinase (PK).

Regulation of pyruvate kinase (PK)

The final regulatory step of glycolysis is the reaction catalyzed by pyruvate kinase. The enzyme converts phosphoenol pyruvate (PEP) to pyruvate. PK can be regulated by phosphorylation and allosteric means. PK is subject to feed-forward activation by fructose 1,6-bisphosphate, which allosterically activates the enzyme, increasing flux in the downward direction. As energy levels in the cell increase, ATP levels will reduce enzyme activity through allosteric inhibition (figure 4.6). PK can also be regulated through phosphorylation. Similar to PFK2, PK is dephosphorylated and active in the fed state but phosphorylated during the fasted state, which renders the enzyme inactive; the phosphorylation is glucagon mediated.

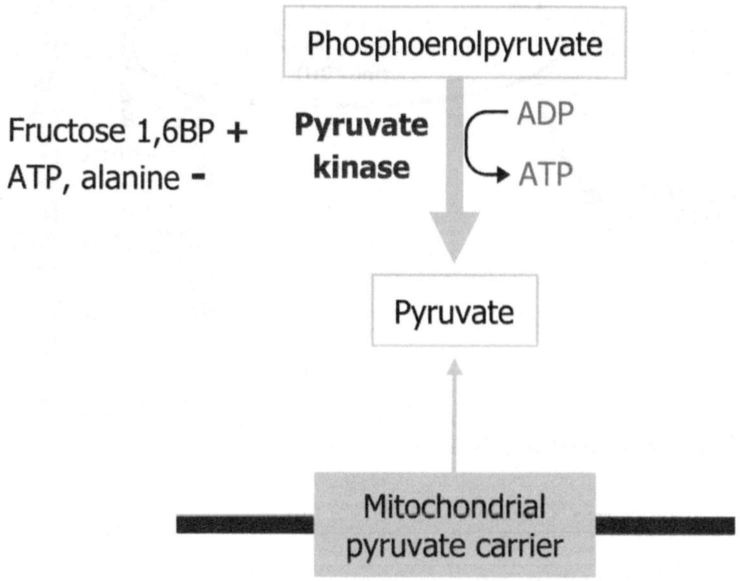

Figure 4.6: Regulation of pyruvate kinase phosphorylation and fructose 1,6-bisphosphate.

Movement of NADH from the cytosol to the mitochondria

The NADH generated in the cytosol by glycolysis must be oxidized back to NAD^+ in order to maintain a pool of NAD^+ needed for glucose oxidation. As NADH oxidation takes place in the mitochondria, and the membrane is not permeable to NADH, two shuttles are used to move cytosolic NADH into the mitochondria. These processes are a way to get energy out of cytoplasmic NADH into the mitochondria.

Glycerol 3-phosphate shuttle

The glycerol 3-phosphate shuttle is the major shuttle used in most tissues to move NADH from the cytosol to the mitochondria for oxidation. In this pathway, NAD^+ is regenerated by glycerol 3-phosphate dehydrogenase, which transfers electrons from NADH to dihydroxyacetonephosphate to generate glycerol 3-phosphate. Glycerol 3-phosphate can diffuse across the mitochondrial membrane where it will donate electrons to membrane bound FAD (bound to succinate dehydrogenase) (figure 4.7).

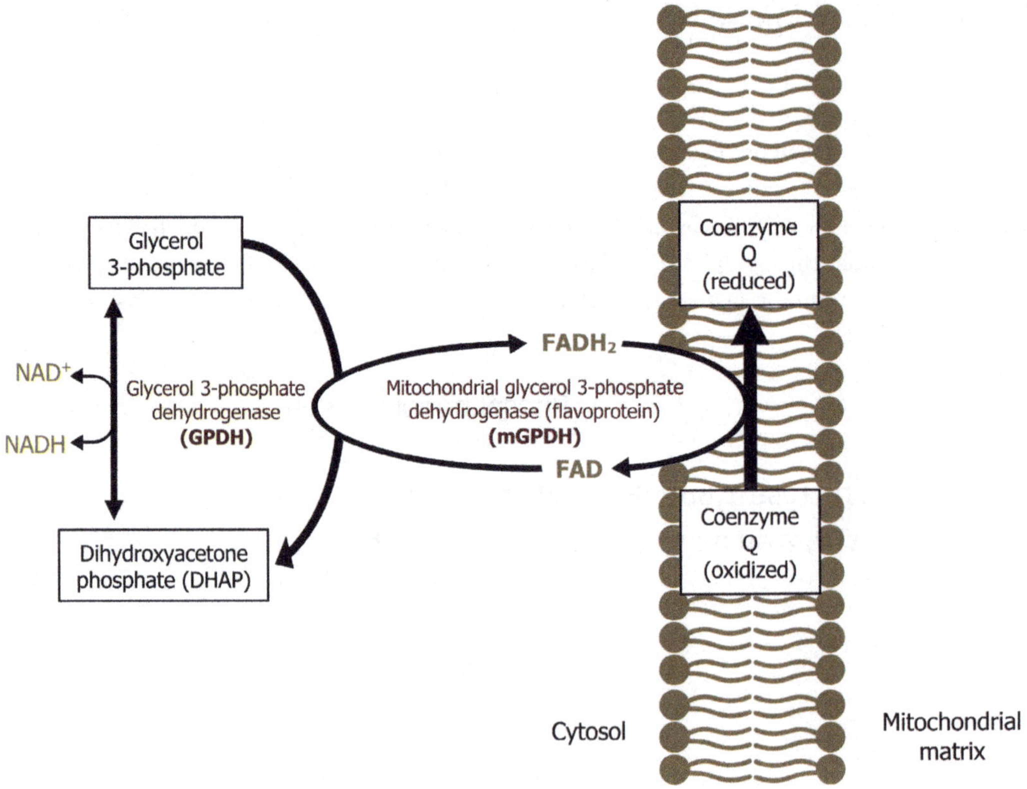

Figure 4.7: Glycerol 3-phosphate shuttle.

Malate-aspartate shuttle

Many tissues also contain the malate-aspartate shuttle, which can also carry cytosolic NADH into the mitochondria. Cytosolic NADH is used to reduce oxaloacetate (OAA) to malate, which can cross the mitochondrial membrane. Once inside the mitochondria, malate can be oxidized to OAA to produce NADH. OAA can't pass through the mitochondrial membrane, so it requires transamination to aspartate, which can be shuttled into the cytosol to regenerate the cycle (figure 4.8).

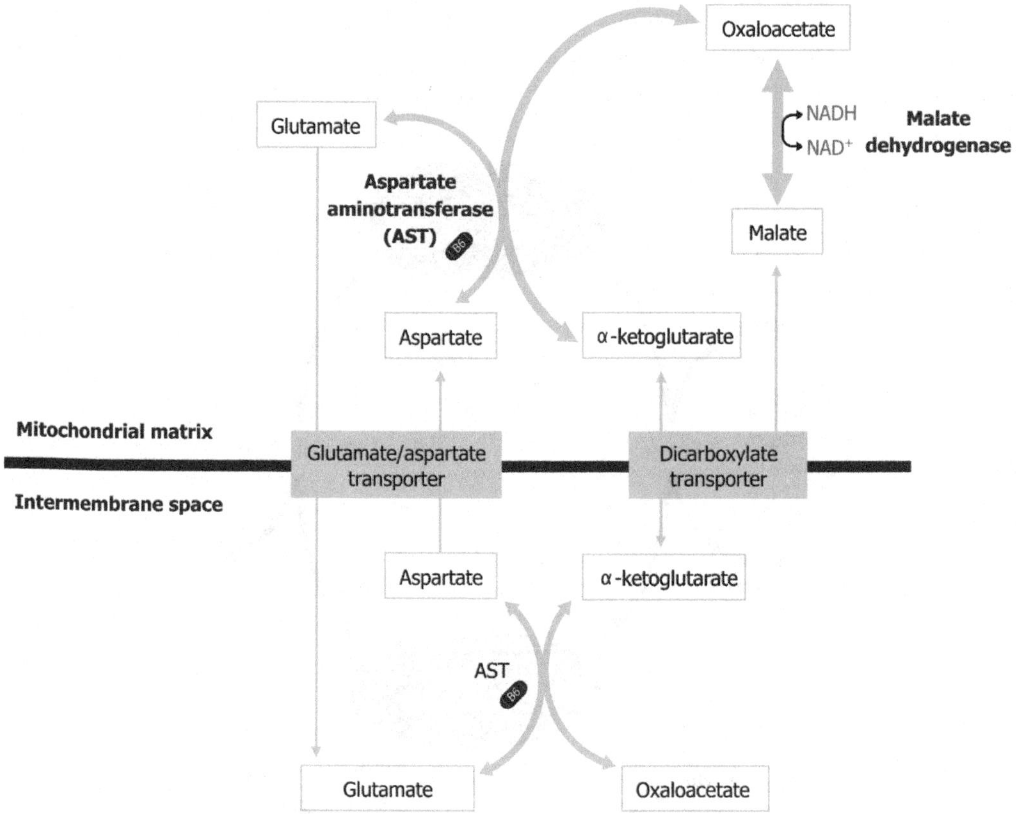

Figure 4.8: Malate-aspartate shuttle.

Pyruvate dehydrogenase complex

Under aerobic conditions, the pyruvate produced by glycolysis will be oxidized to acetyl-CoA using the pyruvate dehydrogenase complex (PDC). This enzyme is a key transition point between cytosolic and mitochondrial metabolism. This complex is composed of three subunits, which require the cofactors thiamine pyrophosphate, lipoic acid, and $FADH_2$; NADH is also required for the reaction to move forward. The enzyme is highly regulated by both covalent and allosteric regulation. Deficiencies of the PDC can be recessive or X-linked (depending on the subunit deficient) and present with symptoms of lactic acidosis after consuming a meal high in carbohydrates. This metabolic deficiency can be managed by delivering a ketogenic diet and bypassing glycolysis all together.

Regulation of the pyruvate dehydrogenase complex (PDC)

The PDC is regulated by allosteric and covalent regulations. The complex itself can be allosterically activated by pyruvate and NAD^+. Elevation of substrate (pyruvate) will enhance flux through this enzyme as will the indication of low energy states as triggered by high NAD^+ levels. The PDC is also inhibited by acetyl-CoA and NADH directly. Product inhibition is a very common regulatory mechanism, and high NADH would signal sufficient energy levels, therefore decreasing activity of the PDC.

The PDC is also regulated through covalent modification. Phosphorylation of the complex will decrease activity of the enzyme.

The enzyme responsible for phosphorylation of the PDC is pyruvate dehydrogenase kinase. The kinase is regulated inversely to the PDC (figure 4.9). The kinase is most active when acetyl-CoA and NADH are high. These compounds will stimulate the kinase to phosphorylate and inactivate the PDC. The PDC can be dephosphorylated by a calcium-mediated phosphatase.

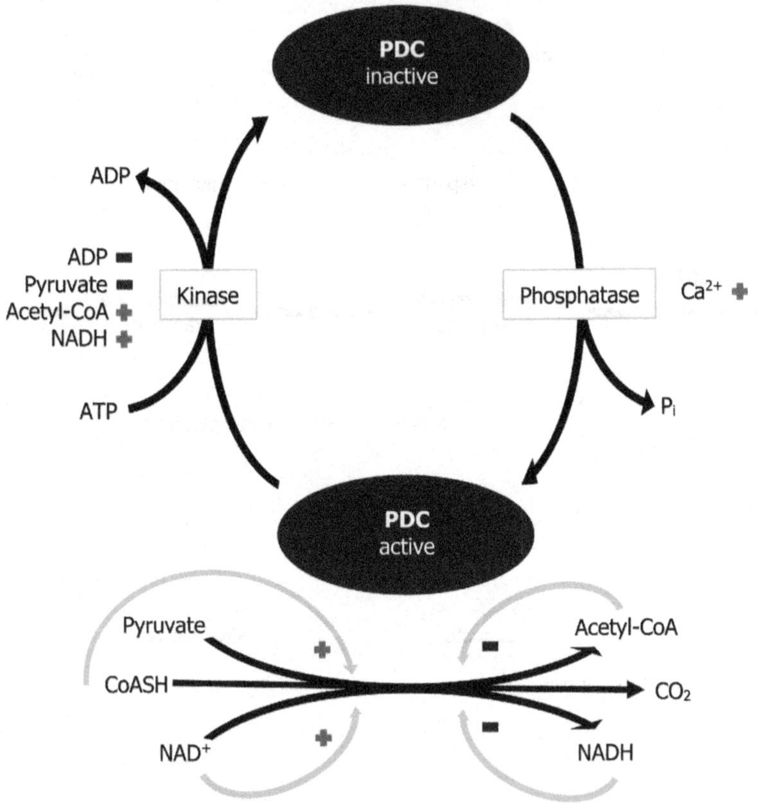

Figure 4.9: Regulation of the pyruvate dehydrogenase complex (PDC).

Summary of pathway regulation

Metabolic pathway	Major regulatory enzyme(s)	Allosteric effectors	Hormonal effects
Glycolysis (pyruvate oxidation)	Glucokinase (liver)	GKRP	
Glycolysis (pyruvate oxidation)	Hexokinase	Glucose 6-P (-)	
Glycolysis (pyruvate oxidation)	PFK-1	Fructose 2,6-BP, AMP (+) Citrate (-)	Insulin/glucagon ratio >1 → dephosphorylation of PFK2 and increased production of F 2,6-BP
Glycolysis (pyruvate oxidation)	Pyruvate kinase	Fructose 1,6-BP (+) ATP, alanine (-)	Insulin/glucagon ratio >1 → dephosphorylation
Pyruvate dehydrogenase complex	PDC	Pyruvate, NAD+ (+) Acetyl-CoA, NADH, ATP (-)	Insulin/glucagon ratio >1 → dephosphorylation

Table 4.1: Summary of pathway regulation.

4.1 References and resources

Text

Ferrier, D. R., ed. *Lippincott Illustrated Reviews: Biochemistry*, 7th ed. Philadelphia: Wolters Kluwer Health/ Lippincott Williams & Wilkins, 2017, Chapter 6: Bioenergetics and Oxidative Phosphorylation: Section V, VI, Chapter 8: Introduction to Metabolism and Glycolysis, Chapter 9: TCA Cycle and Pyruvate Dehydrogenase Complex: Section IIA, IIB, Chapter 11: Glycogen Metabolism: Section V, VI, Chapter 16: Fatty Acid Ketone Body and TAG Metabolism: Section II, IV, V, Chapter 23: Metabolic Effect of Insulin and Glucagon, Chapter 25: Diabetes Mellitus.

Le, T., and V. Bhushan. *First Aid for the USMLE Step 1*, 29th ed. New York: McGraw Hill Education, 2018, 72–78, 85–89.

Lieberman, M., and A. Peet, eds. *Marks' Basic Medical Biochemistry: A Clinical Approach*, 5th ed. Philadelphia: Wolters Kluwer Health/Lippincott Williams & Wilkins, 2018, Chapter 2: The Fed or Absorptive State, Chapter 19: Basic Concepts of Regulation: Section IV.A.1.2, Chapter 20: Cellular Bioenergetics, Chapter 22: Generation of ATP from Glucose: Section I.A.B.C, III, Chapter 24: Oxidative Phosphorylation and the ETC: Section I.E, II, III, Chapter 31: Synthesis of Fatty Acids: Section I.A.B, IV, V.

Figures

Grey, Kindred, Figure 4.1 Summary of glycolysis… 2021. https://archive.org/details/4.1_20210924. CC BY 4.0.

Grey, Kindred, Figure 4.2 Regulatory step committed by hexo or glucokinase… 2021. https://archive.org/details/4.2_20210924. CC BY 4.0.

Grey, Kindred, Figure 4.4 Regulation of glucokinase by glucokinase regulatory protein. 2021. https://archive.org/details/4.4_20210924. CC BY 4.0. Added ion channel by Léa Lortal from Noun Project and sphere by Pablo Rozenberg from Noun Project.

Grey, Kindred, Figure 4.5 Regulation of PFK1 by fructose 2,6-bisphosphate generated by PFK2. 2021. https://archive.org/details/4.5-new. CC BY 4.0.

Grey, Kindred, Figure 4.6 Regulation of pyruvate kinase phosphorylation and fructose 1,6-bisphosphate. 2021. https://archive.org/details/4.6-new. CC BY 4.0.

Grey, Kindred, Figure 4.7 Glycerol 3-phosphate shuttle. 2021. https://archive.org/details/4.7_20210924. CC BY 4.0. Added ion channel by Léa Lortal from the Noun Project.

Grey, Kindred, Figure 4.8 Malate-aspartate shuttle. 2021. https://archive.org/details/4.8_20210924. CC BY 4.0.

Lieberman M, Peet A. Figure 4.3 Comparison of glucokinase and hexokinase kinetics. Adapted under Fair Use from Marks' Basic Medical Biochemistry. 5th Ed. pp 154. Figure 9.4 A comparison between hexokinase I and glucokinase. 2017.

Lieberman M, Peet A. Figure 4.9 Regulation of the PDC. Adapted under Fair Use from Marks' Basic Medical Biochemistry. 5th Ed. pp 471. Figure 23.15 Regulation of pyruvate dehydroenase complex (PDC). 2017.

4.2 Tricarboxylic Acid Cycle (TCA)

The TCA cycle is responsible for generating over half of the ATP from the oxidation of fuels. This is primarily because the substrate for the TCA cycle, acetyl-CoA, is generated by the oxidation of fatty acids, glucose, amino acids, and ketone bodies. With each turn of the TCA cycle, there is a net production of three NADH, $FADH_2$, two CO_2, and one GTP for every acetyl-CoA that enters (figure 4.10).

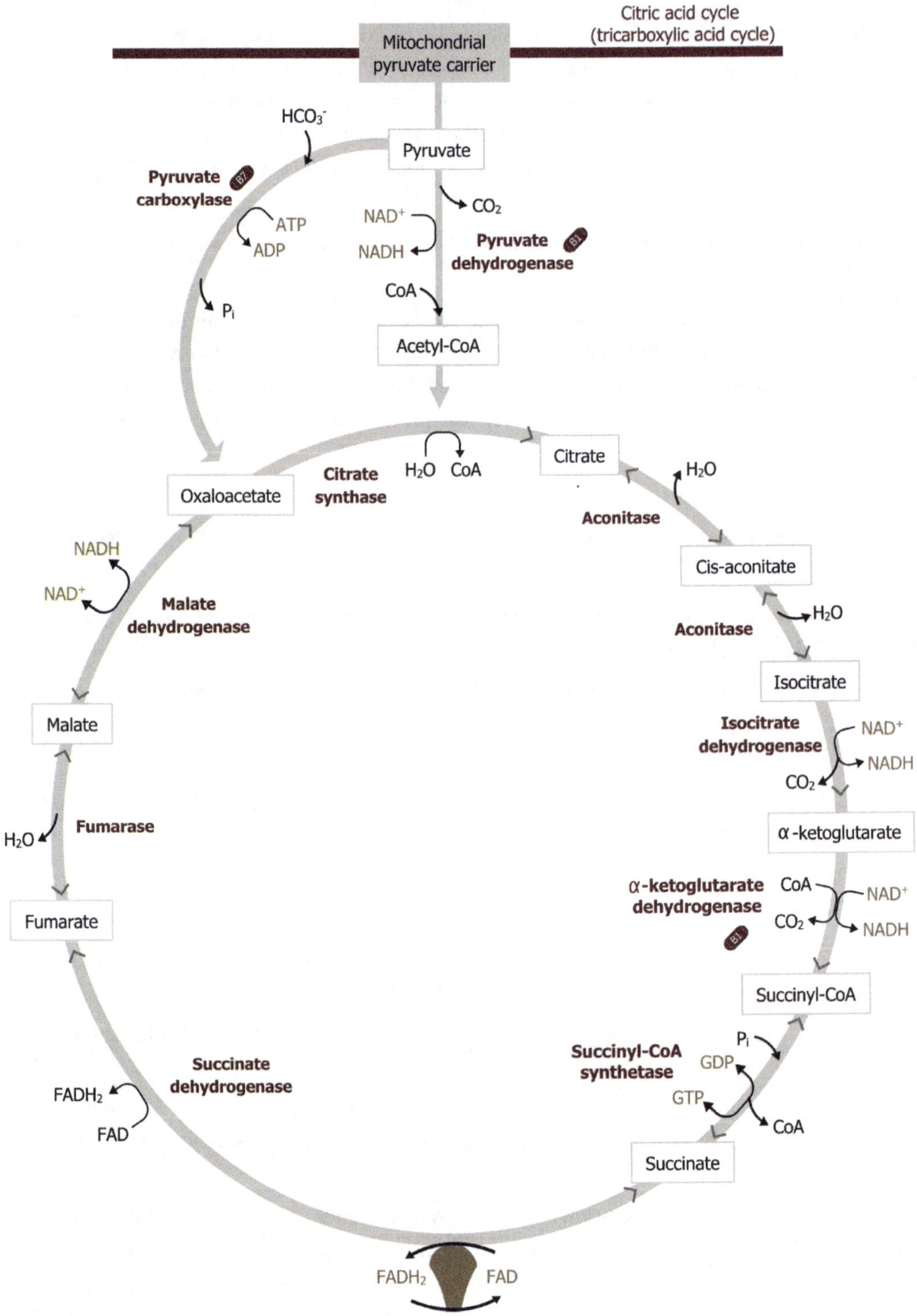

Figure 4.10: Overview of the TCA cycle.

The other major role of the TCA cycle is to provide substrates for other synthetic pathways. Malate is shuttled out of the TCA cycle and used as a substrate for gluconeogenesis and oxaloacetate (OAA) and α-ketoglutarate are used as substrates for amino acid synthesis. Through transamination reactions, these two keto-acids can be converted into aspartate and glutamate, respectively. α-ketoglutarate is also a key substrate for the synthesis of neurotransmitters, and succinyl-CoA is the substrate for heme synthesis. Citrate is also a key compound as it is both an intermediate of the TCA cycle and can be shuttled into the cytosol to provide acetyl-CoA for both cholesterol and fatty acid synthesis (figure 4.11).

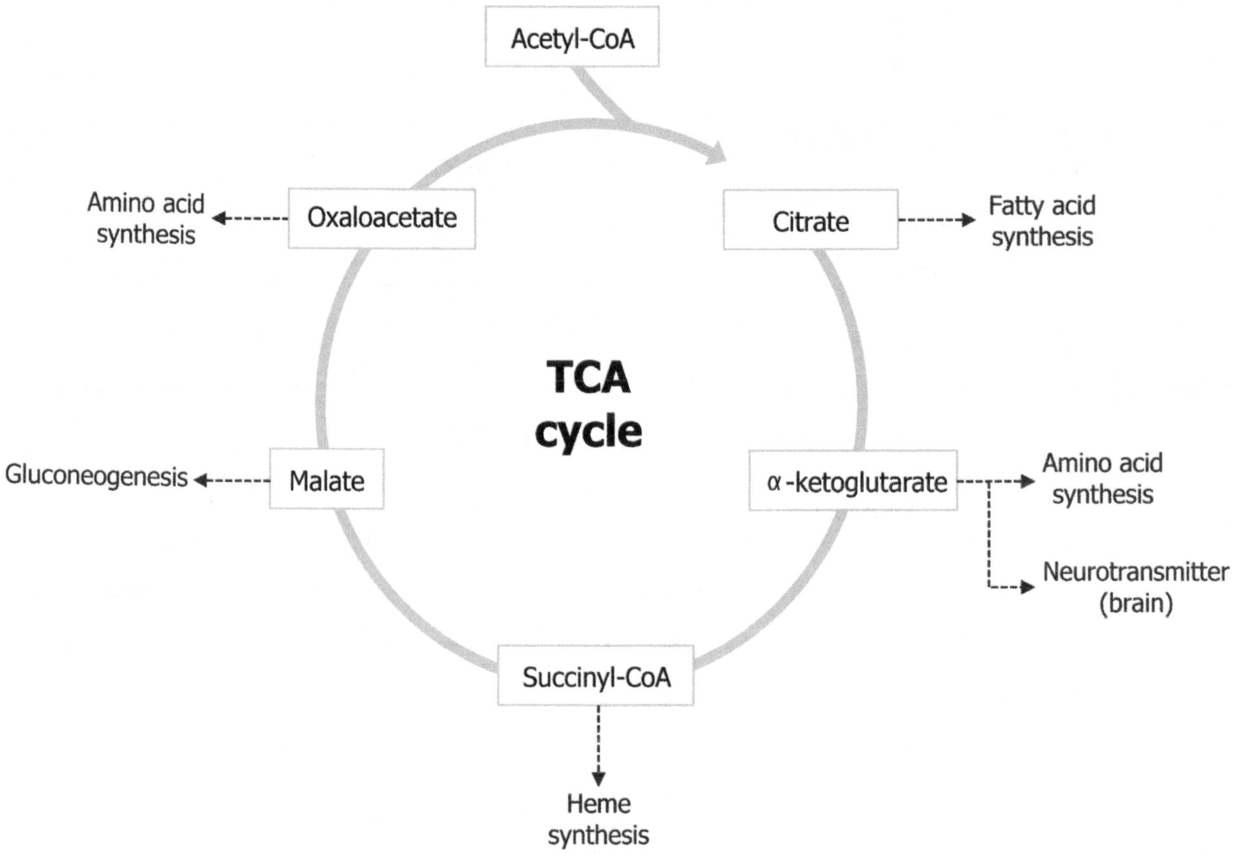

Figure 4.11: Substrates produced by the TCA cycle.

In order to maintain a pool of TCA cycle intermediates, as substrates are removed from the cycle, there are several key reactions (anaplerotic reactions) that are responsible for the addition of intermediates. These reactions are illustrated in figure 4.12. Notice all of these reactions add carbon back to the cycle from amino acids (reactions 1, 2, 3, 4, 5). These will become very important in the discussion of gluconeogenesis where these substrates will provide the majority of carbon for glucose production. Odd chain fatty acid oxidation can also provide carbon in the from of propionyl-CoA (3) although this is not a primary source of TCA cycle intermediates.

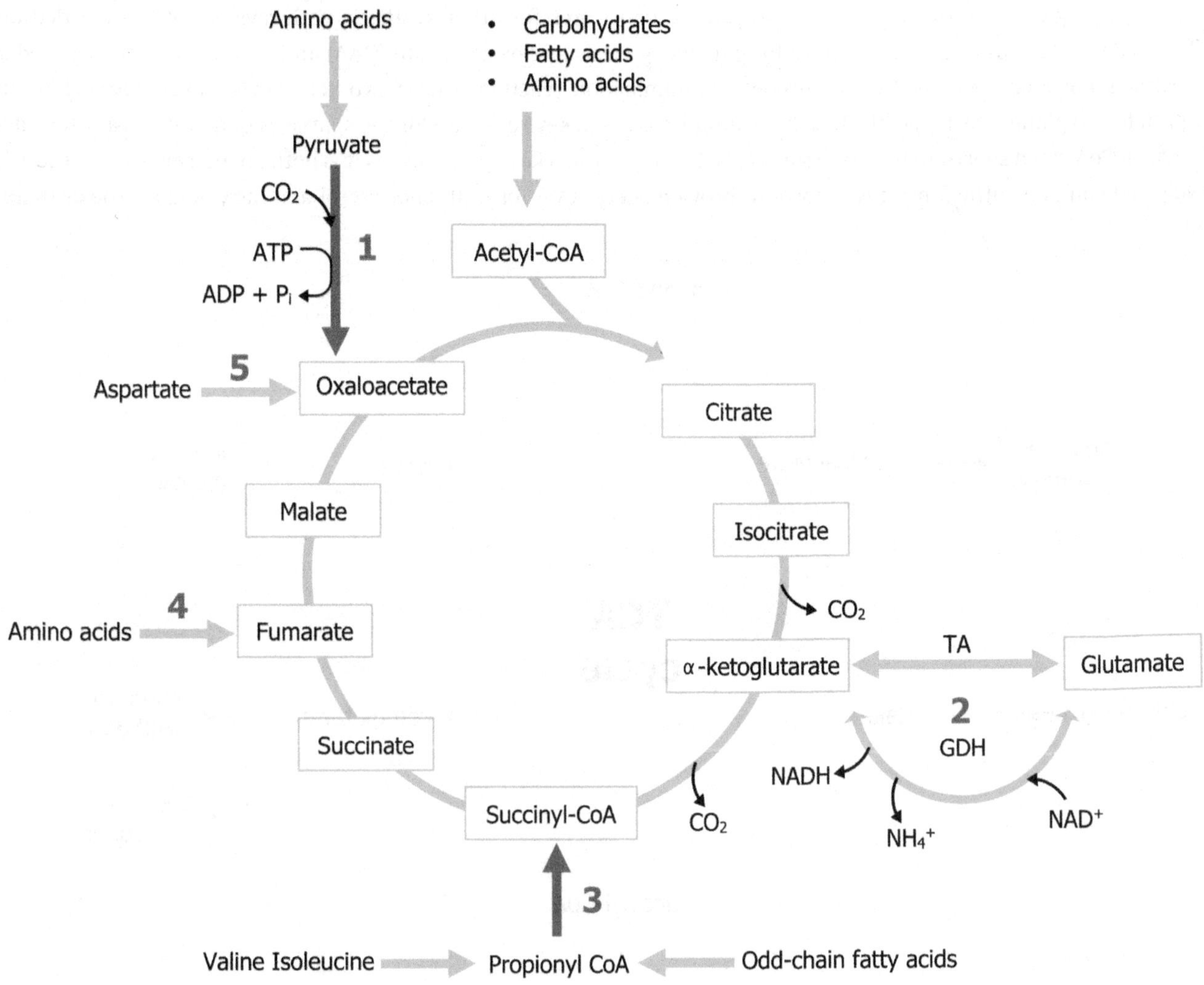

Figure 4.12: Anaplerotic reactions of the TCA cycle.

Regulation of the TCA cycle

Throughout the cycle, there are two key regulatory and irreversible steps to be aware of. The first is the conversion of isocitrate to α-ketoglutarate by isocitrate dehydrogenase, and the second is the conversion of α-ketoglutarate to succinyl-CoA by α-ketoglutarate dehydrogenase. The two key regulatory points are:

Isocitrate dehydrogenase, which can be activated by Ca^{2+} and ADP to increase flux through the cycle, and inhibited by NADH, which would suggest adequate energy in the cell.

Likewise, **α-ketoglutarate dehydrogenase** can be activated by Ca^{2+} and inhibited by NADH (and succinyl-CoA) (figure 4.13).

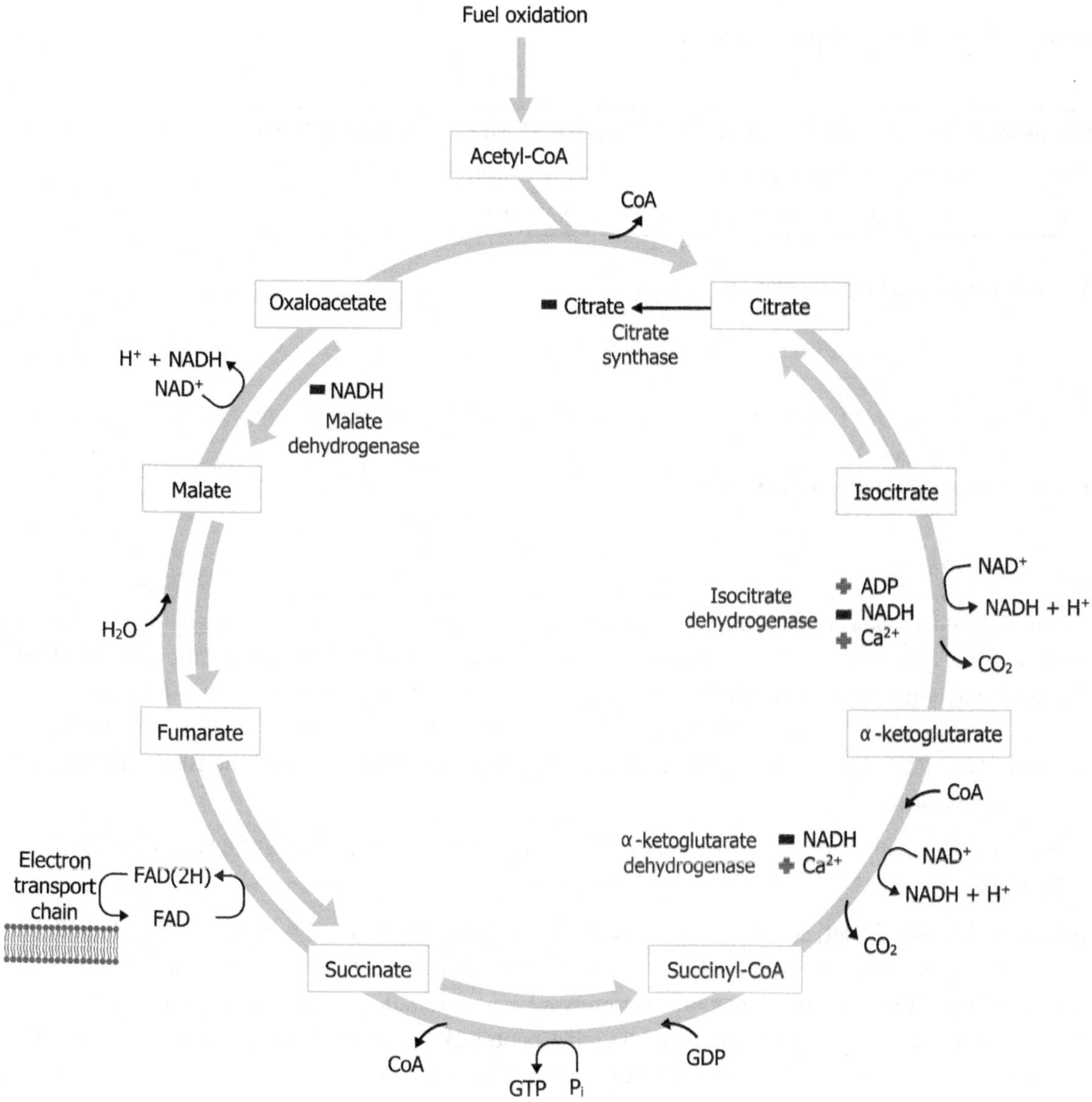

Figure 4.13: Regulation of the TCA cycle.

Malate dehydrogenase can also be inhibited by NADH, however, the reaction is reversible depending on levels of NADH. The oxidation of malate to OAA requires NAD^+, and under certain pathological situations the lack of free NAD^+ within the mitochondria will reduce the rate of this reaction (this is common in the case of alcohol metabolism).

Keep in mind that with the addition of each acetyl-CoA (comprised of 2 carbons) to the TCA cycle, two molecules of CO_2 are released, thus there is no net gain or loss of carbons in the cycle. The process moves forward driven by energetics and substrate availability. The pathway can be active in both the fed and fasted states. In the fed state, acetyl-CoA is generated primarily through glucose oxidation. In contrast, in the fasted state acetyl-CoA is generated primarily from β-oxidation, and the majority of acetyl-CoA is used to synthesize ketones.

Summary of pathway regulation

Metabolic pathway	Major regulatory enzyme(s)	Allosteric effectors	Hormonal effects
TCA cycle	Isocitrate dehydrogenase	ADP, Ca+ (+) NADH (-)	
TCA cycle	α-ketoglutarate dehydrogenase	Ca+ (+) NADH (-)	

Table 4.2: Summary of pathway regulation.

4.2 References and resources

Text

Ferrier, D. R., ed. *Lippincott Illustrated Reviews: Biochemistry*, 7th ed. Philadelphia: Wolters Kluwer Health/ Lippincott Williams & Wilkins, 2017, Chapter 6: Bioenergetics and Oxidative Phosphorylation: Section V, VI, Chapter 8: Introduction to Metabolism and Glycolysis, Chapter 9: TCA Cycle and Pyruvate Dehydrogenase Complex: Section IIA, IIB, Chapter 11: Glycogen Metabolism: Section V, VI, Chapter 16: Fatty Acid Ketone Body and TAG Metabolism: Section II, IV, V, Chapter 23: Metabolic Effect of Insulin and Glucagon, Chapter 25: Diabetes Mellitus.

Le, T., and V. Bhushan. *First Aid for the* USMLE *Step* 1, 29th ed. New York: McGraw Hill Education, 2018, 72–78, 85–89.

Lieberman, M., and A. Peet, eds. *Marks' Basic Medical Biochemistry: A Clinical Approach*, 5th ed. Philadelphia: Wolters Kluwer Health/Lippincott Williams & Wilkins, 2018, Chapter 2: The Fed or Absorptive State, Chapter 19: Basic Concepts of Regulation: Section IV.A.1.2, Chapter 20: Cellular Bioenergetics, Chapter 22: Generation of ATP from Glucose: Section I.A.B.C, III, Chapter 24: Oxidative Phosphorylation and the ETC: Section I.E, II, III, Chapter 31: Synthesis of Fatty Acids: Section I.A.B, IV, V.

Figures

Grey, Kindred, Figure 4.10 Overview of the TCA cycle. 2021. https://archive.org/details/4.10-new. CC BY 4.0.

Grey, Kindred, Figure 4.11 Substrates produced by the TCA cycle. 2021. https://archive.org/details/4.11_20210924. CC BY 4.0.

Lieberman M, Peet A. Figure 4.12 Anaplerotic reactions of the TCA cycle. Adapted under Fair Use from Marks' Basic Medical Biochemistry. 5th Ed. pp 473. Figure 23.18 Major anaplerotic pathways of the tricarboxylic acid (TCA) cycle. 2017.

Lieberman M, Peet A. Figure 4.13 Regulation of the TCA cycle. Adapted under Fair Use from Marks' Basic Medical Biochemistry. 5th Ed. pp 468. Figure 23.11 Major regulatory interaction in the tricarboxylic acid (TCA) cycle. 2017. Added ion channel by Léa Lortal from the Noun Project.

4.3 Electron Transport Chain (ETC)

In the production of NADH and $FADH_2$ by the TCA cycle, β-oxidation or glycolysis is funneled directly into the electron transport chain (ETC) where each of these reduced coenzymes will donate two electrons to electron carriers. As the electrons are passed down their oxidation gradient, some of the energy is lost, but much of this energy is used to pump protons into the intermembrane space of the mitochondria.

The process of oxidative phosphorylation (figure 4.14) involves the coupling of electron transfer with the pumping of protons to generate an electrochemical gradient across the mitochondrial membrane. With the exception of CoQ all proteins are bound to the mitochondria membrane, and electrons are passed between metal containing cytochromes. Complex I and Complex II function in parallel (rather than series) with each other having preference for NADH or $FADH_2$, respectively. Complex II (succinate dehydrogenase) is not required for oxidative phosphorylation because it does not span the mitochondrial membrane (figure 4.14). Electrons are passed down an electrochemical gradient, and molecular oxygen is the final electron acceptor (molecular oxygen).

There are site specific inhibitors of the ETC to be aware of, and these will disrupt electron flow reducing overall ATP production.

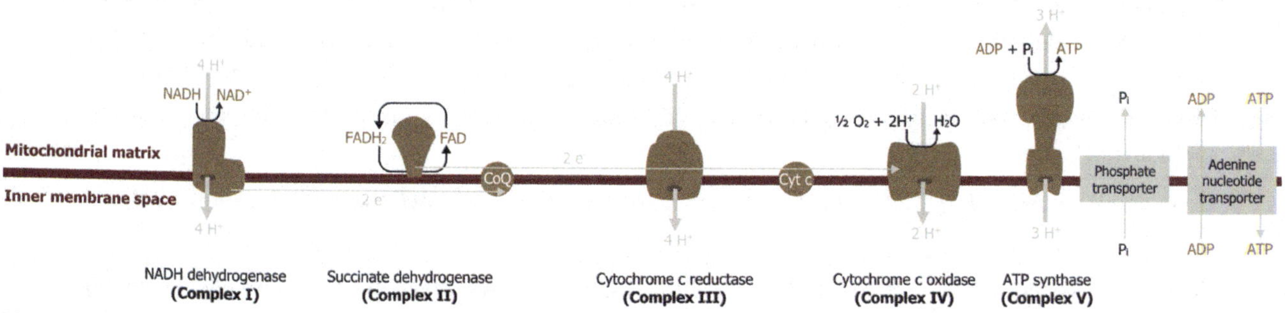

Figure 4.14: Overview of the electron transport chain (ETC).

Inhibitors

Inhibitors block oxidation and reduce both ATP generation and oxygen consumption; this is in contrast to uncouplers, which disrupt the mitochondrial membrane and reduce ATP production but increase oxygen consumption.

A common inhibitor of the ETC is carbon monoxide; this will bind to Complex IV and therefore halt the passing of electrons. Without electrons passing through the complexes, the pumping of protons is diminished and ATP is not produced. Other common inhibitors are cyanide (Complex IV), rotenone (Complex I), antimycin C (Complex III), and oligomycin, which is a Complex V inhibitor.

Uncouplers

Uncoupling of the ETC by the addition of agents such as dinitrophenol have different consequences. Uncouplers disrupt the permeability of the inner membrane (either physically or chemically) and dissipate the proton gradient.

In these cases, the release of protons across the membrane is coupled with the release of heat, rather than harnessed in the form of a phosphate bond. NADH oxidation continues rapidly, oxygen consumption is increased, and ATP production decreases. Valinomycin is another common uncoupler.

Biological uncoupling through the expression of uncoupling proteins (UPC) is also likely. These proteins form a physical pore within the mitochondrial membrane allowing the proton gradient to equilibrate. In brown fat, this nonshivering thermogenesis is a means of generating heat, and other members of this protein family (UPC) are expressed in various tissues but have similar roles.

4.3 References and resources

Text

Ferrier, D. R., ed. *Lippincott Illustrated Reviews: Biochemistry*, 7th ed. Philadelphia: Wolters Kluwer Health/ Lippincott Williams & Wilkins, 2017, Chapter 6: Bioenergetics and Oxidative Phosphorylation: Section V, VI, Chapter 8: Introduction to Metabolism and Glycolysis, Chapter 9: TCA Cycle and Pyruvate Dehydrogenase Complex: Section IIA, IIB, Chapter 11: Glycogen Metabolism: Section V, VI, Chapter 16: Fatty Acid Ketone Body and TAG Metabolism: Section II, IV, V, Chapter 23: Metabolic Effect of Insulin and Glucagon, Chapter 25: Diabetes Mellitus.

Le, T., and V. Bhushan. *First Aid for the USMLE Step 1*, 29th ed. New York: McGraw Hill Education, 2018, 72–78, 85–89.

Lieberman, M., and A. Peet, eds. *Marks' Basic Medical Biochemistry: A Clinical Approach*, 5th ed. Philadelphia: Wolters Kluwer Health/Lippincott Williams & Wilkins, 2018, Chapter 2: The Fed or Absorptive State, Chapter 19: Basic Concepts of Regulation: Section IV.A.1.2, Chapter 20: Cellular Bioenergetics, Chapter 22: Generation of ATP from Glucose: Section I.A.B.C, III, Chapter 24: Oxidative Phosphorylation and the ETC: Section I.E, II, III, Chapter 31: Synthesis of Fatty Acids: Section I.A.B, IV, V.

Figures

Grey, Kindred, Figure 4.14 Overview of the electron transport chain (ETC). 2021. https://archive.org/ details/4.14_20210924. CCBY 4.0.

4.4 Fatty Acid Synthesis

The synthesis of fatty acids is an anabolic pathway that occurs in the cytosol under fed conditions. As glucose is taken up by the liver and the flux through the TCA cycle increases, excess citrate is removed via the citrate shuttle. Once in the cytosol, citrate is cleaved by citrate lyase back into oxaloacetate (OAA) and acetyl-CoA. The OAA can be reduced to malate by cytosolic malate dehydrogenase and decarboxylated by malic enzyme producing pyruvate and NADPH (figure 4.15).

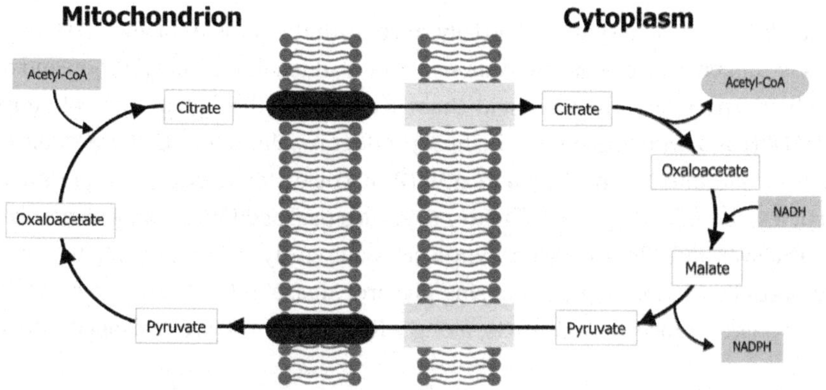

Figure 4.15: Citrate shuttle reaction moves citrate from the mitochondria to the cytosol for fatty acid synthesis.

The NADPH generated through this process is necessary for fatty acid synthesis. This is one of the primary pathways that produces NADPH, and the other is the oxidative portion of the pentose pathway.

The process of fatty acid synthesis starts with the carboxylation of acetyl-CoA to form malonyl-CoA (figures 4.16 and 4.17). The enzyme involved, acetyl-CoA carboxylase, is the regulatory enzyme for this pathway and requires biotin as a cofactor. After the initial priming of fatty acid synthase with acetyl-CoA, all other carbon units are added to the elongating fatty acid chain in the form of malonyl-CoA. You will see later that this intermediate is also a key inhibitor of β-oxidation.

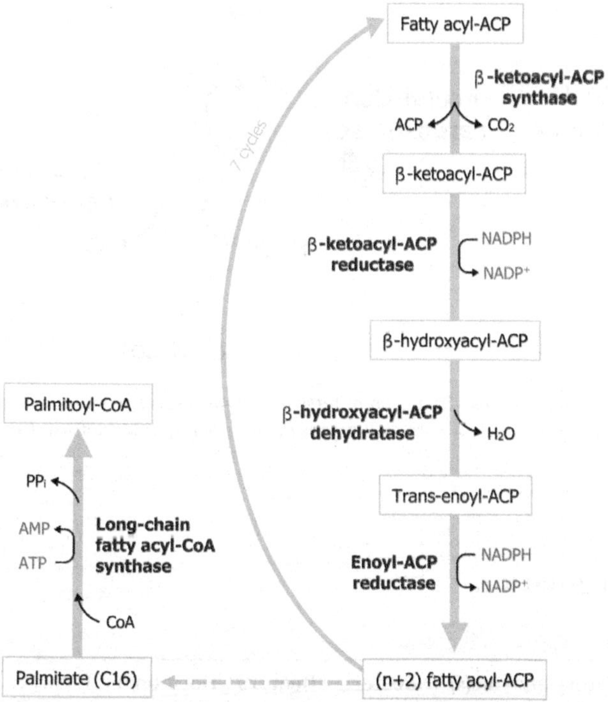

Figure 4.16: Fatty acid synthesis is an iterative process that begins with the transfer of an acetyl moiety from acetyl-CoA to fatty acid synthase; following this activation, carbons are added to the growing chain in the form of malonyl-CoA.

The synthesis of fatty acids by fatty acid synthase initially starts with the transfer of an acetyl moiety from acetyl-CoA to the acyl carrier protein within fatty acid synthase. Malonyl-CoA is added to the acetyl group and decarboxylated to form a four-carbon β-keto chain. From here, the fatty acid chain is elongated through a series of dehydration and reduction reactions, which use NADPH as a reducing agent. The final product is palmitate, a C-16 molecule (figure 4.16). Fatty acids are not stored in the liver and must be packaged into VLDL particles for transport to peripheral tissues for storage. To produce VLDL particles, the newly synthesized fatty acids are packaged into triacylglycerols (TAGs). TAG synthesis can take place in both the liver and adipose tissue. Synthesis requires glycerol 3-phosphate, which can be derived from glycolysis or from the phosphorylation of glycerol using glycerol kinase in the liver. Three fatty acyl-CoA groups react with the glycerol 3-phosphate to form a TAG. TAGs, along with cholesterol, are packaged into VLDLs distributed into circulation (section 6.2).

Regulation of fatty acid synthesis

Acetyl-CoA carboxylase is the regulatory enzyme for fatty acid synthesis. This enzyme is regulated both allosterically and through covalent modification. It is allosterically activated by high levels of citrate and inhibited by its product, fatty acyl-CoA. It can also be inhibited by elevated levels of glucagon, epinephrine, and adenosine monophosphate (AMP)-activated protein kinase phosphorylation. Insulin will stimulate the dephosphorylation and activation of the enzyme such that it can be active in the fed state (figure 4.17).

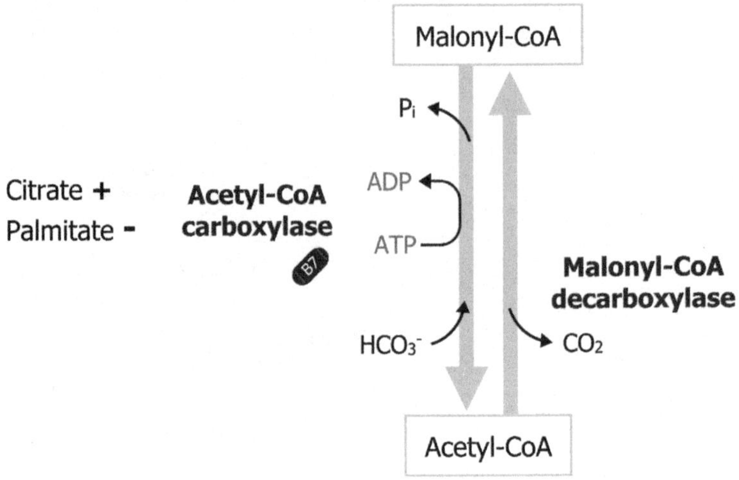

Figure 4.17: Regulatory reaction of fatty acid synthesis. The synthesis of malonyl-CoA by acetyl-CoA carboxylase is highly regulated within the cytosol.

Summary of pathway regulation

Metabolic pathway	Major regulatory enzyme(s)	Allosteric effectors	Hormonal effects
Fatty acid synthesis	Acetyl-CoA carboxylase	Citrate (+)	Insulin ↑
Fatty acid synthesis	Acetyl-CoA carboxylase	Palmitate (-)	Glucagon ↓

Table 4.3: Summary of pathway regulation.

4.4 References and resources

Text

Ferrier, D. R., ed. *Lippincott Illustrated Reviews: Biochemistry*, 7th ed. Philadelphia: Wolters Kluwer Health/ Lippincott Williams & Wilkins, 2017, Chapter 6: Bioenergetics and Oxidative Phosphorylation: Section V, VI, Chapter 8: Introduction to Metabolism and Glycolysis, Chapter 9: TCA Cycle and Pyruvate Dehydrogenase Complex: Section IIA, IIB, Chapter 11: Glycogen Metabolism: Section V, VI, Chapter 16: Fatty Acid Ketone Body and TAG Metabolism: Section II, IV, V, Chapter 23: Metabolic Effect of Insulin and Glucagon, Chapter 25: Diabetes Mellitus.

Le, T., and V. Bhushan. *First Aid for the USMLE Step 1*, 29th ed. New York: McGraw Hill Education, 2018, 72–78, 85–89.

Lieberman, M., and A. Peet, eds. *Marks' Basic Medical Biochemistry: A Clinical Approach*, 5th ed. Philadelphia: Wolters Kluwer Health/Lippincott Williams & Wilkins, 2018, Chapter 2: The Fed or Absorptive State, Chapter 19: Basic Concepts of Regulation: Section IV.A.1.2, Chapter 20: Cellular Bioenergetics, Chapter 22: Generation of ATP from Glucose: Section I.A.B.C, III, Chapter 24: Oxidative Phosphorylation and the ETC: Section I.E, II, III, Chapter 31: Synthesis of Fatty Acids: Section I.A.B, IV, V.

Figures

Grey, Kindred, Figure 4.15 Citrate shuttle reaction moves citrate from the mitochondria to the cytosol for fatty acid synthesis. 2021. https://archive.org/details/4.15-new. CC BY 4.0.

Grey, Kindred, Figure 4.16 Fatty acid synthesis is an iterative process which begins with the transfer of an acetyl moiety from acetyl-CoA to fatty acid synthase, following this activation, carbons are added to the growing chain in the form of malonyl-CoA. 2021. https://archive.org/details/4.16_20210924. CC BY 4.0.

Grey, Kindred, Figure 4.17 Regulatory reaction of fatty acid synthesis. The synthesis of malonyl-CoA by acetyl-CoA carboxylase is highly regulated within the cytosol. 2021. https://archive.org/details/4.17-new. CC BY 4.0.

4.5 Glycogen Synthesis

Glycogen synthesis is the process of storing glucose and occurs primarily in the liver and the skeletal muscle. The metabolic pathways in these tissues are similar, but the utility of glycogen stores is different. Briefly, liver glycogen is catabolized primarily in response to elevated glucagon, and the glucose 6-phosphate generated is dephosphorylated and released into circulation. In contrast, muscle glycogen is only used by the muscle itself; muscle lacks glucose 6-phosphatase and glucose 6-phosphate released from muscle glycogen is oxidized in glycolysis. Although discussed here as a point of comparison, glycogenolysis is a fasted state pathway and occurs in response to glucagon and epinephrine. This will be discussed in section 5.1.

Glycogen synthesis

Initially glucose 6-phosphate, is isomerized to glucose 1-phosphate. UDP-glucose pyrophosphorylase synthesizes UDP-glucose from glucose 1-phosphate and UTP, and this is the source of all the glycosyl residues added to the growing glycogen chain (figure 4.18). Glycogen synthase is the regulatory enzyme for the pathway and is responsible for linking glycosyl residues in a 1,4 linkage. The reaction typically occurs on existing glycogen stores; however, in the absence of any stored glycogen the reaction can occur on the protein primer, glycogenin.

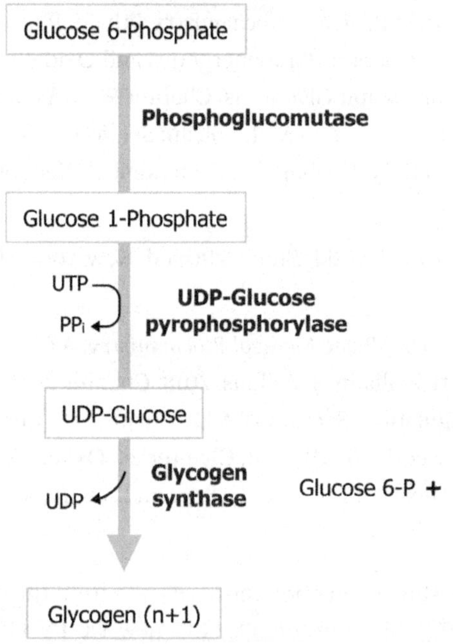

Figure 4.18: Glycogen synthesis.

Regulation of glycogen synthesis

Glycogen synthesis is regulated by a single enzyme, glycogen synthase. This enzyme is primarily regulated through covalent modification. It is active when dephosphorylated and inactive when phosphorylated. The phosphorylation/dephosphorylation is facilitated by glucagon and insulin levels, respectively (table 4.4).

Summary of pathway regulation

Metabolic pathway	Major regulatory enzyme(s)	Allosteric effectors	Hormonal effects
Glycogenesis	Glycogen synthase	Glucose 6-P (+)	Insulin ↑ Glucagon ↓ (liver) Epi ↓ (muscle)
Glycogenolysis (see section 5.1)	Glycogen phosphorylase	AMP (+) muscle Ca^{2+} in muscle	Glucagon ↑ (liver) Epi ↑ (muscle)

Table 4.4: Summary of pathway regulation.

4.5 References and resources

Text

Ferrier, D. R., ed. *Lippincott Illustrated Reviews: Biochemistry*, 7th ed. Philadelphia: Wolters Kluwer Health/ Lippincott Williams & Wilkins, 2017, Chapter 6: Bioenergetics and Oxidative Phosphorylation: Section V, VI, Chapter 8: Introduction to Metabolism and Glycolysis, Chapter 9: TCA Cycle and Pyruvate Dehydrogenase Complex: Section IIA, IIB, Chapter 11: Glycogen Metabolism: Section V, VI, Chapter 16: Fatty Acid Ketone Body and TAG Metabolism: Section II, IV, V, Chapter 23: Metabolic Effect of Insulin and Glucagon, Chapter 25: Diabetes Mellitus.

Le, T., and V. Bhushan. *First Aid for the USMLE Step 1*, 29th ed. New York: McGraw Hill Education, 2018, 72–78, 85–89.

Lieberman, M., and A. Peet, eds. *Marks' Basic Medical Biochemistry: A Clinical Approach*, 5th ed. Philadelphia: Wolters Kluwer Health/Lippincott Williams & Wilkins, 2018, Chapter 2: The Fed or Absorptive State, Chapter 19: Basic Concepts of Regulation: Section IV.A.1.2, Chapter 20: Cellular Bioenergetics, Chapter 22: Generation of ATP from Glucose: Section I.A.B.C, III, Chapter 24: Oxidative Phosphorylation and the ETC: Section I.E, II, III, Chapter 31: Synthesis of Fatty Acids: Section I.A.B, IV, V.

Figures

Grey, Kindred, Figure 4.18 Glycogen synthesis. 2021. https://archive.org/details/4.18_20210924. CC BY 4.0.

5. Fuel for Later

Learning Objectives

Gluconeogenesis and glycogenolysis

- Determine the regulatory states of the key gluconeogenic enzymes (fructose bisphosphatase 1 (FBP1), pyruvate carboxylase/PEPCK, glucose 6-phosphatase) under fed and fasting conditions.
- Relate how gluconeogenesis, the urea cycle, and β-oxidation are interconnected and how defects in one of these pathways can result in the presentation of hypoglycemia.
- Describe the process and regulation of glycogenolysis.
- Compare the use of muscle and liver glycogen stores.

Lipolysis, β-oxidation, and ketogenesis

- Describe the process of β-oxidation and how this connects to ketogenesis and lipolysis.
- Describe the importance of carnitine in the movement of fatty acids into the mitochondria using carnitine palmitoyltransferase.
- Evaluate the role of malonyl-CoA as a regulator of β-oxidation (key enzyme carnitine palmitoyltransferase 1).
- Describe how hormone levels impact lipolysis through the regulation of hormone-sensitive lipase.

Urea cycle and nitrogen metabolism

- Define ketogenic and glucogenic amino acids, and list them as exclusively ketogenic, glucogenic, or both.
- Describe urea cycle regulation by N-acetyl glutamate (NAGS) and substrate availability.
- Relate the activity of the urea cycle to the fed and fasted states.
- Describe the interconversion between keto-acids and amino acids, including the requirement of pyridoxal phosphate (PLP) as a cofactor (transaminase reaction).
- Describe the importance of the reactions catalyzed by (A) glutamine synthetase, (B) glutaminase, and (C) glutamate dehydrogenase.

Glycogenolysis (see section 4.5**)**

- Contrast the regulation and the utility of skeletal muscle versus liver glycogen.
- Evaluate the regulatory status of critical enzymes in the following pathways: glycolysis, glycogen synthesis and degradation, fatty acid synthesis and β-oxidation, and gluconeogenesis.
- Determine how different storage disorders can present with alternative phenotypes.

About this Chapter

In order to maintain glucose homeostasis, mechanisms are in place to supply fuel to essential tissues even under fasted conditions. This section will address how these pathways are interconnected and simultaneously regulated to achieve this goal.

5.1 Gluconeogenesis and Glycogenolysis

Gluconeogenesis and glycogenolysis are the two pathways essential for glucose homeostasis. Figure 5.1 illustrates the time frame and overlap of glycogenolysis and gluconeogenesis. These pathways are activated nearly simultaneously when the insulin to glucagon ratio becomes sufficiently reduced. Over time, the reliance on the pathways changes.

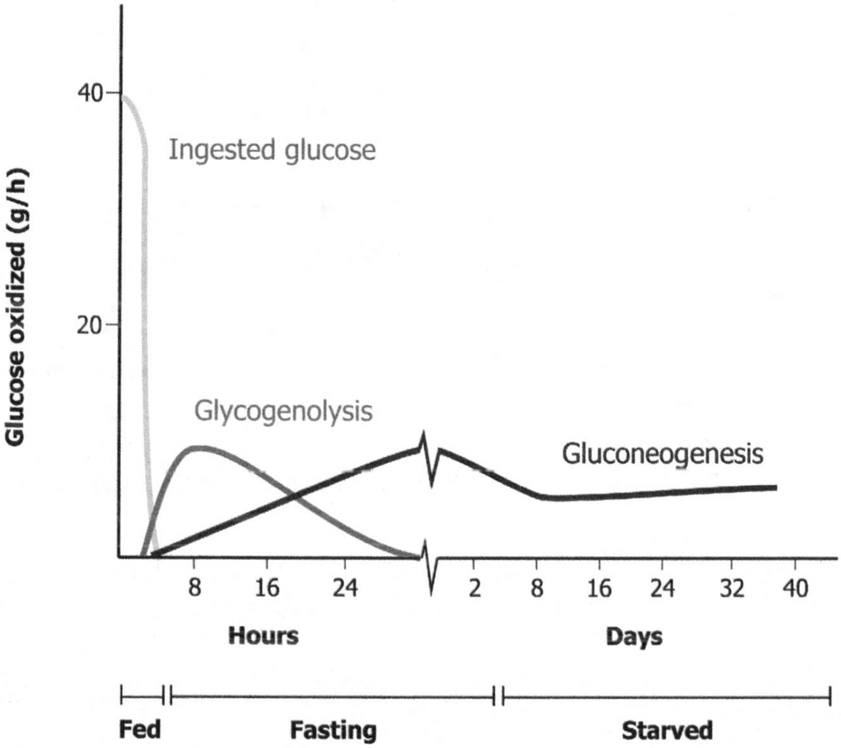

Figure 5.1: Glucose production by glycogenolysis and gluconeogenesis.

Gluconeogenesis (GNG) is an anabolic pathway that produces glucose from lactate, glycerol, or glucogenic amino acids. This pathway is activated primarily in the liver during fasting and is coordinated with the catabolic pathways of β-oxidation and protein catabolism. The pathway follows the reverse of glycolysis with the exception of four unique enzymes, which overcome the irreversible steps of glycolysis (figure 5.2).

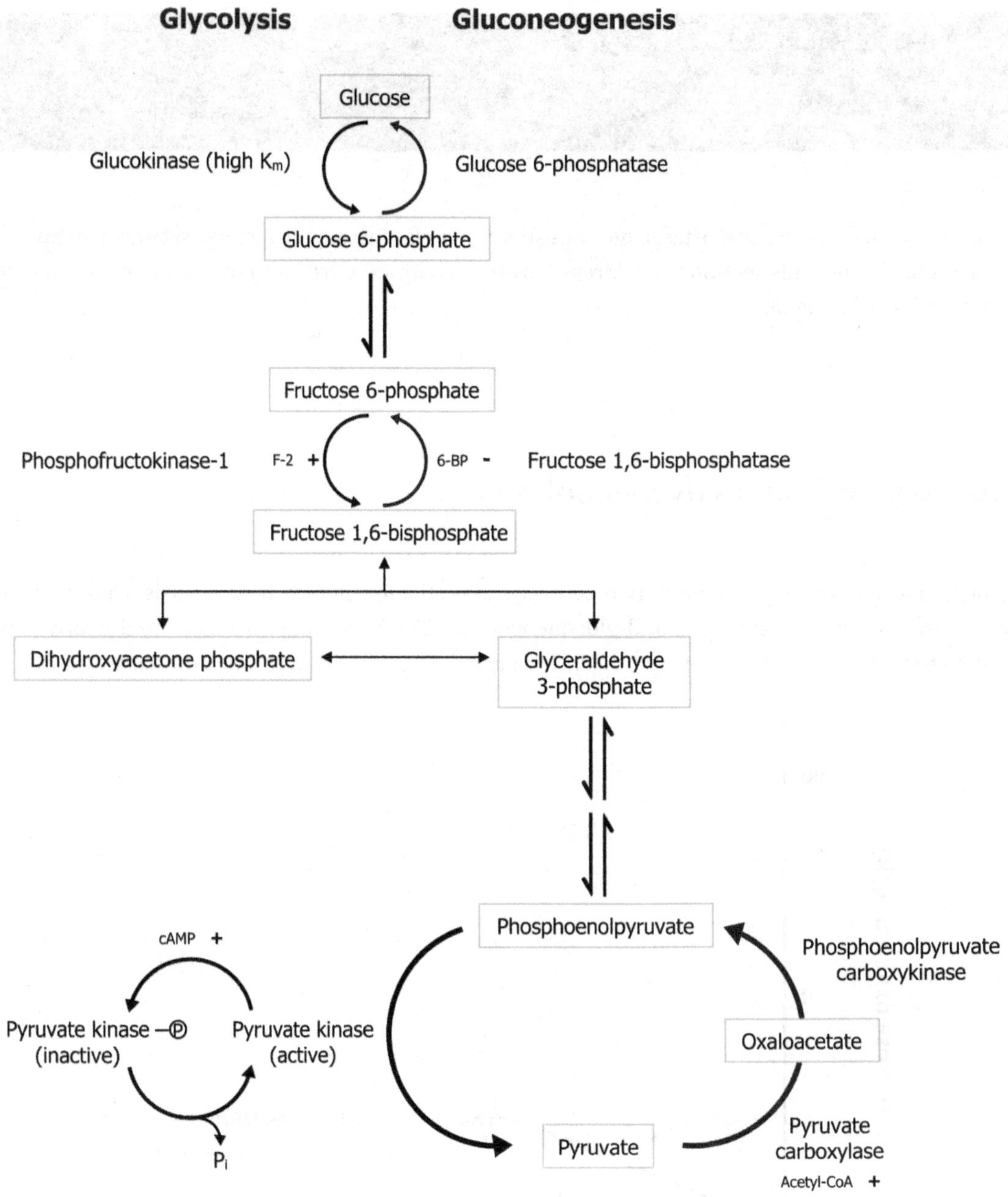

Figure 5.2: Comparison of glycolysis and gluconeogenesis.

Substrates for GNG

Amino acids

The primary substrates for GNG are derived from glucogenic amino acids released through cortisol-mediated protein catabolism. In the fasted state, cortisol is elevated, and it supports fasted state pathways through the activation of protein catabolism – in the skeletal muscle – and by increasing the transcription of enzymes needed for gluconeogenesis (specifically phosphoenol carboxykinase (PEPCK)). As amino acids are released from the skeletal muscle, primarily as glutamine and alanine, they are taken up by the liver. In order to be used for glucose synthesis, they undergo transamination to generate a useful intermediate of the TCA cycle, predominantly α-ketoglutarate and pyruvate (see figures 5.3 and 5.10) . In the case of alanine, this can be transaminated to generate pyruvate. Glutamine will first be deaminated by glutaminase, and the remaining glutamate will be transaminated to form α-ketoglutarate (see figure 5.11). Both pyruvate and α-ketoglutarate will increase substrates in the TCA cycle, ultimately increasing the pool of available malate to be shuttled out of the mitochondria. It is through this process of protein catabolism and transamination that glucogenic amino acids contribute to the synthesis of oxaloacetate (OAA) needed for gluconeogenesis.

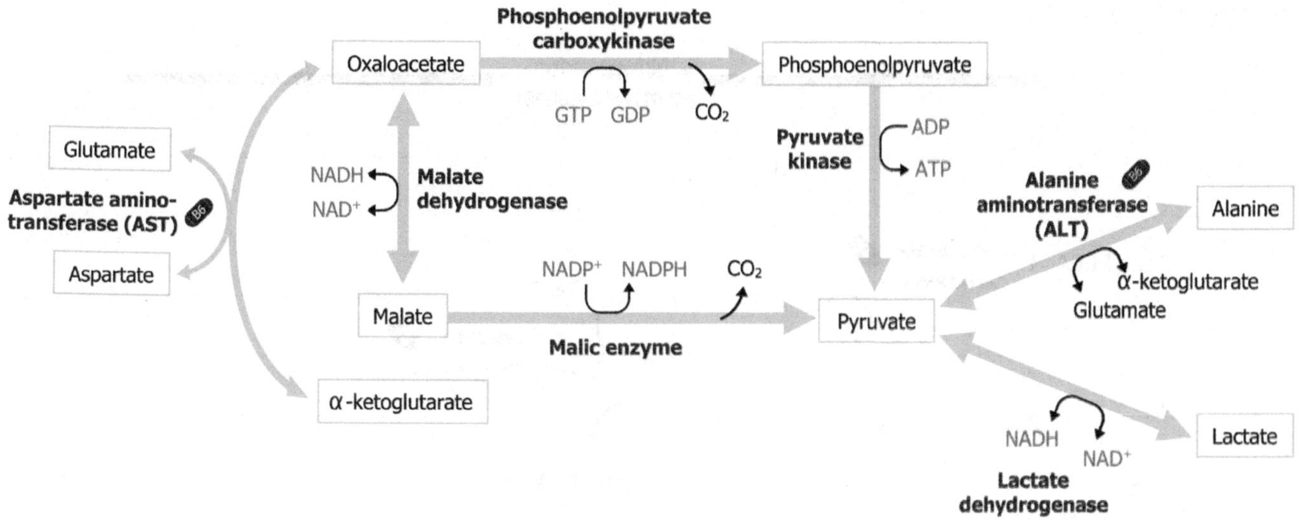

Figure 5.3: Locations of amino acid and lactate entering gluconeogenesis as substrates for the pathway.

Lactate

Lactate is primarily produced through the Cori cycle or from anaerobic glucose oxidation. (Note: The Cori cycle, or lactic acid cycle, refers to the metabolic pathway in which lactate produced by anaerobic glycolysis in the muscle or RBC travels to the liver and is converted to glucose. The glucose returns to the peripheral tissues and is metabolized back to lactate.) Once in the liver, lactate can be oxidized back to pyruvate through the reverse reaction catalyzed by lactate dehydrogenase (figure 5.3).

Glycerol

When lipolysis is stimulated by epinephrine or glucagon, activation of hormone-sensitive lipase in the adipose allows for the hydrolysis of triacylglycerol into three free fatty acid chains and glycerol. The glycerol released into circulation will be taken up by the liver. Once in the liver it can be converted into dihydroxyacetone phosphate (DHAP), a glycolytic intermediate. This is an additional way in which carbons can be obtained for glucose synthesis (figure 5.4).

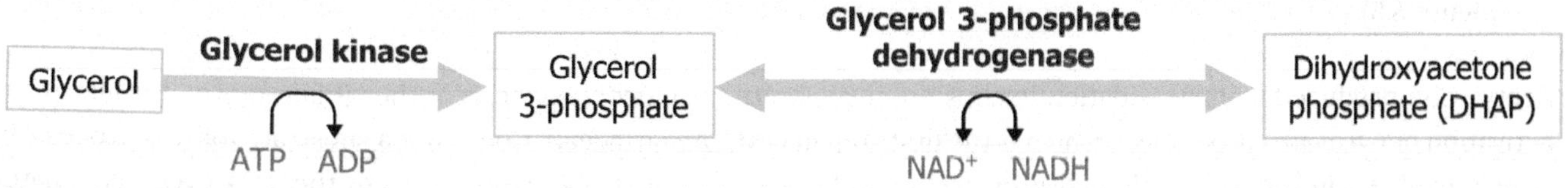

Figure 5.4: Glycerol as a substrate for gluconeogenesis; after phosphorylation to glycerol 3-phosphate it can be converted to DHAP, which can enter directly into glycolysis.

Interconnection of GNG and other metabolic pathways

Gluconeogenesis is heavily reliant on support from other pathways. It requires amino acids for carbon substrates from cortisol-mediated protein catabolism. The ability of those amino acids to be deaminated relies on the ability of the urea cycle to remove ammonia in the form of nontoxic urea, and perhaps most importantly, gluconeogenesis relies on the process of β-oxidation.

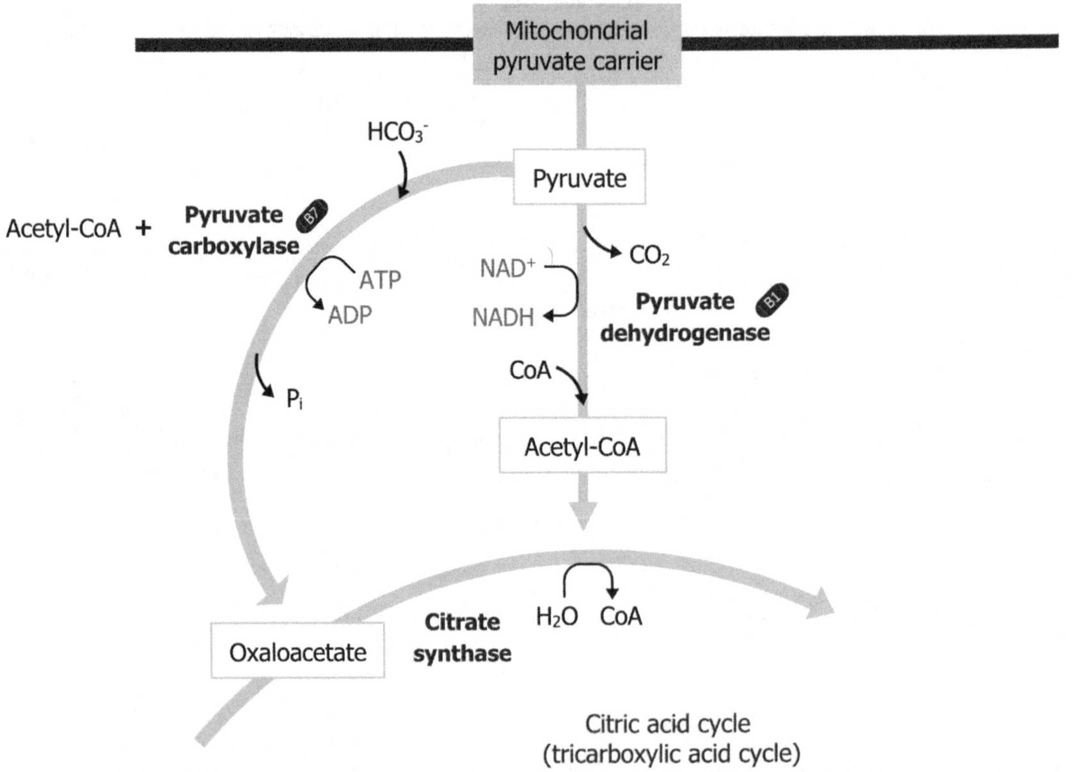

Figure 5.5: Reaction catalyzed by pyruvate carboxylase; this allows the bypass of the irreversible step catalyzed by pyruvate kinase.

β-oxidation

The process of β-oxidation supports gluconeogenesis in two major ways:

1. The NADH and $FADH_2$ generated from β-oxidation is oxidized in the electron transport chain to produce ATP. This ATP provides the needed energy for glucose synthesis. It also supplies energy to the urea cycle for nitrogen disposal.
2. β-oxidation also produces acetyl-CoA. This compound is needed to allosterically activate pyruvate carboxylase (figure 5.5).

Acetyl-CoA produced from β-oxidation itself is not a substrate for gluconeogenesis, rather it is required for allosteric activation of pyruvate carboxylase, which is the first step in GNG. Again, acetyl-CoA is not a substrate for this process; it is fully oxidized in the TCA cycle and provides no additional carbons to be exported from the TCA cycle as malate. Therefore the cell has to rely on amino acid carbon skeletons, glycerol, and lactate as substrates for glucose production (section 5.2).

Regulation of gluconeogenesis

Pyruvate carboxylase and phosphoenol carboxykinase (PEPCK)

Gluconeogenesis is essentially the reverse of glycolysis with four key regulatory steps that allow the bypass of the three irreversible steps of glycolysis (figure 5.2). This initial step of GNG starts in the mitochondria using pyruvate carboxylase (figure 5.5). This enzyme converts pyruvate in the mitochondria to oxaloacetate and requires biotin as a cofactor. This enzyme is allosterically activated by acetyl-CoA. The OAA produced is reduced to malate, which is shuttled out of the mitochondria using the malate-aspartate shuttle. Once in the cytosol, the malate is oxidized back to OAA and decarboxylated by the enzyme phosphoenol carboxykinase (PEPCK) to generate phosphoenol pyruvate (figure 5.3). The combination of these two enzymes, pyruvate carboxylase and PEPCK, allows the cell to bypass the irreversible step catalyzed by pyruvate kinase.

Once phosphoenol pyruvate (PEP) is synthesized, it will continue through the reverse process using the glycolytic enzymes until it reaches its next irreversible conversion.

Fructose 1,6-bisphosphatase (FBP1)

As PEP continues through the reverse of glycolysis, fructose 1,6-bisphosphate is generated. To bypass the irreversible step catalyzed by phosphofructokinase 1 (PFK1) in glycolysis, the enzyme fructose 1,6-bisphosphatase (FBP1) is present and dephosphorylates fructose 1,6-bisphosphate to produce fructose 6-phosphate. This enzyme, FBP1, is inhibited by AMP and fructose 2,6-bisphosphate (figure 5.2).

Like glycolysis, there is an additional regulation here by the bifunctional enzyme phosphofructokinase 2 (PFK2)/fructose 2,6-bisphosphatase (figure 4.1). This bifunctional enzyme functions as a kinase in the fed state (PFK2) and generates fructose 2,6-bisphosphate that allosterically activates PFK1. In the fasted state the enzyme is phosphorylated by glucagon-activated protein kinase A, and this actives the phosphatase activity of the enzyme. The enzyme dephosphorylates fructose 2,6-bisphosphate and therefore reduces the allosteric activation of PFK1 facilitating the reverse reaction by fructose 1,6-bisphosphatase (figure 5.2).

Glucose 6-phosphatase

Finally, glucose 6-phosphatase is required to dephosphorylate glucose 6-phosphate so it can be released from the liver. This is a key step for both glycogenolysis and gluconeogenesis, and deficiencies in this enzyme can lead to severe bouts of fasting hypoglycemia.

Glycogenolysis

In contrast to glycogen synthesis, glycogenolysis is the release of glucose 6-phosphate from glycogen stores. It can occur in both the liver and the skeletal muscle but under two different conditions (figures 5.6 and 5.7). As noted above, this is a pathway active in the fasted state.

- In the **liver**, glycogenolysis is the initial source of glucose for the maintenance of blood glucose levels when glucagon levels start to increase. The glucose 6-phosphate generated from liver glycogenolysis is dephosphorylated and released into the blood stream.
- In **skeletal muscle**, glycogenolysis provides glucose only for the skeletal muscle, and this fuel is not released into the blood stream as skeletal muscle lacks glucose 6-phosphatase, the enzyme needed to dephosphorylate glucose. Therefore, skeletal muscle glycogen is primarily used under anaerobic exercise conditions when oxidizing fatty acids is not rapid enough to produce ATP for the exercising tissue.

Regulation of glycogenolysis

Hepatic glycogenolysis

In the liver, glucagon will initiate glycogenolysis through a GPCR-mediated signaling cascade. This leads to the activation of adenylyl cyclase and an increase in cAMP. cAMP activates protein kinase A, which phosphorylates and activates glycogen phosphorylase. Glycogen phosphorylase will initiate glycogen degradation. Also under these conditions, using the same mechanism, glycogen synthase will be phosphorylated and inactivated, ensuring glycogen synthesis is not occurring at the same time (figure 5.6).

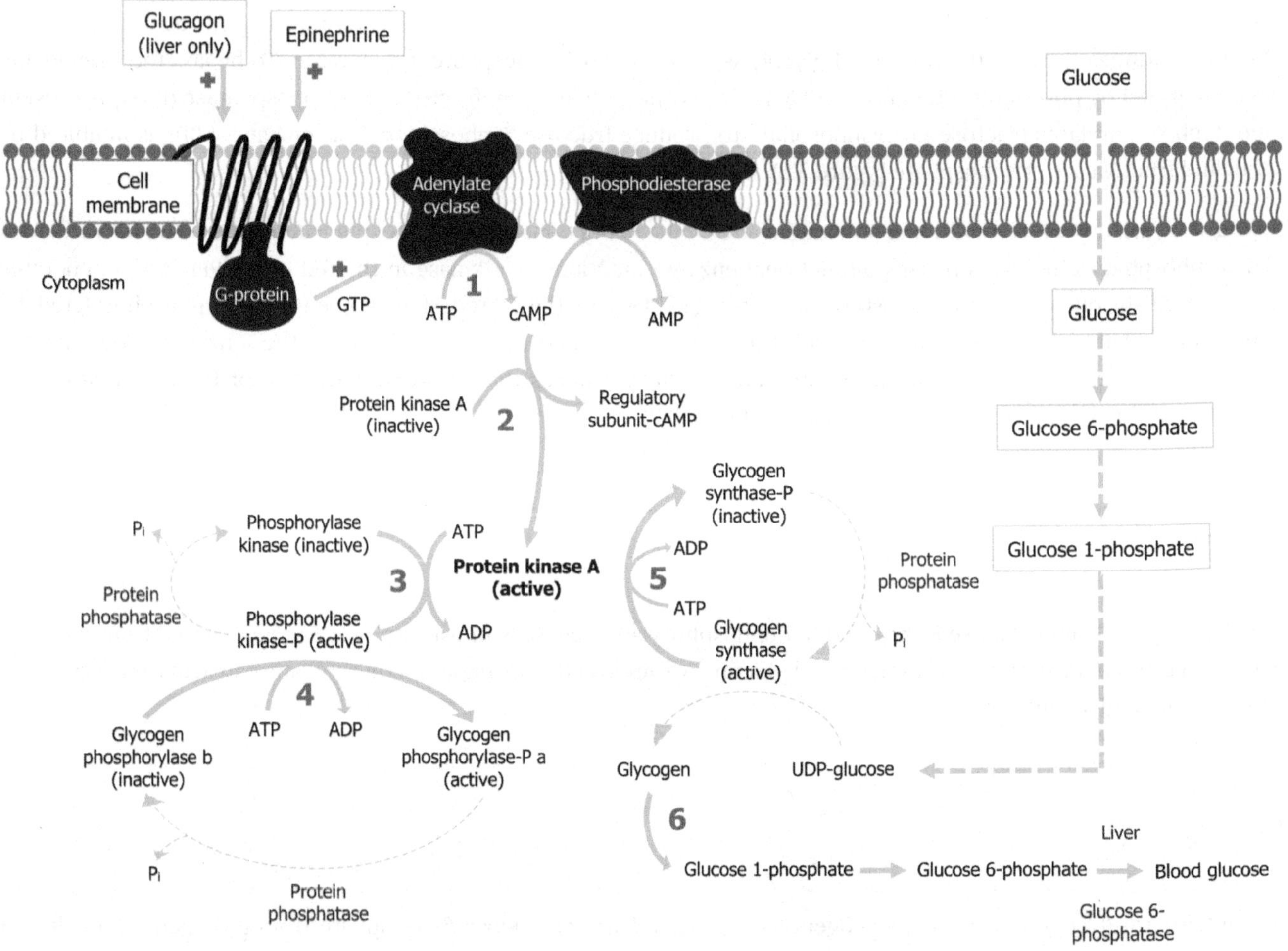

Figure 5.6: Hepatic glycogenolysis by epinephrine.

Epinephrine can also enhance hepatic glycogenolysis by binding an α-agonist receptor. This initiates the cleavage of phosphatidylinositol 4,5-bisphosphate (PIP_2) into inositol 1,4,5-triphosphate (IP_3) and diacylglyerol (DAG) by phospholipase C. IP_3 stimulates Ca^{2+} release from endoplasmic reticulum and results in both:

1. phosphorylation and activation of glycogen phosphorylase and
2. phosphorylation and inactivation of glycogen synthase.

In all cases, the glucose 6-phosphate released from glycogen stores is dephosphorylated by glucose 6-phosphatase and released from the liver.

Skeletal muscle glycogenolysis

Skeletal muscle glycogen is not impacted by glucagon but responds to AMP, Ca^{2+}, and epinephrine (figure 5.7).

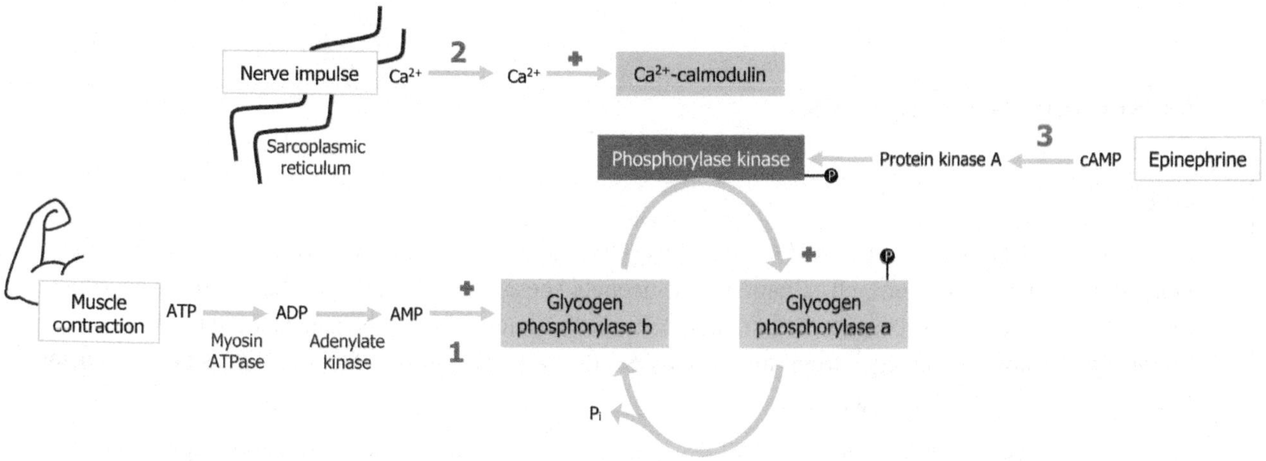

Figure 5.7: Skeletal muscle glycogenolysis.

- The primary regulator of this process is AMP. Elevated AMP will allosterically activate glycogen phosphorylase independent of phosphorylation.
- Next, glycogen phosphorylase can be activated by Ca^{2+}. Similar to the above cascade, calcium will activate the Ca^{2+} calmodulin complex, which will in turn activate phosphorylase kinase, ultimately leading to the phosphorylation and activation of glycogen phosphorylase.
- Finally, epinephrine can also stimulate skeletal muscle glycogenolysis through an increase in cAMP (the cascade of events is the same as glucagon-stimulated hepatic glycogenolysis).

Summary of pathway regulation

Metabolic pathway	Major regulatory enzyme(s)	Allosteric effectors	Hormonal effects
Gluconeogenesis	Fructose 1,6-bisphosphatase (FBP1)	Citrate (+) Fructose 2,6-BP, AMP (-)	Glucagon ↑ decreases F 2,6-BP by reducing activation of PFK1
Gluconeogenesis	Pyruvate carboxylase Phosphoenolpyruvate carboxykinase	Acetyl-CoA (+)	Cortisol-mediated enhanced transcription
Glycogenolysis	Glycogen phosphorylase	AMP (+) muscle CaB^{2+} (+) in muscle	Glucagon ↑ (liver) Epi ↑ (muscle)

Table 5.1: Summary of pathway regulation.

5.1 References and resources

Text

Ferrier, D. R., ed. *Lippincott Illustrated Reviews: Biochemistry*, 7th ed. Philadelphia: Wolters Kluwer Health/ Lippincott Williams & Wilkins, 2017, Chapter 10: Gluconeogenesis: Section II, III, IV, Chapter 11: Glycogen Metabolism: Section V, VI, Chapter 16: Fatty Acid Ketone Body and TAG Metabolism: Section III, IV, V, Chapter 19: Removal of Nitrogen from Amino Acids: Section V, VI, Chapter 23: Metabolic Effect of Insulin and Glucagon, Chapter 25: Diabetes Mellitus.

Le, T., and V. Bhushan. *First Aid for the USMLE Step 1*, 29th ed. New York: McGraw Hill Education, 2018, 78, 82, 86, 89–90.

Lieberman, M., and A. Peet, eds. *Marks' Basic Medical Biochemistry: A Clinical Approach*, 5th ed. Philadelphia: Wolters Kluwer Health/Lippincott Williams & Wilkins, 2018, Chapter 3: The Fasted State, Chapter 19: Basic Concepts in Regulation, Chapter 24: Oxidative Phosphorylation and the ETC, Chapter 26: Formation of Glycogen, Chapter 28: Gluconeogenesis, Chapter 30: Oxidation of Fatty Acids, Chapter 34: Integration of Carbohydrate and Lipid Metabolism, Chapter 36: Fate of Amino Acids Nitrogen: Urea Cycle.

Figures

Ferrier D. Figure 5.1 Glucose production by glycogenolysis and gluconeogenesis. Adapted under Fair Use from Lippincott Illustrated Reviews Biochemistry. 7th Ed. pp 329. Figure 24.11 Sources of blood glucose after ingestion of 100 g of glucose. 2017.

Grey, Kindred, Figure 5.2 Comparison of glycolysis and gluconeogenesis. 2021. https://archive.org/details/5.2-new. CC BY 4.0.

Grey, Kindred, Figure 5.3 Locations of amino acid and lactate entering gluconeogenesis as substrates for the pathway. 2021. https://archive.org/details/5.3_20210924. CC BY 4.0.

Grey, Kindred, Figure 5.4 Glycerol as a substrate for gluconeogenesis, after phosphorylation to glycerol 3 -phosphate it can be converted to DHAP which can enter directly into glycolysis. 2021. https://archive.org/details/5.4_20210924. CC BY 4.0.

Grey, Kindred, Figure 5.5 Reaction catalyzed by pyruvate carboxylase, this allows the by pass of the irreversible step catalyzed by pyruvate kinase. 2021. https://archive.org/details/5.5_20210924. CC BY 4.0.

Grey, Kindred, Figure 5.7 Skeletal muscle glycogenolysis. 2021. https://archive.org/details/5.7_20210924. CC BY 4.0. Added Muscle by Pascal Heß from the Noun Project.

Lieberman M, Peet A. Figure 5.6 Hepatic glycogenolysis by epinephrine. Adapted under Fair Use from Marks' Basic Medical Biochemistry. 5th Ed. pp 534. Figure 26.7 Regulation of glycogen synthesis and degradation in the liver. 2017. Added ion channel by Léa Lortal from the Noun Project.

5.2 Lipolysis, β-oxidation, and Ketogenesis

The processes of lipolysis, β-oxidation, and ketogenesis work in concert within the cell but should be considered distinct pathways.

Lipolysis

Lipolysis is the release of fatty acids from adipose tissue where they are stored as triacylglycerols (TAGs). This process is mediated by increasing levels of glucagon and epinephrine, which bind G-protein coupled receptors on the adipose tissue and activate lipolysis This cell-signaling cascade phosphorylates and activates hormone-sensitive lipase, the regulatory enzyme for lipolysis. Once phosphorylated (through hormone-mediated increase in cAMP) this enzyme will hydrolyze TAGs to three long-chain fatty acids (LCFAs) and glycerol. The LCFAs are released into the bloodstream and will circulate bound to albumin (fatty acids are hydrophobic and require a protein carrier). LCFAs will be taken up and oxidized by peripheral tissues and the liver under fasted conditions. The glycerol will also be released and used as a substrate for hepatic gluconeogenesis (section 5.1) (figure 5.6).

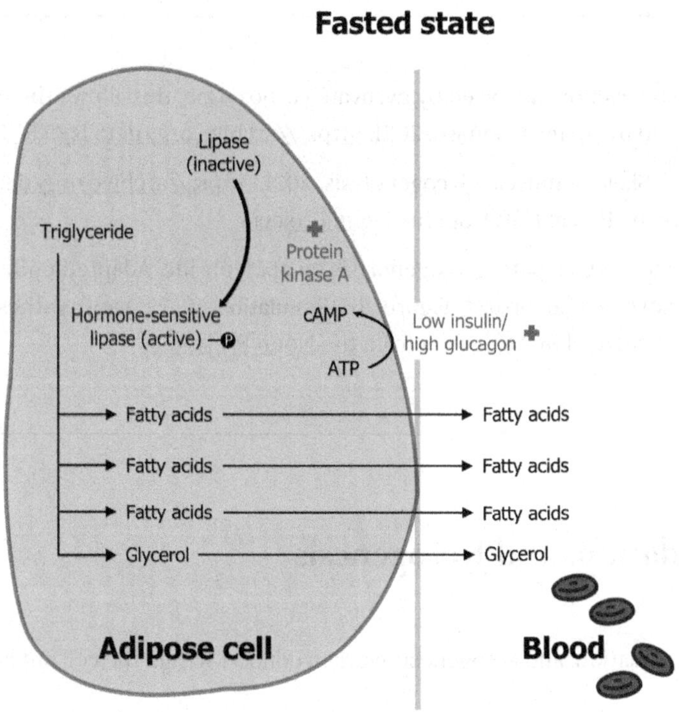

Figure 5.8: Process of lipolysis.

β-oxidation (oxidation of free fatty acids)

Fatty acid oxidation is a high energy yielding process. It can support the cellular energy needs during fasting and under conditions when excess energy is needed (exercise). After uptake from circulation, the LCFAs must be transferred into the mitochondria where β-oxidation occurs. Initially, the LCFAs are activated to acyl-CoA derivatives in the cytosol by acyl-CoA synthetase. The fatty acyl-CoA can then be transferred across the mitochondrial membranes using a series of transport proteins: carnitine palmitoyltransferase 1 and 2 (CPT1 and CPT2) (figure 5.9).

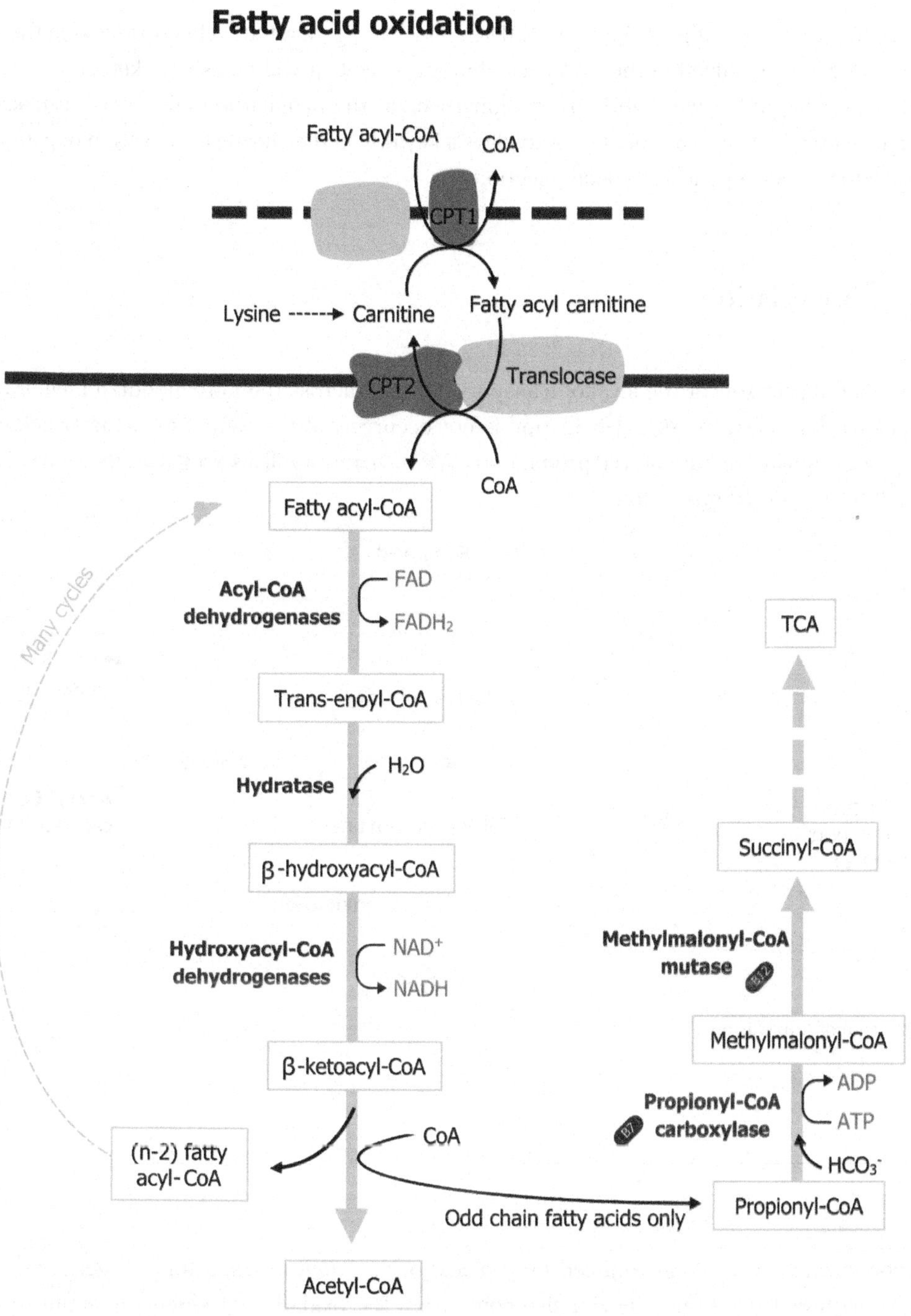

Figure 5.9: Overview of LCFA transport into the mitochondria and β-oxidation.

CPT1 sits on the outer mitochondrial membrane and transfers the fatty acyl-CoA to carnitine. Fatty acyl carnitine is transferred into the mitochondrial matrix through CPT2, and the carnitine is released and recycled. Only long-chain fatty acyl-CoAs require carnitine as a carrier; short- and medium-chain fatty acids can move into the mitochondria without the assistance of these transporters. Once in the matrix, the fatty acyl-CoA is now ready to undergo β-oxidation (figure 5.9).

β-oxidation is an iterative process that involves a series of enzymes that preferentially oxidize different length fatty acids (long, medium, and short). The full β-oxidation spiral consists of four steps that result in the generation of acetyl-CoA,

NADH, and $FADH_2$ for each cycle (figure 5.9). The NADH and $FADH_2$ generated will be oxidized in the ETC to produce ATP. The acetyl-CoA can be oxidized in the TCA cycle, but more likely it will be used in ketogenesis. Oxidation of odd chain fatty acids will result in the generation of propionyl-CoA as the final carbon unit, which can also be oxidized in the TCA cycle. The acetyl-CoA from β-oxidation also plays a key role in the allosteric activation of pyruvate carboxylase, which is necessary for gluconeogenesis to occur (section 5.1).

Regulation of β-oxidation

β-oxidation is regulated primarily at the level of transport of LCFAs across the mitochondrial membrane. Malonyl-CoA will inhibit CPT1 therefore ensuring that β-oxidation is not occurring at the same time as fatty acid synthesis (figure 5.10; section 4.4). Additionally, the rate of ATP production (ATP/ADP ratio) will also regulate the rate of NADH and $FADH_2$ produced through β-oxidation (figure 5.10).

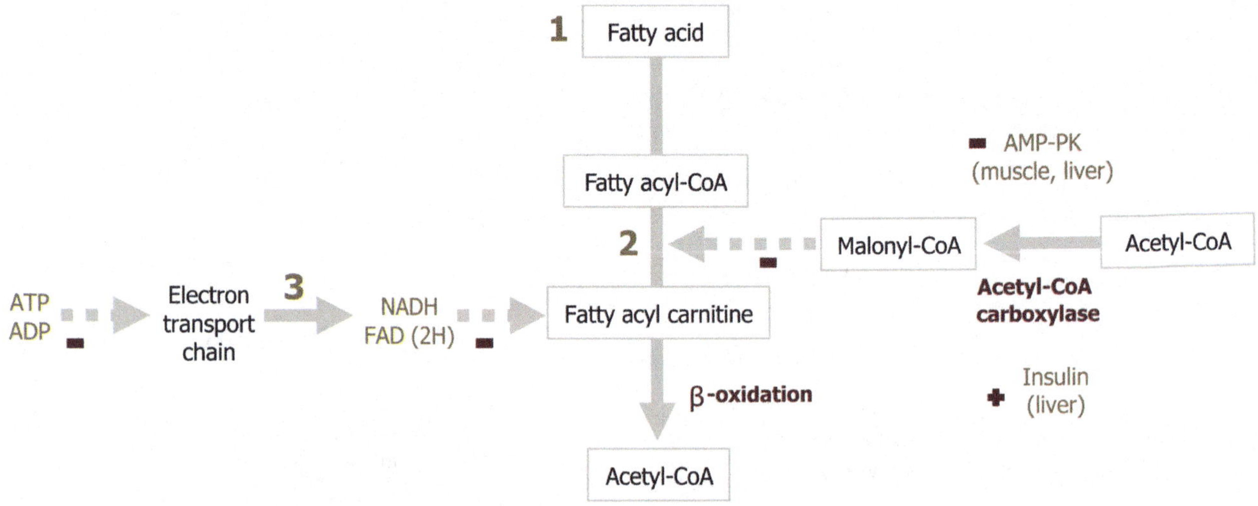

Figure 5.10: Regulation of β-oxidation.

Ketogenesis

As mentioned above, the acetyl-CoA produced by β-oxidation is primarily used for ketogenesis – the synthesis of ketone bodies. Substrates for ketogenesis can also come from the oxidation of ketogenic amino acids. In the fasted state, the process of β-oxidation generates a significant amount of acetyl-CoA, and although some of this substrate can be oxidized in the TCA cycle, we need to consider the other metabolic processes occurring. First, the significant amount of NADH generated through β-oxidation reduces flux through the TCA cycle by decreasing the activity of both α-ketoglutarate dehydrogenase and isocitrate dehydrogenase. Second, the process of gluconeogenesis is occurring, and intermediates of the TCA cycle, specifically malate, are actively being moved out of the mitochondria. The combination of these two processes reduces the TCA cycle activity allowing for an accumulation of acetyl-CoA. As acetyl-CoA levels elevate in the mitochondria, this will drive the thiolase reaction to generate acetoacetyl-CoA from two acetyl-CoA molecules (figure 5.11).

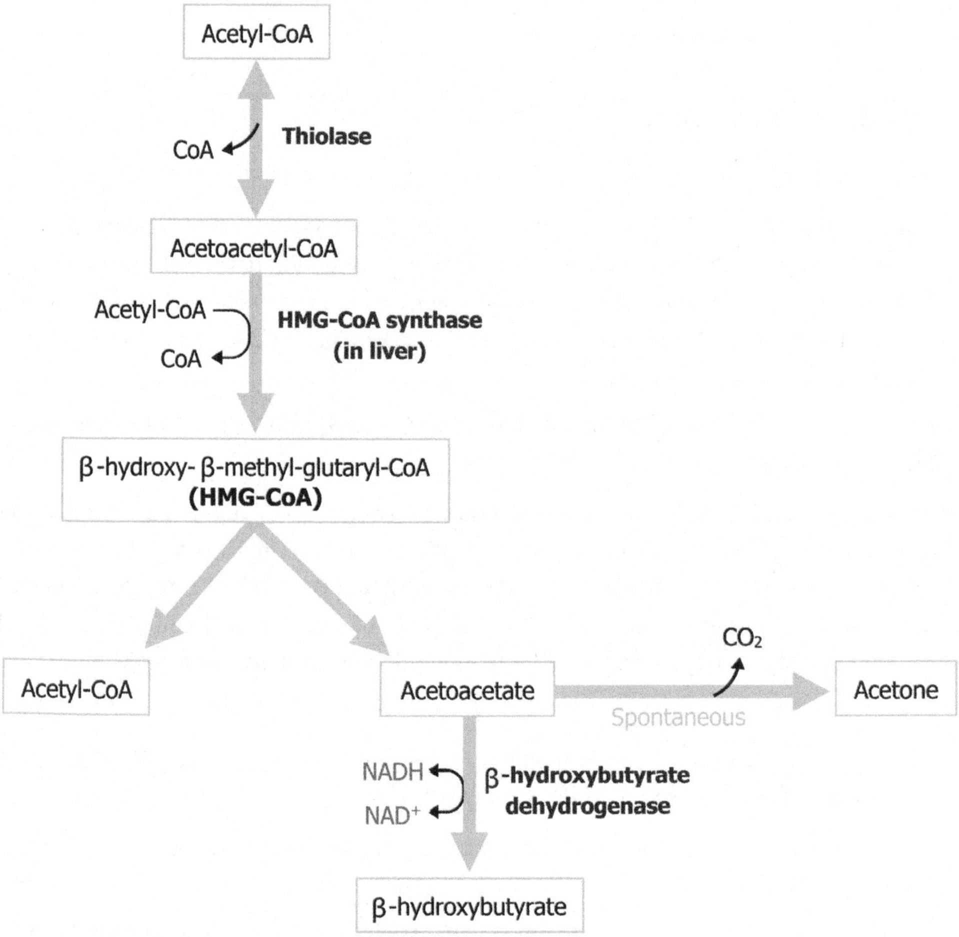

Figure 5.11: Overview of ketone body formation.

This compound is the substrate for HMG-CoA synthase, which generates 3-hydroxy-3-methyl glutaryl-CoA (HMG-CoA). HMG-CoA is then accepted by HMG-CoA lyase where an acetyl-CoA group is removed to generate acetoacetate. Acetoacetate can either undergo spontaneous decarboxylation to acetone, which can be exhaled, or it can be reduced to β-hydroxybutyrate using NADH. Acetoacetate and β-hydroxybutyrate are the two primary ketone bodies in circulation, and the ratio of the two is dependent on levels of NADH (figure 5.11). These two ketone bodies can be used as fuel in most tissues with the exception of the liver, which lacks thiophorase, the enzyme needed to metabolize these substrates. Ketone oxidation is not a primary fuel source, as fatty acid oxidation is preferred, but it can supply energy to some peripheral tissues. The brain can also oxidize ketones but only under extreme situations, such as starvation states.

Summary of pathway regulation

Metabolic pathway	Major regulatory enzyme	Allosteric effectors	Hormonal effects
Lipolysis	Hormone-sensitive lipase	None	Epi ↑ Insulin ↓
β-oxidation	Carnitine palmitoyltransferase	Malonyl-CoA (-)	None

Table 5.2: Summary of pathway regulation.

5.2 References and resources

Text

Ferrier, D. R., ed. *Lippincott Illustrated Reviews: Biochemistry*, 7th ed. Philadelphia: Wolters Kluwer Health/ Lippincott Williams & Wilkins, 2017, Chapter 10: Gluconeogenesis: Section II, III, IV, Chapter 11: Glycogen Metabolism: Section V, VI, Chapter 16: Fatty Acid Ketone Body and TAG Metabolism: Section III, IV, V, Chapter 19: Removal of Nitrogen from Amino Acids: Section V, VI, Chapter 23: Metabolic Effect of Insulin and Glucagon, Chapter 25: Diabetes Mellitus.

Le, T., and V. Bhushan. *First Aid for the USMLE Step 1*, 29th ed. New York: McGraw Hill Education, 2018, 78, 82, 86, 89–90.

Lieberman, M., and A. Peet, eds. *Marks' Basic Medical Biochemistry: A Clinical Approach*, 5th ed. Philadelphia: Wolters Kluwer Health/Lippincott Williams & Wilkins, 2018, Chapter 3: The Fasted State, Chapter 19: Basic Concepts in Regulation, Chapter 24: Oxidative Phosphorylation and the ETC, Chapter 26: Formation of Glycogen, Chapter 28: Gluconeogenesis, Chapter 30: Oxidation of Fatty Acids, Chapter 34: Integration of Carbohydrate and Lipid Metabolism, Chapter 36: Fate of Amino Acids Nitrogen: Urea Cycle.

Figures

Grey, Kindred, Figure 5.8 Process of lipolysis. 2021. https://archive.org/details/5.6_20210924. CC BY 4.0. Added red blood cells by Lucas Helle from the Noun Project.

Grey, Kindred, Figure 5.9 Overview of LCFA transport into the mitochondria and β-oxidation. 2021. https://archive.org/details/5.7_20210924_202109. CC BY 4.0.

Grey, Kindred, Figure 5.10 Regulation of β-oxidation. 2021. https://archive.org/details/5.8_20210924. CC BY 4.0.

Grey, Kindred, Figure 5.11 Overview of ketone body formation. 2021. https://archive.org/details/5.9-deleted. CC BY 4.0.

5.3 Nitrogen Metabolism and the Urea Cycle

Amino acids play key roles as precursors to nitrogen-containing compounds (such as nucleotides and neurotransmitters), as substrates for protein synthesis, and as an oxidizable substrate for energy production (or storage). Unlike carbohydrate and lipid metabolism, we must be concerned with the fates of both the carbon- and nitrogen-containing moieties when discussing the metabolism of amino acids. In the case of amino acids, nitrogen is released as ammonia (NH_3), and at physiological pH the majority of ammonia is present as an ammonium ion (NH_4^+). (It is important to note that only ammonia can cross cellular membranes.) The majority of ammonia is incorporated into urea (in the liver) and excreted by the kidney, while the remaining carbon-containing skeleton is oxidized or utilized in other anabolic pathways (i.e., gluconeogenesis).

Transport of nitrogen via amino acids

The amino acid pool is continually in flux and can be influenced by both dietary protein consumption as well as normal protein turnover within the tissues. Given that the major site of nitrogen disposal is the liver, a mechanism for transport of excess amino acid nitrogen from the peripheral tissues to the liver is in place. Both alanine and glutamine play an essential role as nontoxic carriers of ammonia from peripheral tissues to the liver (figures 5.12 and 5.13). To generate alanine and glutamine for transport, amino acids can undergo transamination reactions.

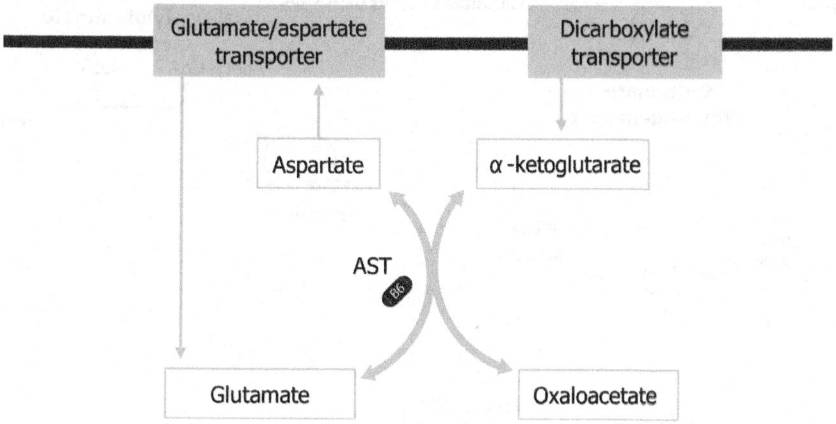

Figure 5.12: Transamination reaction.

Transamination: The movement of nitrogen

Amino transferases are a family of enzymes (which require pyridoxal phosphate; PLP) as a cofactor to help transfer nitrogen from amino acids on to keto-acid backbones. These enzymes do not free ammonia, but will transfer nitrogen from an amino group to a keto-group in an exchange or transferase reaction. Alanine aminotransferase (ALT) and aspartate aminotransferase (AST) are common and clinically relevant transferases. AST will preferentially accept aspartate and transaminate it in a reaction with α-ketoglutarate (the keto-acid of glutamate) to generate oxaloacetate (OAA) (the keto-acid of aspartate) and glutamate (figures 5.12 and 5.13).

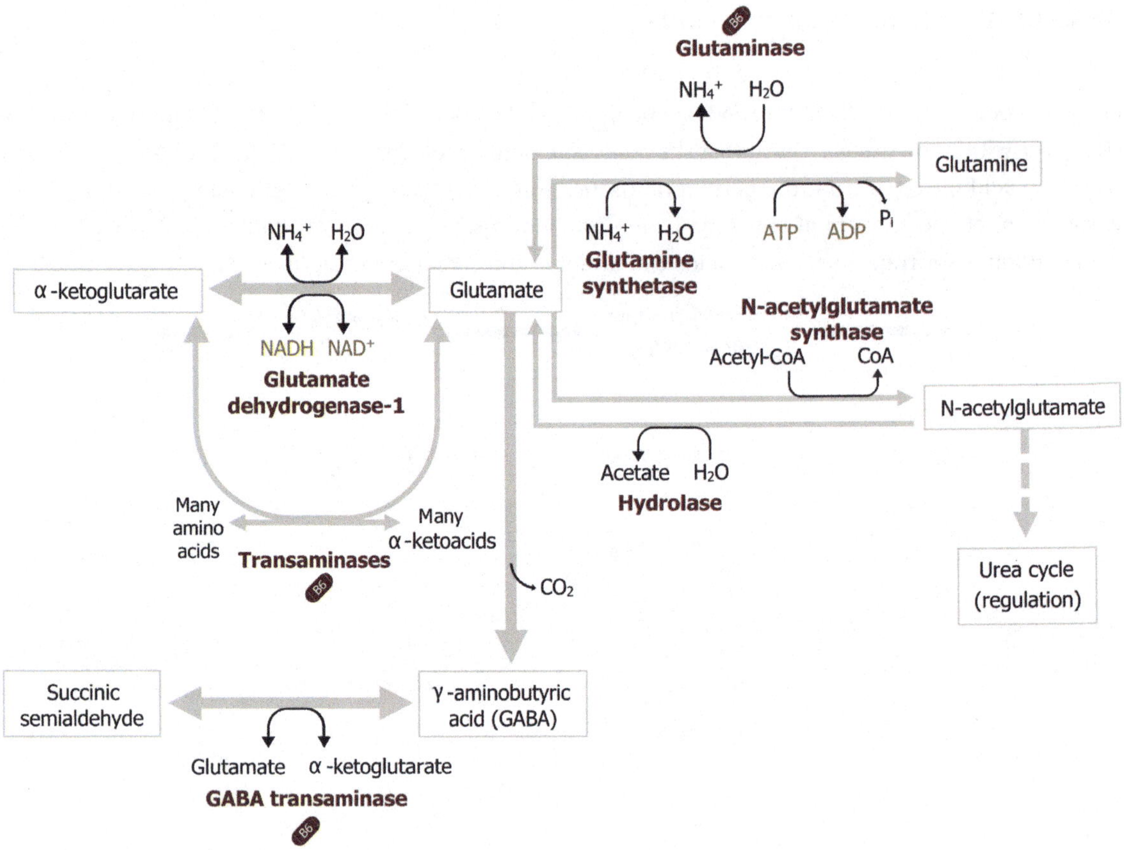

Figure 5.13: Reactions catalyzed by glutamate dehydrogenase, glutaminase, and glutamine synthetase.

Glutamate dehydrogenase, glutamine synthetase, and glutaminase

In addition to transaminases, there are three other enzymes that play essential roles in nitrogen transport. Glutamate dehydrogenase (GDH) is present in most tissues and is one of the few enzymes able to fix or free ammonia. In figure 5.14, in the skeletal muscle, glutamate dehydrogenase is illustrated fixing ammonia to α-ketoglutarate to generate glutamate, while in the liver it is shown freeing ammonia in the reverse reaction. The direction of the reaction will be influenced by several factors including cellular needs, the levels of NAD^+ or $NADP^+$, and levels of ammonia (figure 5.14).

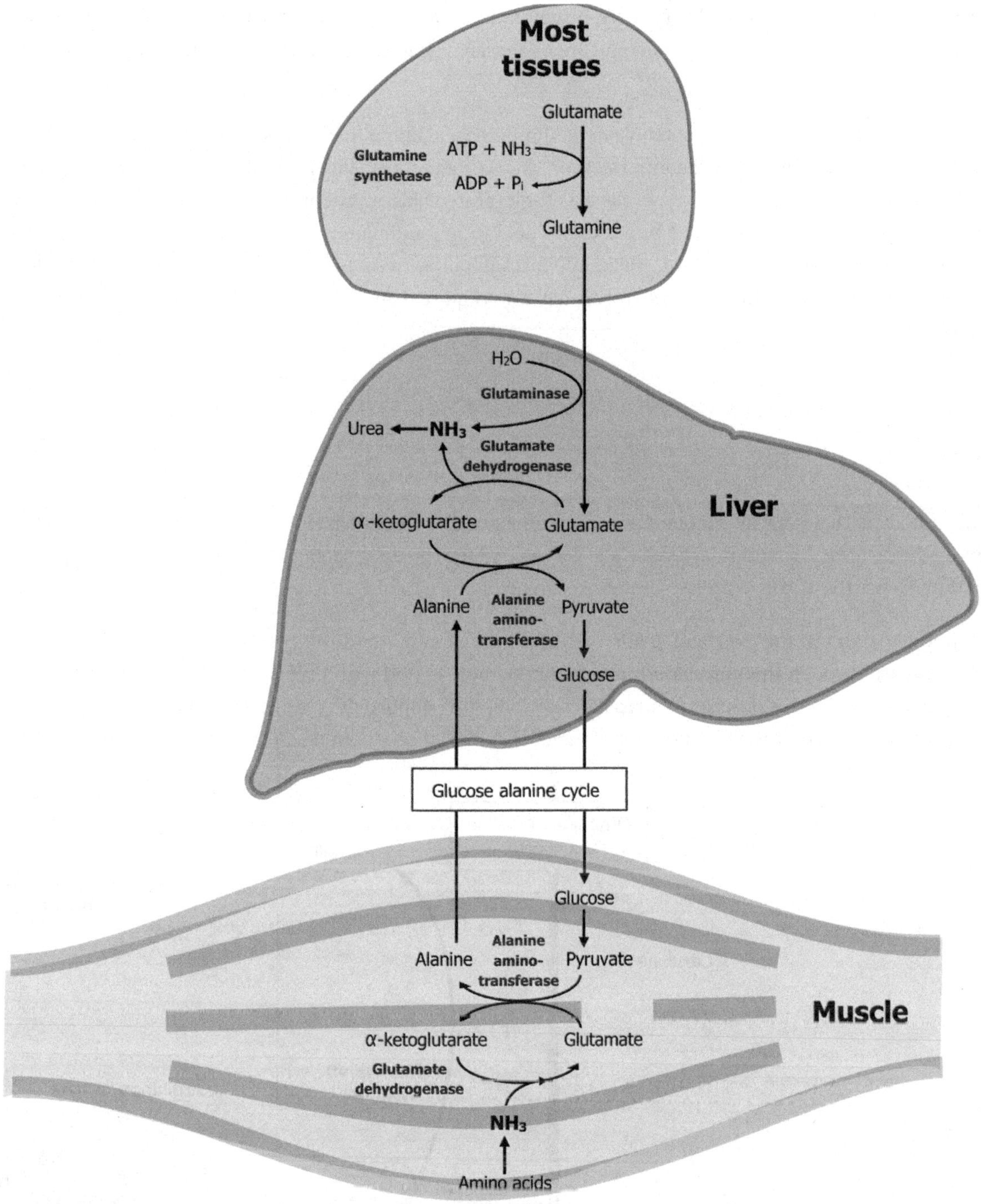

Figure 5.14: Movement of ammonia from peripheral tissues to the liver.

In peripheral tissues, glutamate generated from transamination or from the GDH reaction can be used to fix an additional ammonia to generate glutamine. This reaction, catalyzed by glutamine synthetase, facilitates the synthesis and subsequent movement of excess nitrogen from peripheral tissues to the liver (figure 5.14).

In skeletal muscle, the alanine-glucose cycle is commonly used for the transport of nitrogen from the skeletal muscle to the liver. In this process, ammonia from amino acid degradation is transaminated to form glutamate. Alanine aminotransferase (AST) will transaminate glutamate with pyruvate to generate alanine (and α-ketoglutarate). The alanine is released and transported to the liver where it will undergo another transamination to generate pyruvate, which is used as a substrate for glucose production (gluconeogenesis). The glucose is released from the liver and oxidized by the skeletal muscle.

The other key enzyme in nitrogen metabolism is glutaminase. Glutaminase, is active in the liver and responsible for deaminating glutamine as it is shuttled into the liver. The free ammonia can enter into the urea cycle, and the remaining glutamate can be transaminated to generate α-ketoglutarate. This is in contrast to glutamine synthetase, which is primarily used by peripheral tissues as a means of generating glutamine to remove ammonia from the tissues to the liver (figure 5.14). Nitrogen metabolism, unlike glucose metabolism, is fairly consistent in the fed and fasted states. Excess dietary amino acids, which are not stored, will also require deamination, and the carbons can be stored as either glycogen or fat.

Urea cycle

Ammonia freed in the liver by glutaminase (or glutamate dehydrogenase) will readily enter the urea cycle to be incorporated into urea. A functioning urea cycle is essential for the disposal of nitrogen from catabolic processes, and if dysfunction occurs the accumulation of ammonia can be life threatening.

The urea cycle occurs in the liver and spans both the mitochondria and the cytosolic compartments. The initial free ammonia diffuses through the mitochondrial membrane and is fixed with carbon dioxide (in the form of bicarbonate) during the initial step in this process (figures 5.15 and 5.16). It is important to remember that the synthesis of urea is an anabolic process that requires ATP. Therefore deficiencies in ATP production can inhibit nitrogen disposal as well.

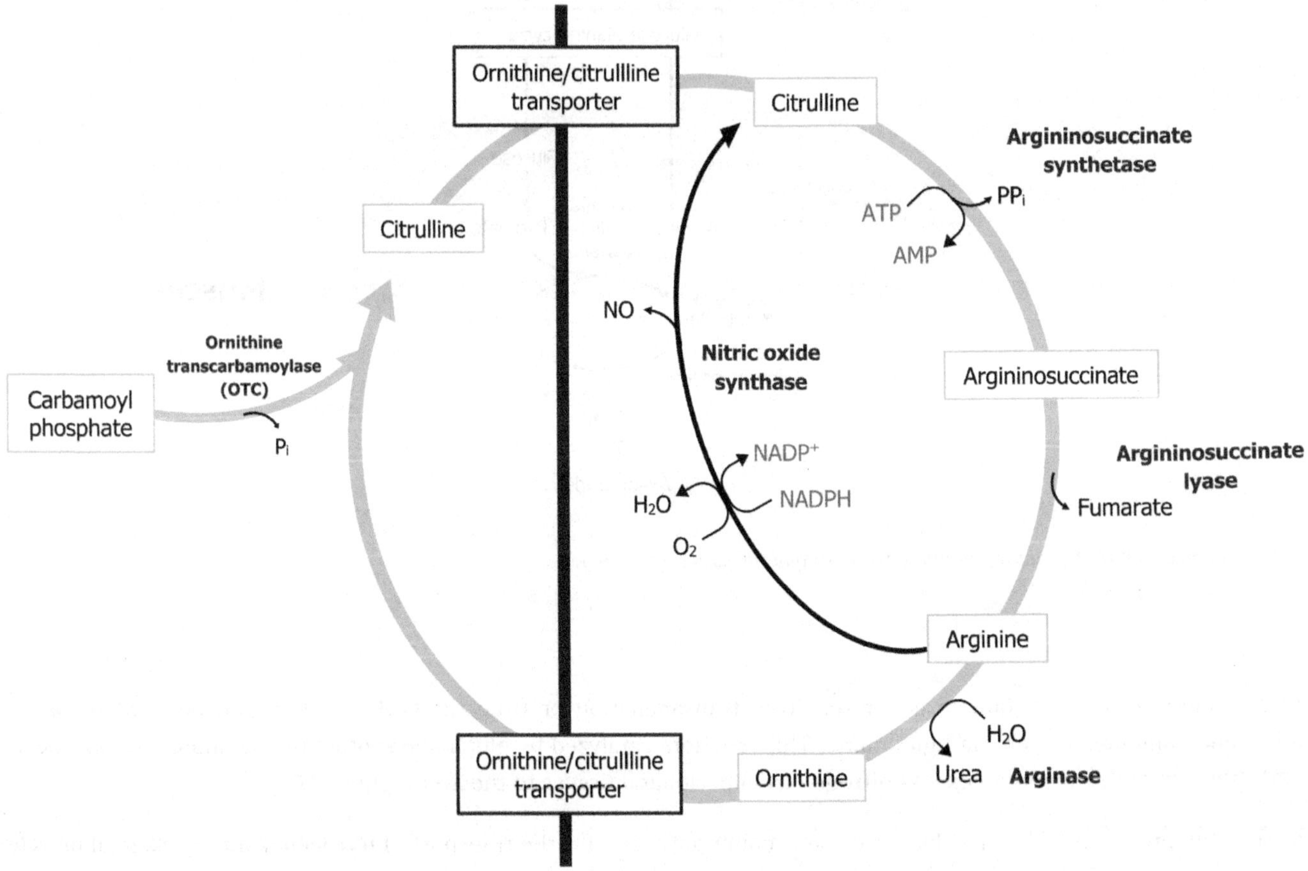

Figure 5.15: Overview of the urea cycle; the pathway spans both the mitochondria and cytosol.

The product of this pathway, urea, is made of two nitrogenous groups with the first coming from the free ammonia released by glutaminase. The second nitrogen is added later in the cycle by aspartate (figures 5.16 and 5.17).

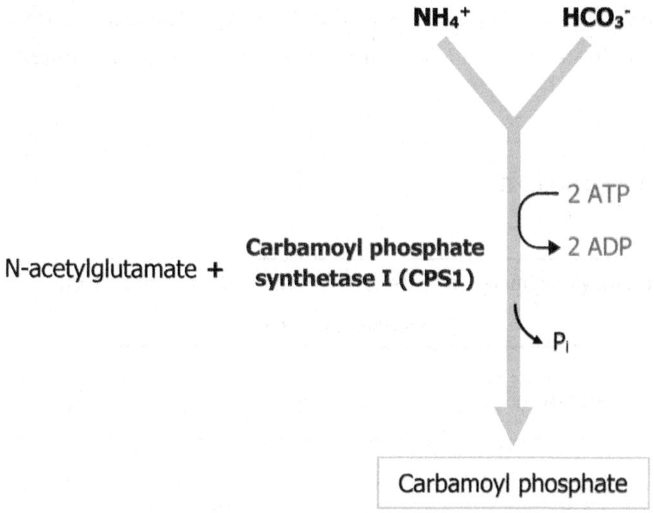

Figure 5.16: Key regulatory step in the urea cycle. CPS1 is activated by N-acetylglutamate.

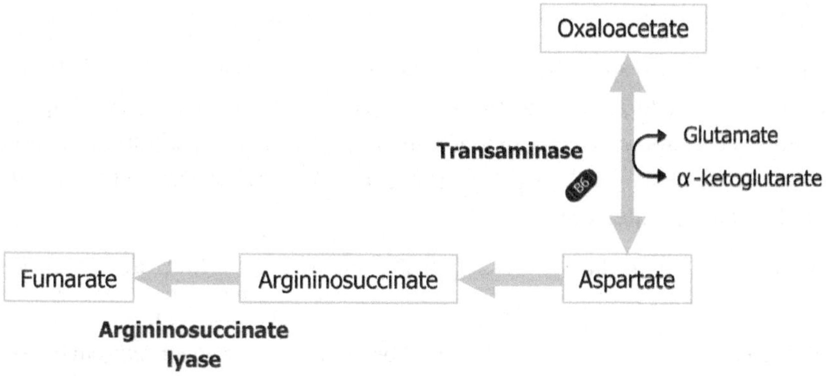

Figure 5.17: Entry of the second nitrogen into the urea cycle; aspartate donates the second nitrogen for the synthesis of urea.

Regulation of the urea cycle

This pathway is predominantly regulated at one key enzyme, carbamoyl phosphate synthetase 1 (figure 5.16). This enzyme requires N-acetylglutamate (NAGS) as an allosteric activator. The synthesis of NAGS is enhanced by arginine, which is an intermediate of the urea cycle. Therefore the cycle provides positive feedback on itself. As flux through the urea cycle increases, and synthesis of arginine increases, this will enhance NAGS production and increase synthesis of carbamoyl phosphate.

Unlike the other pathways discussed, the urea cycle functions independent of hormonal control as it functions to dispose of nitrogen either from excess dietary sources or from protein catabolism/turnover. In the fasted state this is especially important as the carbon skeletons produced are required as substrates for gluconeogenesis (see figure 5.3). In the fed state, amino acids can be deaminated and contribute to the carbon pool (see figures 4.12 and 4.13).

In summary, the process of nitrogen movement from the peripheral tissues to the liver is essential. It involves transamination reactions to produce alanine, and the synthesis of glutamine (by glutamine synthetase) to generate two nontoxic carriers of ammonia. Once transported to the liver, again, transamination coupled with the reactions of glutaminase and glutamate dehydrogenase will allow for ammonia to be freed and enter into the urea cycle.

Summary of pathway regulation

Metabolic pathway	Major regulatory enzyme(s)	Allosteric effectors	Hormonal effects
Urea cycle	CPS I	N-acetylglutamate (+)	

Table 5.3: Summary of pathway regulation.

5.3 References and resources

Text

Ferrier, D. R., ed. *Lippincott Illustrated Reviews: Biochemistry*, 7th ed. Philadelphia: Wolters Kluwer Health/ Lippincott Williams & Wilkins, 2017, Chapter 10: Gluconeogenesis: Section II, III, IV, Chapter 11: Glycogen Metabolism: Section V, VI, Chapter 16: Fatty Acid Ketone Body and TAG Metabolism: Section III, IV, V, Chapter 19: Removal of Nitrogen from Amino Acids: Section V, VI, Chapter 23: Metabolic Effect of Insulin and Glucagon, Chapter 25: Diabetes Mellitus.

Le, T., and V. Bhushan. *First Aid for the USMLE Step 1*, 29th ed. New York: McGraw Hill Education, 2018, 78, 82, 86, 89–90.

Lieberman, M., and A. Peet, eds. *Marks' Basic Medical Biochemistry: A Clinical Approach*, 5th ed. Philadelphia: Wolters Kluwer Health/Lippincott Williams & Wilkins, 2018, Chapter 3: The Fasted State, Chapter 19: Basic Concepts in Regulation, Chapter 24: Oxidative Phosphorylation and the ETC, Chapter 26: Formation of Glycogen, Chapter 28: Gluconeogenesis, Chapter 30: Oxidation of Fatty Acids, Chapter 34: Integration of Carbohydrate and Lipid Metabolism, Chapter 36: Fate of Amino Acids Nitrogen: Urea Cycle.

Figures

Grey, Kindred, Figure 5.12. Figure 5.12: Transamination reaction. 2021. CC BY 4.0. Added Liver by Liam Mitchell from the Noun Project and Muscle by Laymik from the Noun Project.

Grey, Kindred, Figure 5.13 Reactions catalyzed by glutamate dehydrogenase, glutaminase and glutamine synthetase. 2021. https://archive.org/details/5.11_20210924. CC BY 4.0.

Grey, Kindred, Figure 5.14 Movement of ammonia from peripheral tissues to the liver. 2021. https://archive.org/details/5.12_20210924. CC BY 4.0.

Grey, Kindred, Figure 5.15 Overview of the urea cycle, the pathway spans both the mitochondria and cytosol. 2021. https://archive.org/details/5.13_20210924. CC BY 4.0.

Grey, Kindred, Figure 5.16 Key regulatory step in the urea cycle. CPS1 is activated by N-acetyl glutamate. 2021. https://archive.org/details/5.14_20210924. CC BY 4.0.

Grey, Kindred, Figure 5.17 Entry of the second nitrogen into the urea cycle; aspartate donates the second nitrogen for the synthesis of urea. 2021. https://archive.org/details/5.15_20210924. CC BY 4.0.

6. Lipoprotein Metabolism and Cholesterol Synthesis

Learning Objectives

- Describe the structure and composition (including associated apoproteins) of the plasma lipoproteins (chylomicrons, VLDL, IDL, LDL, and HDL).
- Compare and contrast the functions of the various lipoprotein particles with respect to their composition, synthesis, transport, and uptake.
- Describe the regulation of cholesterol biosynthesis by the following factors: energy availability, hormones, food intake, and pharmacological manipulation.
- Predict the effect of changes of plasma cholesterol levels on the intracellular synthesis of cholesterol and the transcriptional regulation of genes that are involved in cholesterol homeostasis.
- Predict the consequence of defects in the LDL receptor on plasma lipid levels, receptor number, and the activity of enzymes involved in cellular cholesterol metabolism.

About this Chapter

Cholesterol synthesis and lipoprotein metabolism are several of the most clinically relevant metabolic pathways. Dyslipidemias are a common medical concern, and understanding how to interpret and treat these disorders is fundamental to clinical practice. This section will describe the role, metabolism, and regulation of lipoproteins within circulation.

6.1 Cholesterol Synthesis

Cholesterol is a key component of cell membranes and is an essential precursor for steroid hormone synthesis. All twenty-seven carbons are derived from acetyl-CoA, and the initial synthesis involves the condensation of acetyl-CoA to mevalonate (figure 6.1).

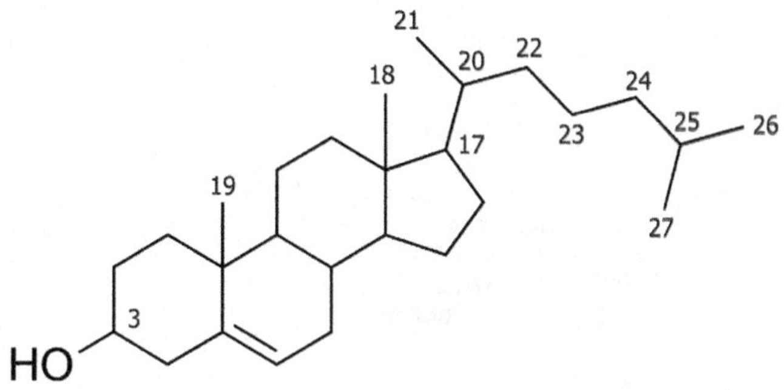

Figure 6.1: Structure of cholesterol.

Cholesterol synthesis takes place in the cytosol, and the acetyl-CoA needed can be obtained from several sources such as β-oxidation of fatty acids, the oxidation of ketogenic amino acids, such as leucine and lysine, and the pyruvate dehydrogenase reaction (acetyl-CoA shuttled out of the mitochondria is in the form of citrate, which is cleaved into acetyl-CoA and pyruvate by citrate lyase). The process of cholesterol synthesis involves four stages (figure 6.2); however, only the first stage is regulated and will be focused on here.

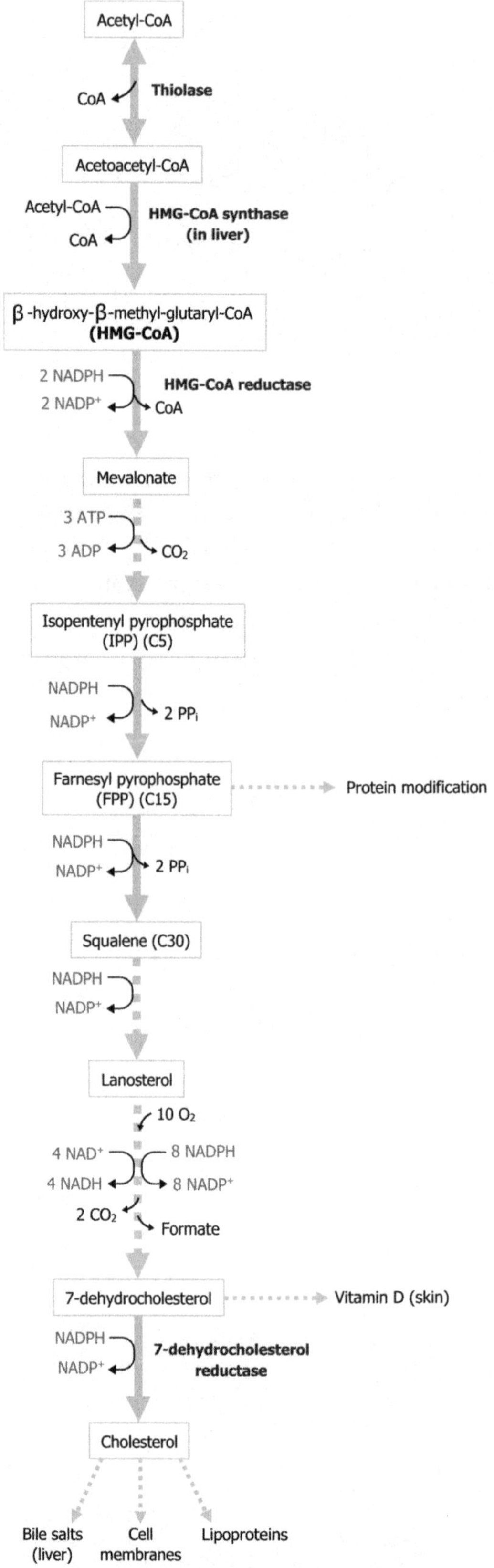

Figure 6.2: Cholesterol synthetic pathway.

Synthesis of mevalonate from acetyl-CoA

The first stage of cholesterol synthesis leads to the production of the intermediate mevalonate. The synthesis of mevalonate is the committed, rate-limiting step in cholesterol formation. In this reaction, two molecules of acetyl-CoA condense, forming acetoacetyl-CoA, which then condenses with a third molecule of acetyl-CoA to yield the six-carbon compound β-hydroxy-β-methylglutaryl-CoA (HMG-CoA) (figure 6.3) (the cytosolic HMG-CoA synthase in this reaction is distinct from the mitochondrial HMG-CoA synthase that catalyzes a similar reaction involved in production of ketone bodies). The committed step and major point of regulation of cholesterol synthesis involves reduction of HMG-CoA to mevalonate, in a reaction that is catalyzed by HMG-CoA reductase.

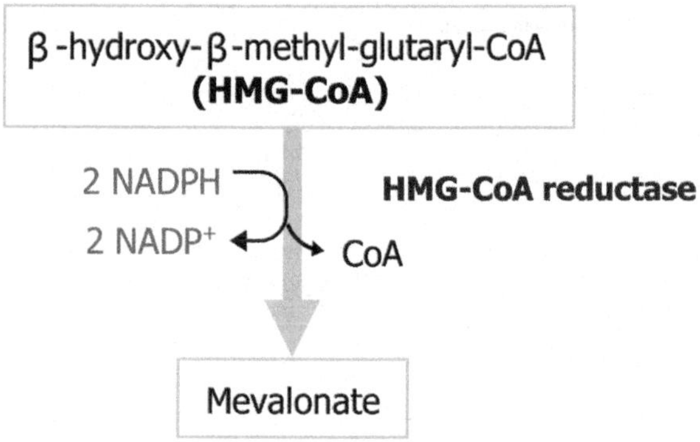

Figure 6.3: Regulatory step catalyzed by HMG-CoA reductase.

The subsequent steps of the pathway proceed largely unregulated, and mevalonate is used to synthesize isoprenoid units (five-carbon units). These five-carbon chains are joined in a head-to-tail fashion generating squalene, thirty-carbons, which undergoes a cyclization reaction after epoxidation. The cyclized product, lanosterol, undergoes several reactions to generate the final product, cholesterol.

Regulation of cholesterol synthesis

The major regulatory enzyme for cholesterol synthesis is HMG-CoA reductase. This enzyme is tightly controlled by many different types of regulation and can be influenced by hormonal changes as well as cellular needs (figure 6.4). This is also one of the primary pharmacological targets for the management of hypercholesterolemia. The statins are direct inhibitors of this enzyme.

Transcriptional control

A

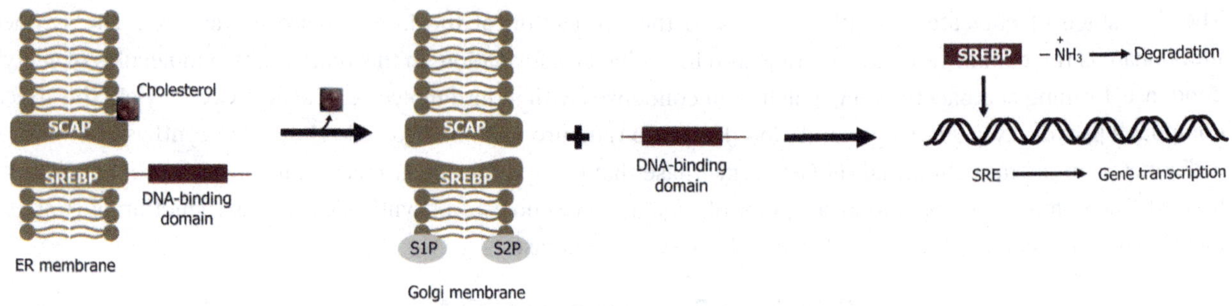

B

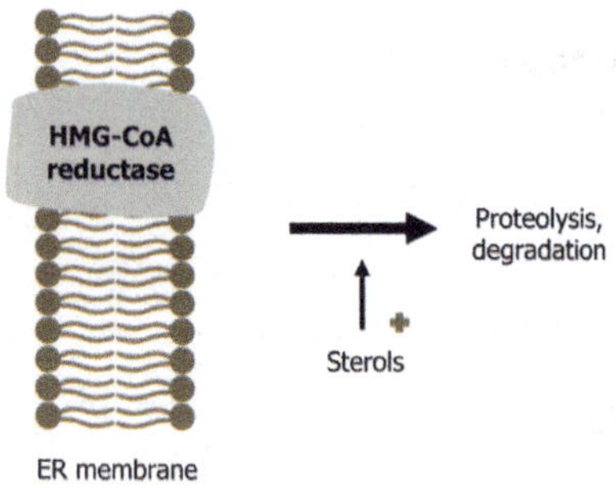

C

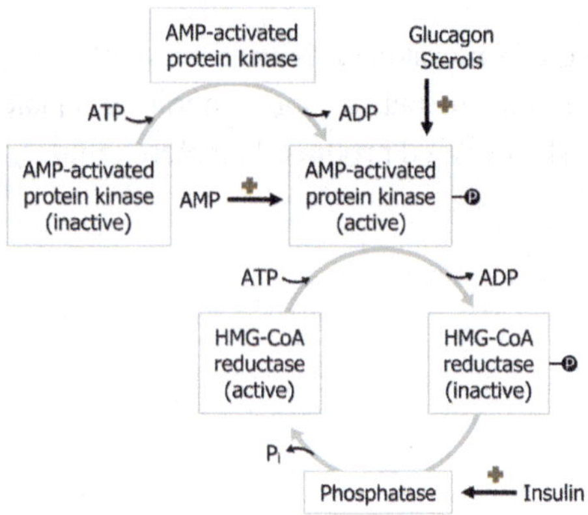

Figure 6.4: Regulation of cholesterol synthesis.

The rate of synthesis of HMG-CoA reductase messenger RNA (mRNA) is controlled by one of the family of sterol-regulatory element-binding proteins (SREBPs). SREBPs are integral proteins of the endoplasmic reticulum (ER). When cholesterol levels in the cell are high, the SREBP is bound to SCAP (SREBP cleavage activating protein) in the ER membrane. When cholesterol levels drop, the sterol leaves its SCAP-binding site, and the SREBP:SCAP complex is transported to the Golgi apparatus. Within the Golgi, two proteolytic cleavages occur, which release the N-terminal transcription factor domain from the Golgi membrane. Once released, the active amino terminal component travels to the nucleus to bind to sterol-regulatory elements (SREs). Binding to this upstream element enhances transcription of the HMG-CoA reductase gene. The soluble SREBPs are rapidly turned over and need to be continuously produced to stimulate reductase mRNA transcription effectively. As cholesterol levels in the cell increase, due to de novo synthesis, cholesterol will bind to SCAP and prevent translocation of the complex to the Golgi, leading to a decrease in transcription of the reductase gene and thus less reductase protein being produced (figure 6.4).

Proteolytic degradation of HMG-CoA reductase

The amount of HMG-CoA reductase can also be influenced by proteolytic degradation. The membrane domains of HMG-CoA reductase contain sterol-sensing regions, which are similar to those in SCAP. As levels of cholesterol (or its derivatives) increase in the cell, this causes a change in the oligomerization state of the membrane domain of HMG-CoA reductase, rendering the enzyme more susceptible to proteolysis. This, in turn, decreases the activity of the enzyme.

Regulation by covalent modification

Much like other anabolic enzymes, the activity of HMG-CoA reductase can be influenced by phosphorylation. Elevated glucagon levels increase phosphorylation of the enzyme, thereby inactivating it, whereas hyperinsulinemia increases the activity of the reductase by activating phosphatases, which dephosphorylate the reductase. Increased levels of intracellular sterols may also increase phosphorylation of HMG-CoA reductase, thereby reducing its activity as well (feedback suppression).

Adenosine monophosphate (AMP)-activated protein kinase can also phosphorylate and inactivate HMG-CoA reductase. Thus, cholesterol synthesis decreases when ATP levels are low and increases when ATP levels are high, similar to what occurs with fatty acid synthesis (recall that acetyl-CoA carboxylase is also phosphorylated and inhibited by the AMP-activated protein kinase; section 4.4.)

Several fates of cholesterol

Almost all mammalian cells are capable of producing cholesterol. Most of the biosynthesis of cholesterol occurs within liver cells, although the gut, the adrenal cortex, and the gonads (as well as the placenta in pregnant women) also produce significant quantities of the sterol. A small portion of hepatic cholesterol is used for the synthesis of hepatic membranes, but the bulk of synthesized cholesterol is secreted from the hepatocyte as one of three compounds: cholesterol esters, biliary cholesterol (cholesterol found in the bile), or bile acids.

Cholesterol esterification and transport

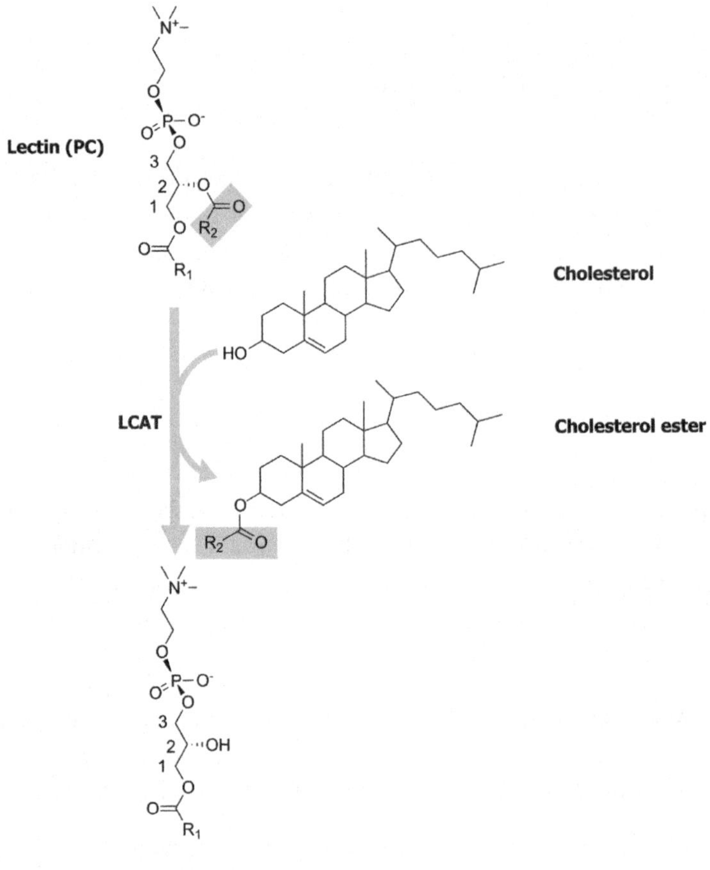

Figure 6.5: Esterification of cholesterol by LCAT.

Cholesterol is an amphipathic molecule (containing both polar and nonpolar regions), and in its native state it can freely diffuse through membranes. In order to be stored in cells, cholesterol must be modified by increasing its hydrophobicity. Cholesterol ester production in the liver is catalyzed by acyl-CoA-cholesterol acyl transferase (ACAT). ACAT catalyzes the transfer of a fatty acid from coenzyme A to the hydroxyl group on carbon 3 of cholesterol. (This is similar to the reaction catalyzed by lecithin:cholesterol acyltransferase within the plasma associated with HDLs; figure 6.5.) Regardless of whether the additional group is an acyl chain or phosphatidylcholine, the resulting cholesterol esters are more hydrophobic than free cholesterol. The liver packages some of the esterified cholesterol into the hollow core of lipoproteins, primarily VLDL. VLDL is secreted from the hepatocyte into the blood and transports the cholesterol esters (triacylglycerols, phospholipids, apoproteins, etc.) to the tissues that require greater amounts of cholesterol than they can synthesize de novo. These tissues then use the cholesterol for the synthesis of membranes, the formation of steroid hormones, and the biosynthesis of vitamin D.

Synthesis of specialized products

The hepatic cholesterol pool serves as a source of cholesterol for the synthesis of the relatively hydrophilic bile acids and their salts. These derivatives of cholesterol are effective detergents because they contain both polar and nonpolar regions. They are introduced into the biliary ducts of the liver. They are stored and concentrated in the gallbladder and later discharged into the gut in response to the ingestion of food. Finally, cholesterol is the precursor of all five classes of steroid hormones: glucocorticoids, mineralocorticoids, androgens, estrogens, and progestins. Cholesterol and steroid hormones are transported through the blood from their sites of synthesis to their target organs. Because of their hydrophobicity, they must be complexed with a serum protein. Serum albumin can act as a nonspecific carrier for the steroid hormones, but there are specific carriers as well (section 2.1).

6.1 References and resources

Text

Ferrier, D. R., ed. *Lippincott Illustrated Reviews: Biochemistry*, 7th ed. Philadelphia: Wolters Kluwer Health/ Lippincott Williams & Wilkins, 2017, Chapter 15: Metabolism of Dietary Lipids, Chapter 18: Cholesterol and Steroid Metabolism.

Le, T., and V. Bhushan. *First Aid for the USMLE Step 1*, 29th ed. New York: McGraw Hill Education, 2018, 92–94.

Lieberman, M., and A. Peet, eds. *Marks' Basic Medical Biochemistry: A Clinical Approach*, 5th ed. Philadelphia: Wolters Kluwer Health/Lippincott Williams & Wilkins, 2018, Chapter 29: Digestion and Transport of Dietary Lipids, Chapter 32: Cholesterol Absorption: Synthesis, Metabolism and Fate Section.

Figures

Grey, Kindred, Figure 6.1 Structure of cholesterol. 2021. Chemical structure by Henry Jakubowski. https://archive.org/details/6.1_20210924. CC BY 4.0.

Grey, Kindred, Figure 6.2 Cholesterol synthetic pathway. 2021. https://archive.org/details/6.2_20210924. CC BY 4.0

Grey, Kindred, Figure 6.3 Regulatory step catalyzed by HMG-CoA reductase. 2021. https://archive.org/details/6.3_20210924. CC BY 4.0.

Grey, Kindred, Figure 6.5 Esterification of cholesterol by LCAT. 2021. Chemical structure by Henry Jakubowski. https://archive.org/details/6.5_20210924. CC BY 4.0.

Lieberman M, Peet A. Figure 6.4 Regulation of cholesterol synthesis. Adapted under Fair Use from Marks' Basic Medical Biochemistry. 5th Ed. pp 647. Figure 32.6 Regulation of 3-hydroxymethylglutryl coenzyme A (HMG-CoA reductase activity. 2017. Added squiggle by Made by Made from the Noun Project and ion channel by Léa Lortal from the Noun Project.

6.2 Lipid Transport

Most of the lipids found in the body fall into the categories of fatty acids and triacylglycerols (TAGs); glycerophospholipids and sphingolipids; eicosanoids; cholesterol, bile salts, and steroid hormones; and fat-soluble vitamins. These lipids have very diverse chemical structures and functions. However, they are related by a common property, their relative insolubility in water.

As such, a transport system for distribution of major lipids is in place to aid in the movement of these compounds. This system involves the family of lipoproteins, which have distinct roles in carrying dietary lipids, lipids synthesized through de novo mechanism in the liver, and for reverse cholesterol transport (figure 6.6).

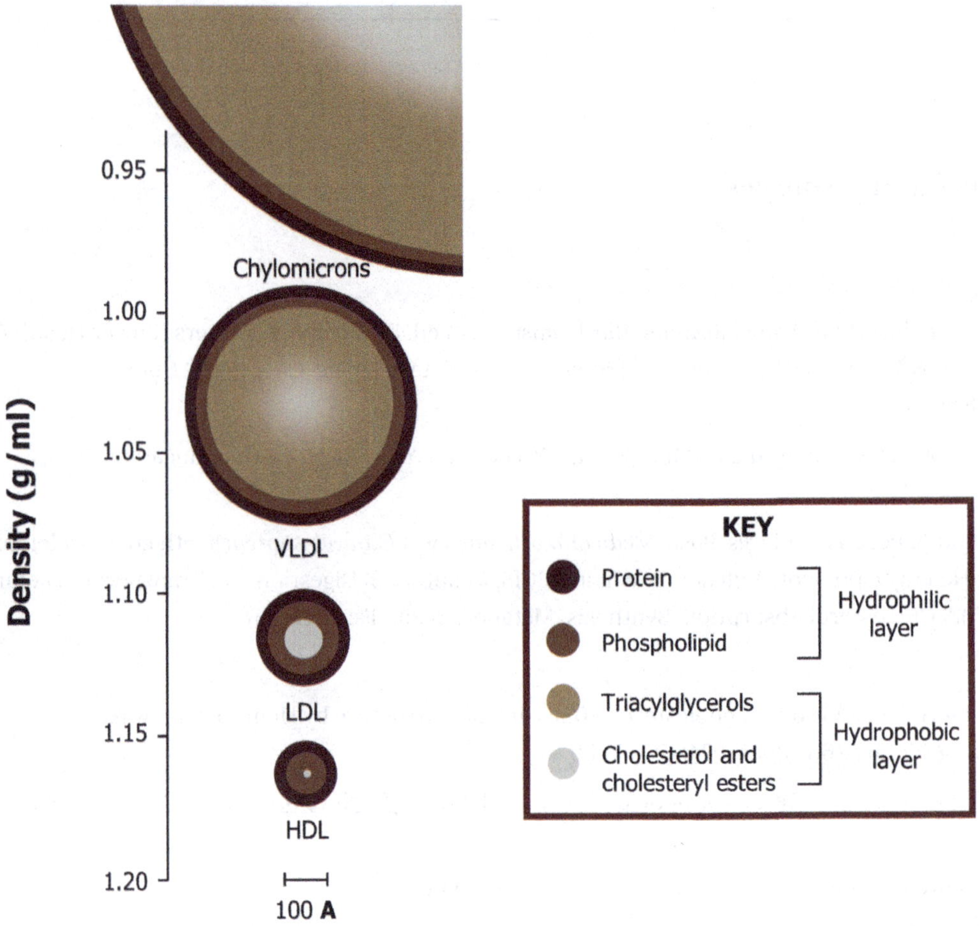

Figure 6.6: Overview of lipoprotein size and structure.

In addition to the lipid components of lipoproteins, they contain protein components termed apoproteins. The complement of apoproteins on each lipoprotein is unique and is a distinguishing characteristic of each family of lipoproteins. The apoproteins ("apo" describes the protein within the shell of the particle in its lipid-free form) not only add to the hydrophilicity and structural stability of the particle, but they have other functions as well: (1) They activate certain enzymes required for normal lipoprotein metabolism, and (2) they act as ligands on the surface of the lipoprotein that target specific receptors on peripheral tissues that require lipoprotein delivery for their innate cellular functions.

Chylomicrons: Transport of dietary lipids

Fatty acids, which are stored as TAGs, serve as fuels, providing the body with its major source of energy. TAGs are the major dietary lipids and are digested in the lumen of the intestine. The initial digestive products, free fatty acids and 2-monoacylglycerol, are reconverted to TAGs in intestinal epithelial cells, packaged in lipoproteins known as chylomicrons, and secreted into the lymph (figure 6.7).

Chylomicrons are the largest lipoproteins and contain cholesterol and fat-soluble vitamins, in addition to their major component, dietary TAGs. The major apoprotein associated with chylomicrons as they leave the intestinal cells is ApoB-48. (The B-48 apoprotein is structurally and genetically related to the B-100 apoprotein synthesized in the liver that serves as a major protein of VLDL.) Microsomal transfer protein (MTP) aids in the loading of apoB-48 protein onto the chylomicron before the nascent chylomicron is secreted. Nascent chylomicrons are secreted by the intestinal epithelial cells into the chyle of the lymphatic system and enter the blood through the thoracic duct. Nascent chylomicrons begin to enter the blood within one to two hours after the start of a meal; as the meal is digested and absorbed, they continue to enter the blood for many hours. Chylomicron maturation occurs in circulation as they accept additional apoproteins from high-density lipoprotein (HDL) (figures 6.7 and 6.10).

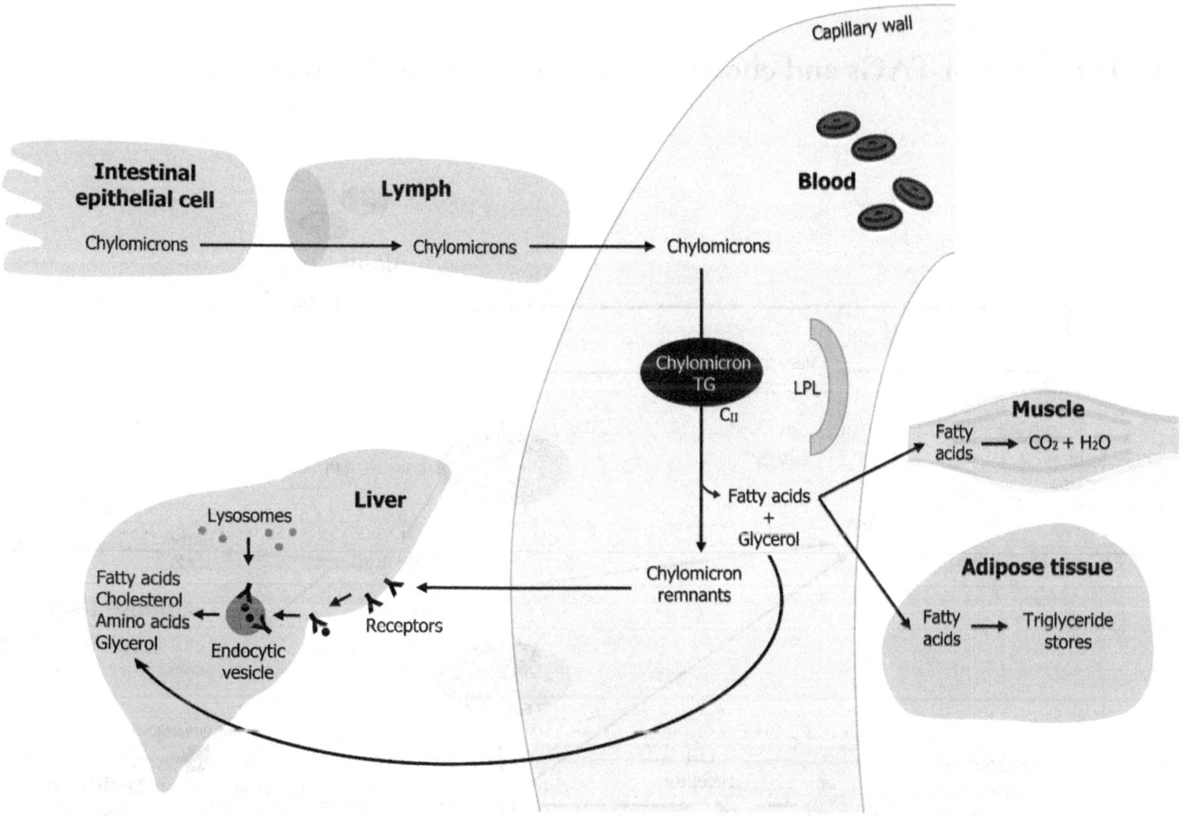

Figure 6.7: Transport of dietary lipids via chylomicrons.

HDL predominantly transfers apoproteins E and CII to the nascent chylomicrons. ApoE is recognized by membrane receptors, and this interaction allows apoE-bearing lipoproteins to enter these cells by endocytosis; once inside the cell the particle is broken down through a lysosomal-mediated process. ApoCII acts as an activator of lipoprotein lipase (LPL), the enzyme on capillary endothelial cells, which digests the TAGs of the chylomicrons and VLDLs in the blood.

Fate of chylomicrons

The TAGs transported by chylomicrons are hydrolyzed by lipoprotein lipase (LPL), an enzyme present on endothelial cells that line the capillary walls. ApoCII on the chylomicron will interact with LPL and activate the enzyme. Insulin stimulates the synthesis and secretion of LPL so that after a meal, when triglyceride levels increase in circulation, LPL is upregulated (through insulin release) to facilitate the hydrolysis of fatty acids from the triglyceride.

Therefore, adipose LPL is more active after a meal, when chylomicron levels are elevated in the blood. The fatty acids released from TAGs by LPL are eventually repackaged in the adipose tissue and stored as TAGs within the tissue.

The portion of a chylomicron that remains in the blood after LPL action is known as a chylomicron remnant. The remnant has returned (or lost) many of the apoC molecules bound to the mature chylomicron, exposing apoE. The remaining remnant binds to apoE receptors on hepatocytes, and is taken up by the process of endocytosis. Lysosomes fuse with the endocytic vesicles, and the chylomicron remnants are degraded by lysosomal enzymes. The products released through this degradation process (e.g., amino acids, fatty acids, cholesterol, etc.) can be recycled within the cell.

VLDL: Transport of TAGs and cholesterol synthesized in the liver

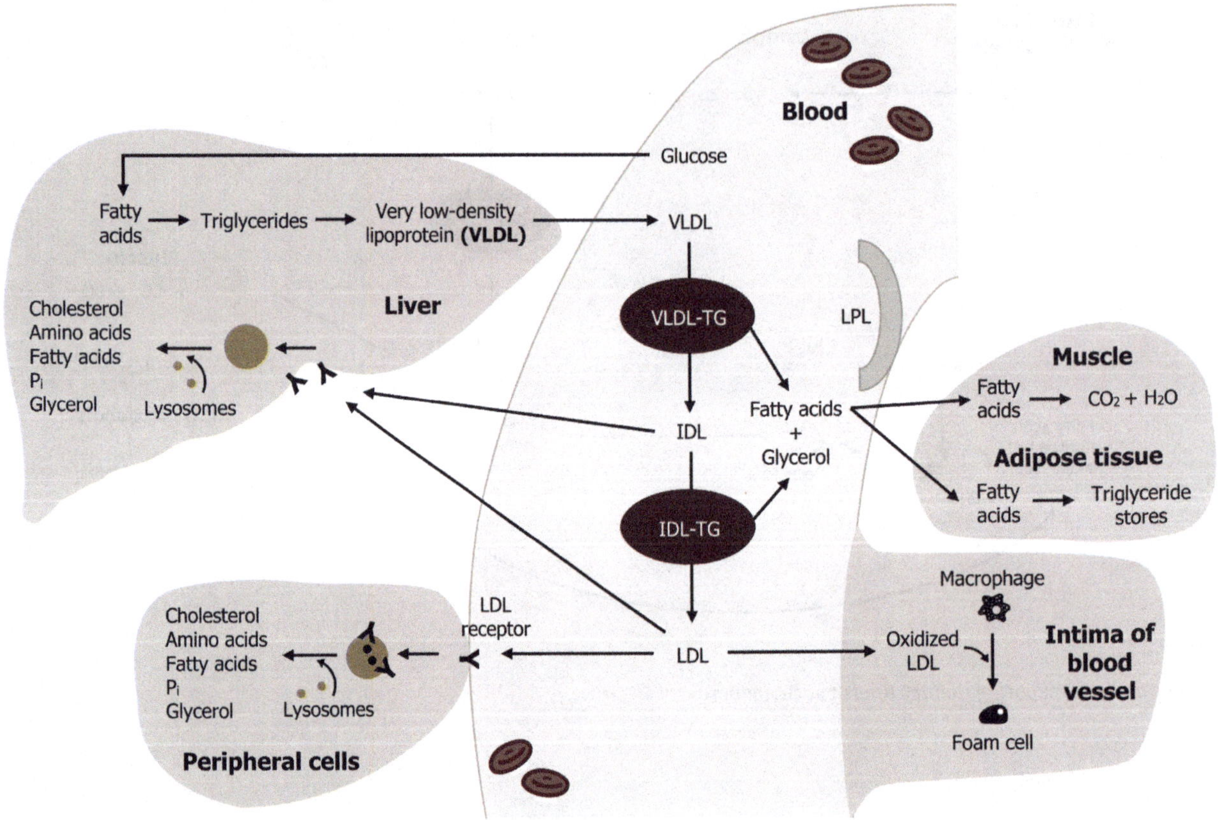

Figure 6.8: Transport of TAGs from de novo synthesis using VLDL.

Very low-density lipoprotein (VLDL) is produced in the liver, mainly from lipogenesis. Lipogenesis is an insulin-stimulated process through which excess glucose is converted to fatty acids (section 4.4), which are subsequently esterified to glycerol to form TAGs. TAGs produced in the smooth endoplasmic reticulum of the liver are packaged with cholesterol, phospholipids, and proteins (synthesized in the rough endoplasmic reticulum) to form VLDLs. Apart from their initial origin, VLDLs and chylomicrons are very similar with respect to maturation and activity. The VLDL particles acquire apoB-100 through an MTP-mediated reaction before being released into circulation. Within circulation, VLDLs also interact with HDL and acquire ApoCII and ApoE (figure 6.8). Like chylomicrons, VLDLs are also hydrolyzed by lipoprotein lipase (LPL), and the released fatty acids can be taken up by muscle and other tissues to be oxidized. After a meal, these fatty acids are also taken up by adipose tissue and stored as TAGs. In summary, the process of dietary versus de novo lipid transport has many parallels, which are compared in figure 6.9.

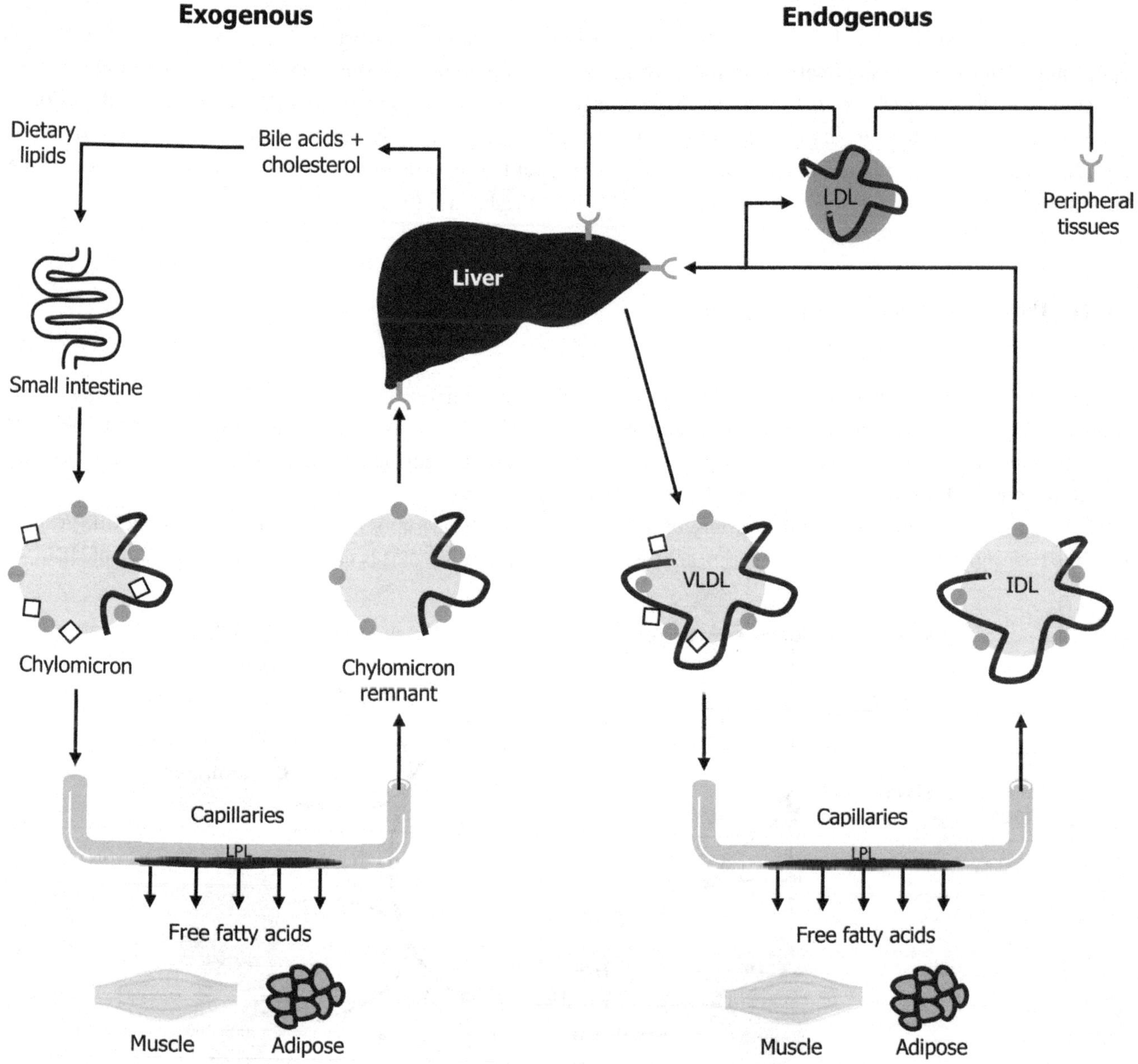

Figure 6.9: Comparison of the role of chylomicrons and VLDLs in lipid transport.

Although VLDLs and chylomicrons have similar roles in the cell, it is important to keep them distinct. The comparison between the transport of exogenous lipids and endogenous lipids is illustrated in figure 6.9. Because the fatty acids stored in adipose tissue come both from chylomicrons and VLDL, we produce our major fat stores both from dietary fat (which is transported by chylomicrons) and dietary sugar (which can be synthesized into TAGs and packaged into VLDL). An excess of dietary protein also can be used to produce the fatty acids for VLDL synthesis. Clinically, measured triacylglycerols (under fasting conditions) will largely reflect the VLDL contribution.

Fate of VLDL

Much like the conversion of chylomicrons to chylomicron remnants, LPL converts VLDL to an intermediate-density lipoprotein (IDL). IDLs, having relatively low TAG content, are taken up by the liver through endocytosis, and degraded lysosomes as discussed above. IDL may also be converted to low-density lipoprotein (LDL) by further digestion of TAGs. Endocytosis of LDL occurs in peripheral tissues (and the liver) and is the major means of cholesterol transport and delivery to peripheral tissues. LDLs taken up by peripheral tissues will help increase the amount of intracellular cholesterol and therefore influence the regulation of HMG-CoA reductase (figure 6.11).

HDL: Reverse cholesterol transport

The primary function of high-density lipoprotein (HDL) is to transport excess cholesterol obtained from peripheral tissues to the liver. HDL also has other roles integral to lipid transport such as exchanging proteins and lipids with chylomicrons and VLDL. HDL particles can be created by several mechanisms, however, nascent HDLs are primarily secreted from the liver and intestine as a relatively small particles whose shell, like that of other lipoproteins, contains phospholipids, free cholesterol, and a variety of apoproteins, specifically apoAI, apoAII, apoCI, and apoCII. Very low levels of triacylglycerols or cholesterol esters are found in the hollow core of this early, or nascent, version of HDL.

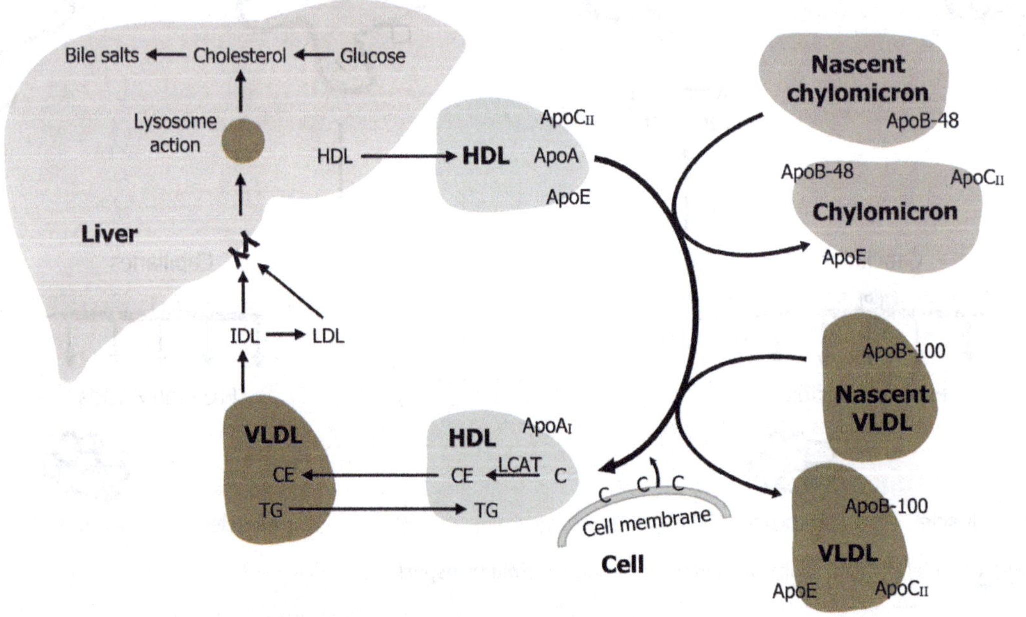

Figure 6.10: Interaction of chylomicrons and VLDL with HDL in circulation.

HDLs can also be generated through budding of apoA from chylomicrons and VLDL particles or from free apoAI, which may be shed from other circulating lipoproteins. In this case, the apoAI acquires cholesterol and phospholipids from other lipoproteins and cell membranes, forming a nascent-like HDL particle within the circulation (figure 6.10).

Fate of HDL

In the process of maturation, the nascent HDL particles accumulate phospholipids and cholesterol from cells lining the blood vessels. As the central hollow core of nascent HDL progressively fills with cholesterol esters, HDL takes on a more globular shape to eventually form the mature HDL particle. A major benefit of HDL particles derives from their ability to remove cholesterol from cholesterol-laden cells and to return the cholesterol to the liver, a process known as reverse cholesterol transport. This is particularly beneficial in vascular tissue; by reducing cellular cholesterol levels in the subintimal space, the likelihood that foam cells (lipid-laden macrophages that engulf oxidized LDL cholesterol) will form within the blood vessel wall is reduced.

Reverse cholesterol transport requires a movement of cholesterol from cellular stores to the lipoprotein particle. Cells contain the protein ABCA1 (ATP-binding cassette protein 1) that uses ATP hydrolysis to move cholesterol from the inner leaflet of the membrane to the outer leaflet. Once the cholesterol has reached the outer membrane leaflet, the HDL particle can accept it. To trap the cholesterol within the HDL core, the HDL particle acquires the enzyme lecithin-cholesterol acyltransferase (LCAT) from the circulation (figure 6.10). LCAT catalyzes the transfer of a fatty acid from the 2-position of lecithin (phosphatidylcholine) in the phospholipid shell of the particle to the 3-hydroxyl group of cholesterol, forming a cholesterol ester. The cholesterol esters form the core of the HDL particle and are no longer free to return to the cell.

Mature HDL particles can bind to specific receptors on hepatocytes (such as the apoE receptor), but the primary means of clearance of HDL from the blood is through its uptake by the scavenger receptor SR-B1. This receptor is present on many cell types, and once the HDL particle is bound to the receptor, its cholesterol and cholesterol esters are transferred into the cells. When depleted of cholesterol and its esters, the HDL particle dissociates from the SR-B1 receptor and reenters the circulation.

HDL interactions with other particles

As previously mentioned, HDL plays a key role in the maturation of both chylomicrons and VLDL. First, HDL transfers apoE and apoCII to chylomicrons and to VLDL. The apoCII stimulates the degradation of the TAGs of chylomicrons and VLDL by activating LPL. After digestion of the chylomicrons and the VLDL TAGs, apoE and apoCII are transferred back to HDL.

Another key interaction HDL has with VLDL allows for the redistribution of cholesterol between the two lipoproteins. When HDL obtains free cholesterol from cell membranes, HDL either transports the free cholesterol and cholesterol esters directly to the liver or it can exchange its cholesterol for TAGs in an interaction with VLDL. The cholesterol esterase transfer protein (CETP) resides in circulation and exchanges TAGs from VLDLs with cholesterol-esters from HDL. The greater the concentration of triacylglycerol-rich lipoproteins in the blood, the greater the rate of these exchanges. The CETP exchange pathway may partially explain the observation that whenever triacylglycerol-rich lipoproteins are present in the blood in high concentrations, the amount of cholesterol reaching the liver via cholesterol-enriched VLDL and VLDL remnants increases (figure 6.10), and is consistent with a proportional reduction in the total amount of cholesterol and cholesterol esters that are transferred directly to the liver via HDL.

Lipoprotein receptor-mediated endocytosis

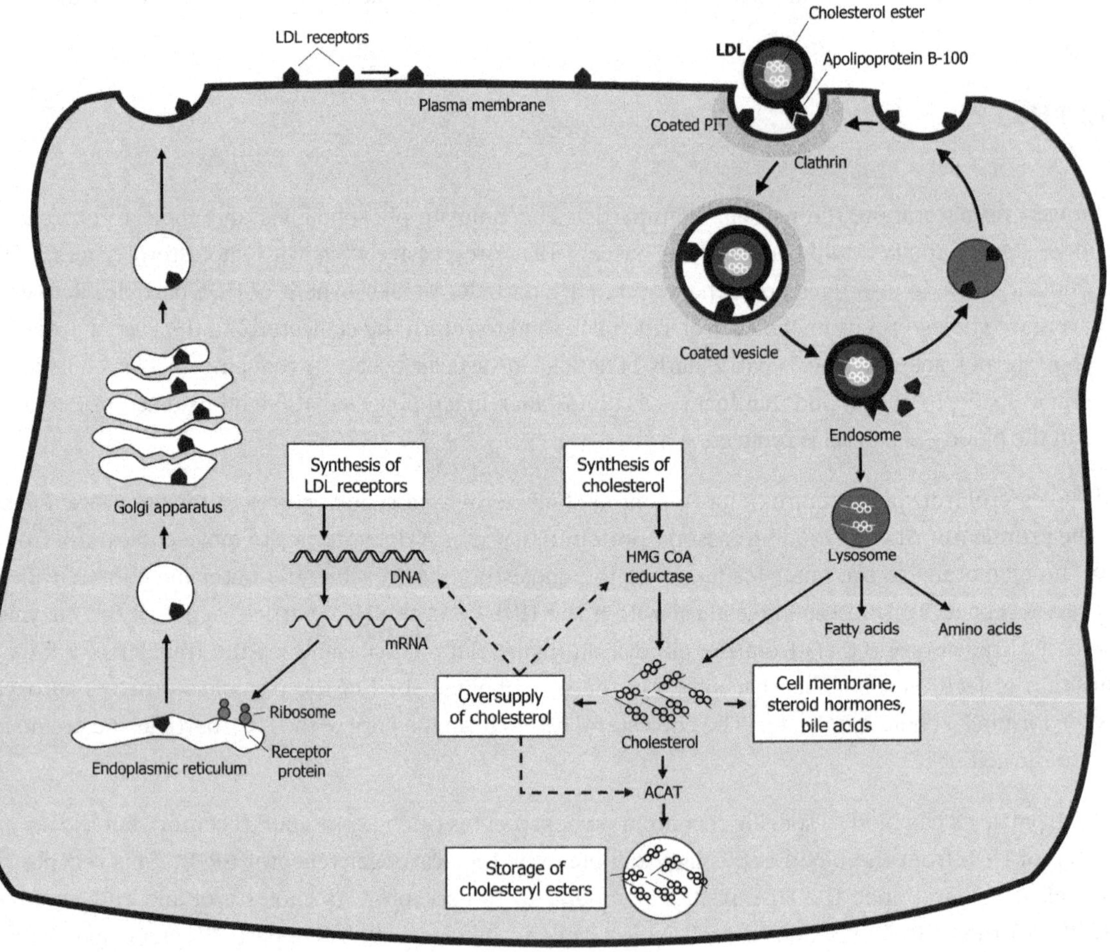

Figure 6.11: Uptake of LDL and regulation of cholesterol synthesis.

As VLDLs mature to LDLs, these lipoproteins can be taken up through an interaction of the ApoB100 with the LDL receptors on the cell surface. The receptors for LDL are found in clathrin-coated pits within the cell membrane of the target cells. Upon receptor ligand interaction, the plasma membrane in the vicinity of the receptor-LDL complex invaginates and fuses to form an endocytic vesicle. These vesicles then fuse with lysosomes, and the cholesterol esters of LDL are hydrolyzed to form free cholesterol, which is rapidly re-esterified through the action of ACAT. This rapid re-esterification is necessary to avoid the damaging effect of high levels of free cholesterol on cellular membranes.

The synthesis of the LDL receptor itself is regulated by feedback inhibition as intracellular levels of cholesterol increase. One probable mechanism for this feedback regulation involves one or more of the SREBPs described earlier. These proteins or the cofactors that are required for the full expression of genes that code for the LDL receptor are also capable of sensing the concentration of cholesterol (and its derivatives) within the cell. When sterol levels are high, the process that leads to the binding of the SREBP to the SRE of these genes is suppressed. The rate of synthesis from mRNA for the LDL receptor is reduced under these circumstances. This, in turn, appropriately reduces the amount of cholesterol that can enter these cholesterol-rich cells by receptor-mediated endocytosis (down-regulation of receptor synthesis). When the intracellular levels of cholesterol decrease, these processes are reversed, and cells act to increase their cholesterol levels. Both synthesis of cholesterol from acetyl-CoA and synthesis of LDL receptors are stimulated. An increased number of receptors (up-regulation of receptor synthesis) results in an increased uptake of LDL cholesterol from the blood, with a subsequent reduction of LDL cholesterol levels. At the same time, the cellular cholesterol pool is replenished (figure 6.11).

6.2 References and resources

Text

Ferrier, D. R., ed. *Lippincott Illustrated Reviews: Biochemistry*, 7th ed. Philadelphia: Wolters Kluwer Health/ Lippincott Williams & Wilkins, 2017, Chapter 15: Metabolism of Dietary Lipids, Chapter 18: Cholesterol and Steroid Metabolism.

Le, T., and V. Bhushan. *First Aid for the USMLE Step 1*, 29th ed. New York: McGraw Hill Education, 2018, 92–94.

Lieberman, M., and A. Peet, eds. *Marks' Basic Medical Biochemistry: A Clinical Approach*, 5th ed. Philadelphia: Wolters Kluwer Health/Lippincott Williams & Wilkins, 2018, Chapter 29: Digestion and Transport of Dietary Lipids, Chapter 32: Cholesterol Absorption: Synthesis, Metabolism and Fate Section.

Figures

Ferrier D. Figure 6.6 Overview of lipoprotein size and structure. Adapted under Fair Use from Lippincott Illustrated Reviews Biochemistry. 7th Ed. pp 227. Figure 18.13 Plasma lipoprotein particles exhibit a range of sizes and densities, and typical values are shown. 2017.

Ferrier D. Figure 6.11 Uptake of LDL and regulation of cholesterol synthesis. Adapted under Fair Use from Lippincott Illustrated Reviews Biochemistry. 7th Ed. pp 233. Figure 18.20 Cellular uptake and degradation of low-density lipoprotein (LDL) particles. 2017. Added squiggle by Made by Made from the Noun Project.

Lieberman M, Peet A. Figure 6.7 Transport of dietary lipids via chylomicrons. Adapted under Fair Use from Marks' Basic Medical Biochemistry. 5th Ed. pp 601. Figure 29.11 Fate of chylomicrons. 2017. Added Liver by Liam Mitchell from the Noun Project, Muscle by Laymik from the Noun Project, and red blood cells by Lucas Helle from the Noun Project.

Lieberman M, Peet A. Figure 6.8 Transport of TAGs from de novo synthesis using VLDL. Adapted under Fair Use from Marks' Basic Medical Biochemistry. 5th Ed. pp 680. Figure 32.12 Fate of very-low-desnity lipoprteins (VLDL). 2017. Added macrophage by Léa Lortal from the Noun Project, Liver by Liam Mitchell from the Noun Project, and red blood cells by Lucas Helle from the Noun Project.

Lieberman M, Peet A. Figure 6.10 Interaction of chylomicrons and VLDL with HDL in circulation. Adapted under Fair Use from Marks' Basic Medical Biochemistry. 5th Ed. pp 683. Figure 32.15 Functions and fate of high-density lipoprotein (HDL). 2017. Added Liver by Liam Mitchell from the Noun Project.

Loscalzo J. Figure 6.9 Comparison of the role of chylomicrons and VLDLs in lipid transport. Adapted under Fair Use from Harrison's Cardiovascular Medicine 2 ed. online. Figure 31.2 The exogenous and endogenous lipoprotein metabolic pathways. 2013. Added Small Intestine by PJ Witt from the Noun Project, Liver by Liam Mitchell from the Noun Project, and Muscle by Laymik from the Noun Project.

7. Pentose Phosphate Pathway (PPP), Purine and Pyrimidine Metabolism

Learning Objectives

- Describe the role of NADPH produced by the pentose phosphate pathway in metabolism and regulation of glucose 6-phosphate dehydrogenase.
- Determine the utility of the oxidative and nonoxidative portions of the pentose phosphate pathway (PPP) and how these pathways interface with glycolysis.
- Describe the amino acid composition of glutathione (GSH) and understand the role of GSH in attenuating oxidative damage.
- Describe how the pentose phosphate pathway and the process of DNA replication interface with the biosynthesis of purine and pyrimidine nucleotides.
- Evaluate the central role of 5-phosphoribosyl-1-pyrophosphate (PRPP) in nucleotide metabolism.
- Describe the purine salvage pathway, specifically the reaction catalyzed by hypoxanthine-guanine phosphoribosyltransferase (HGPRT).
- Identify the key regulatory steps in both purine and pyrimidine synthesis, and evaluate flux through each pathway depending on levels of allosteric activators and inhibitors.
- Describe conditions that lead to elevated orotic acid, and interpret urine orotic acid concentration for the diagnosis of defects of the urea cycle or pyrimidine biosynthesis.

About this Chapter

As we have seen previously, glucose can be diverted to several different pathways depending on metabolic needs. One of these pathways is the pentose phosphate pathway, which plays an integral role in producing both NADPH and the five-carbon sugar ribose. NADPH provides the cell with an energy source for reductive biosynthesis and detoxification of free radicals, while ribose is an essential component in the synthesis of both purine and pyrimidine nucleotides. Aberrations (increases or decreases) in either of these metabolic pathways, PPP or nucleotide synthesis, can result in the common clinical presentations of anemia, jaundice, or gout.

7.1 Pentose Phosphate Pathway

The pentose phosphate pathway (PPP – also known as the hexose monosphosphate shunt) is a cytosolic pathway that interfaces with glycolysis. In this pathway, no ATP is directly produced from the oxidation of glucose 6-phosphate; instead the oxidative portion of the PPP is coupled to the production of NADPH. In addition to generating NADPH, which is essential for detoxification reactions and fatty acid synthesis, it also produces five-carbon sugars required for nucleotide synthesis.

Oxidative and nonoxidative functions

There are two parts of the pathway that are distinct and can be regulated independently. The first phase, or oxidative phase, consists of two irreversible oxidations that produce NADPH. As noted above, NADPH is required for reductive detoxification and fatty acid synthesis. (NADPH is not oxidized in the ETC.) In the red blood cell, this is extremely important as the PPP pathway provides the only source of NADPH. NADPH is essential to maintain sufficient levels of reduced glutathione in the red blood cell. Glutathione is a tripeptide commonly used in tissues to detoxify free radicals and reduce cellular oxidation.

The nonoxidative phase of the pathway allows for the conversion of ribulose 5-phosphate into ribose 5-phosphate, which is needed for nucleotide synthesis (figure 7.1). All of these interconversions in the nonoxidative pathway are reversible and use the enzymes transketolase or transaldolase to move two-carbon or three-carbon units on to other sugar moieties to generate a variety of sugar intermediates. Transketolase requires thiamine pyrophosphate (TPP) as a cofactor. This is of clinical relevance as TPP levels can be measured by addressing the activity of transketolase in a blood sample. A reduction in transketolase activity is an indicator of a thiamine deficiency.

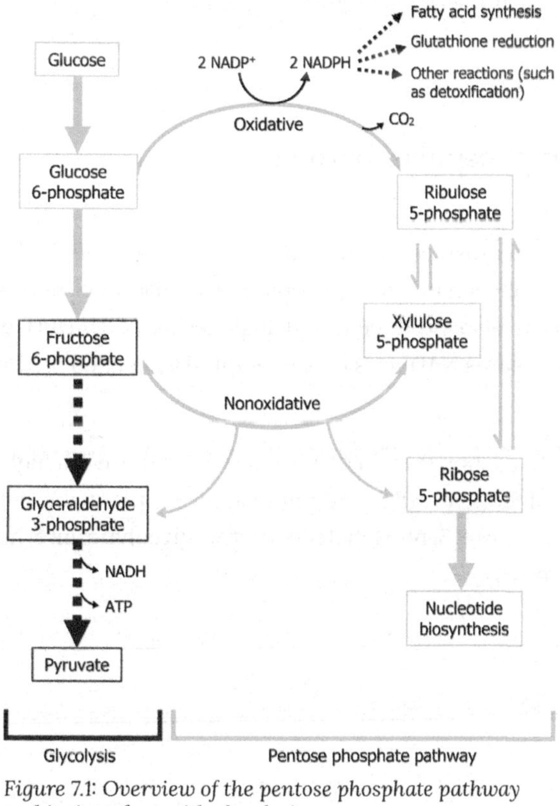

Figure 7.1: Overview of the pentose phosphate pathway and its interface with glycolysis.

Any compounds unused by the nonoxidative pathway will eventually be converted to fructose 6-phosphate or glyceraldehyde 3-phosphate, both of which will re-enter the glycolytic pathway (figures 7.1 and 7.2).

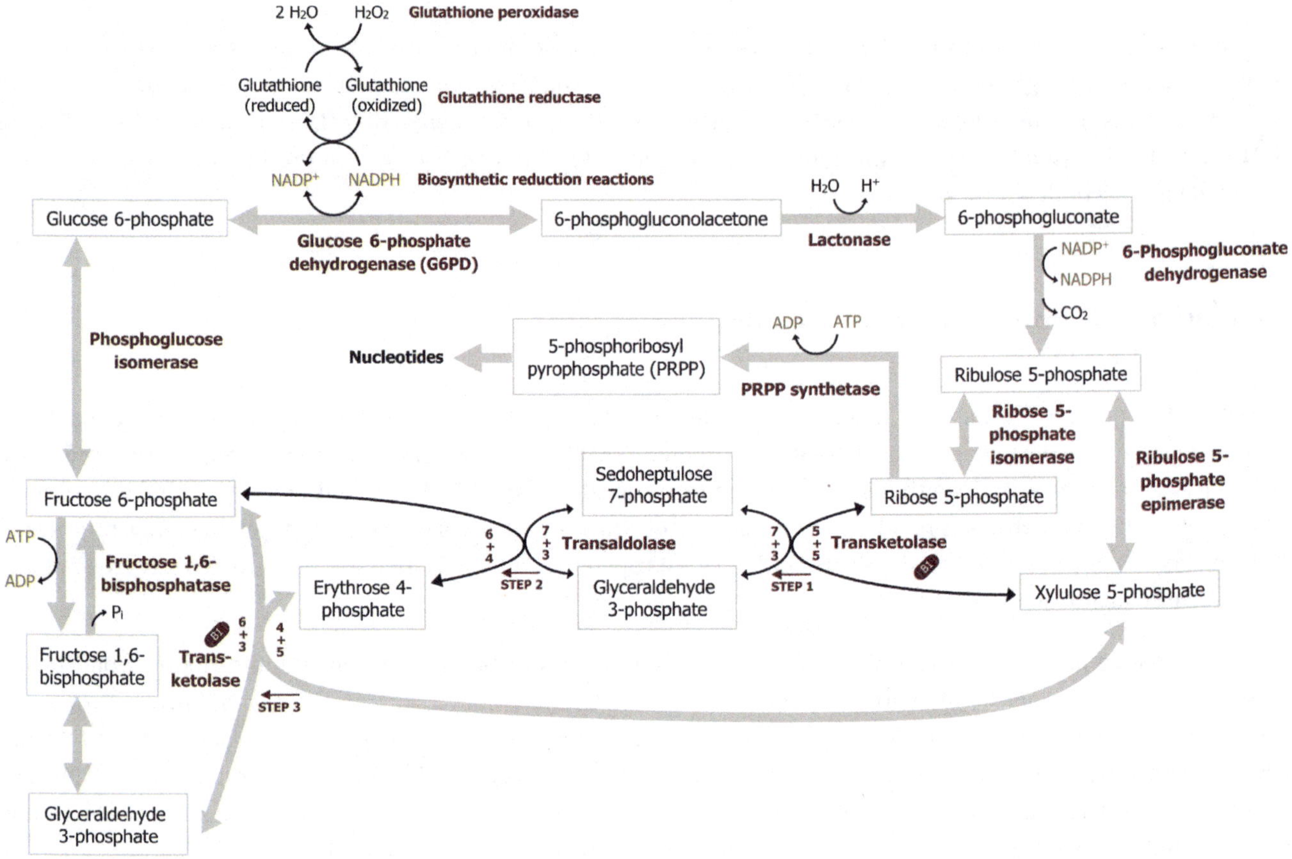

Figure 7.2: Pentose phosphate pathway and its connection to glycolysis and glutathione synthesis.

Regulation of the pentose phosphate pathway

The key regulatory enzyme for the pentose phosphate pathway is within the oxidative portion. Glucose 6-phosphate dehydrogenase oxidizes glucose 6-phosphate to 6-phosphogluconolactone, and is regulated by negative feedback. In this two-step reaction NADPH is also produced, and high levels of NADPH will inhibit the activity of glucose 6-phosphate dehydrogenase. This ensures NADPH is only generated as needed by the cell; this is the primary regulatory mechanism within the pathway.

The nonoxidative phase is not regulated; however, in conditions where there is a high demand for nucleotide production (such as in the case for highly proliferative cells), the nonoxidative part of the pathway can function independently of the oxidative phase to produce ribose 5-phosphate from the glycolytic intermediates fructose 6-phosphate and glyceraldehyde 3-phosphate (figure 7.2).

Requirement of the pentose phosphate pathway in RBCs

The two essential products of this pathway are NADPH and ribose 5-phosphate. NADPH is a high-energy compound often used for reductive biosynthesis as it cannot be oxidized in the ETC. It is also used by many tissues to scavenge (and detoxify) reactive oxygen species (ROS) before causing cellular damage. This is especially important in red blood cells; RBCs lack malic enzyme, making this the only pathway that can generate NADPH. A lack of NADPH in RBCs (such as due to a glucose 6-phosphate dehydrogenase deficiency) can cause excessive hemolysis, leading to the clinical presentation of jaundice (figure 7.3).

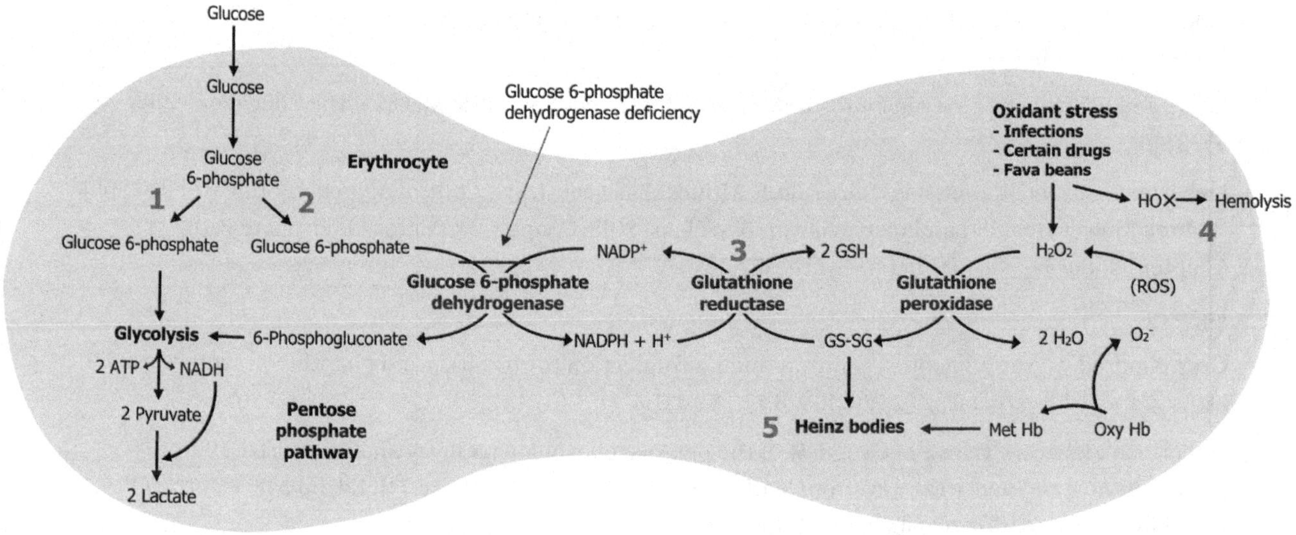

Figure 7.3: NADPH in the red blood cell as a means of reducing glutathione.

Glutathione (GSH) is a tripeptide compound consisting of glutamate, cysteine, and glycine. It plays a key role in scavenging reactive oxygen species (ROS), which cause both DNA and cellular/protein damage. Reduction of GSH in the red blood cell is done exclusively through a series of oxidation reduction reactions using NADPH. The loss of NADPH in RBCs therefore increases ROS and can lead to hemolysis (figure 7.3).

Summary of pathway regulation

Metabolic pathway	Major regulatory enzyme	Allosteric effectors	Hormonal effects
Pentose phosphate pathway	Glucose 6-phosphate dehydrogenase	NADPH (-)	None

Table 7.1: Summary of pathway regulation.

7.1 References and resources

Text

Ferrier, D. R., ed. *Lippincott Illustrated Reviews: Biochemistry*, 7th ed. Philadelphia: Wolters Kluwer Health/ Lippincott Williams & Wilkins, 2017, Chapter 13: Pentose Phosphate Pathway and NAPDH, Chapter 22: Nucleotide Metabolism.

Le, T., and V. Bhushan. *First Aid for the USMLE Step 1*, 29th ed. New York: McGraw Hill Education, 2018, 35–37, 79.

Lieberman, M., and A. Peet, eds. *Marks' Basic Medical Biochemistry: A Clinical Approach*, 5th ed. Philadelphia: Wolters Kluwer Health/Lippincott Williams & Wilkins, 2018, Chapter 27: Pentose Phosphate Pathway, Chapter 39: Purine and Pyrimidine Synthesis.

Figures

Grey, Kindred, Figure 7.2 Pentose pathway and its connection to glycolysis and glutathione synthesis. 2021. https://archive.org/details/7.2_20210926. CC BY 4.0.

Lieberman M, Peet A. Figure 7.1 Overview of the pentose phosphate pathway and its interface with glycolysis. Adapted under Fair Use from Marks' Basic Medical Biochemistry. 5th Ed. pp 543. Figure 27.1 Overview of the pentose phosphate pathway. 2017.

Lieberman M, Peet A. Figure 7.3 NADPH in the red blood cell as a means of reducing glutathione. Adapted under Fair Use from Marks' Basic Medical Biochemistry. 5th Ed. pp 549. Figure 27.7 Hemolysis caused by reactive oxygen species (ROS). 2017.

7.2 Nucleotide Synthesis

Nucleotides are the fundamental building blocks essential for the synthesis of DNA and RNA. Each nucleotide contains three functional groups: a sugar, a base, and phosphate (figure 7.4).

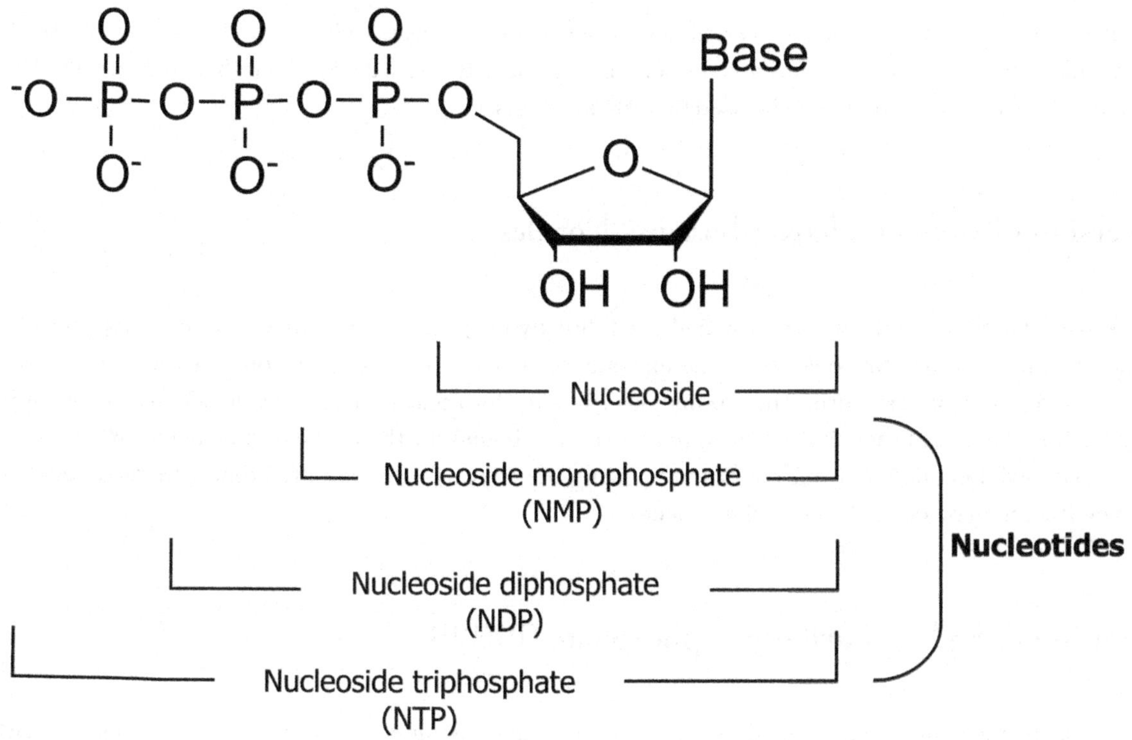

Figure 7.4: Basic structure of nucleotides.

Nucleotides can be divided into two groups: pyrimidines and purines. The family of pyrimidines includes thymine (T), cytosine (C), and uracil (U), which is only incorporated into RNA. These compounds contain a single-ringed nitrogenous base that pairs with a purine nucleotide counterpart. Thymine pairs with adenine forming two hydrogen bonds, in contrast to cytosine, which pairs with guanine to form three hydrogen bonds. Purines, both guanine (G) and adenine (A), are double-ringed structures and more difficult to break down in the body. As such, the salvage pathway for purine metabolism is of importance (figure 7.5).

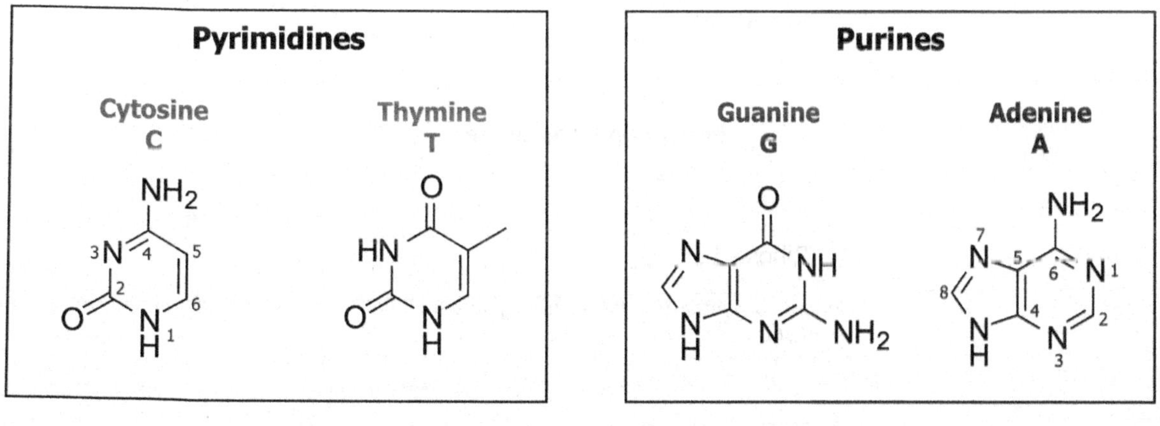

Figure 7.5: Overview of purine and pyrimidine bases.

Nucleotide synthesis will be described below, but one of the fundamental requirements of the synthesis of either purines or pyrimidines is the need for a five-carbon sugar (ribose). This sugar is generated through glucose oxidation via the pentose phosphate pathway.

For purines synthesis, the base is synthesized and attached to the sugar, while for pyrimidine synthesis, the sugar group is added after the base is produced. In either case, ribose is the added sugar, and this must be converted to the deoxyribose form before the bases can be used for DNA synthesis.

Conversion of ribose to deoxyribose nucleotides

All bases are synthesized in the ribose form and used directly for transcription. They can be converted to the deoxy form, which is needed for DNA replication. The enzyme, ribonucleotide reductase, converts the diphosphate form of a ribose base to the deoxybase form. The enzyme has two sites for regulation: an enzyme activity site and a substrate specificity site. The enzyme activity site must have ATP/ADP bound for the enzyme to be active, while the substrate specificity site will bind different nucleotides influencing the enzyme substrate preference, therefore altering which base is being acted upon depending on cellular needs.

Generation of 5-phosphoribosyl-1-phosphate (PRPP)

Ribose 5-phosphate is not used directly for either purine or pyrimidine synthesis, rather it is used to synthesize the "active pentose" – 5-phosphoribosyl-1-pyrophosphate (PRPP). The conversion is catalyzed by the enzyme phosphoribosyl-1-pyrophosphate (PRPP) synthase. PRPP is the activated five-carbon sugar used for nucleotide synthesis and provides both the sugar and phosphate group to nucleotides (figure 7.6).

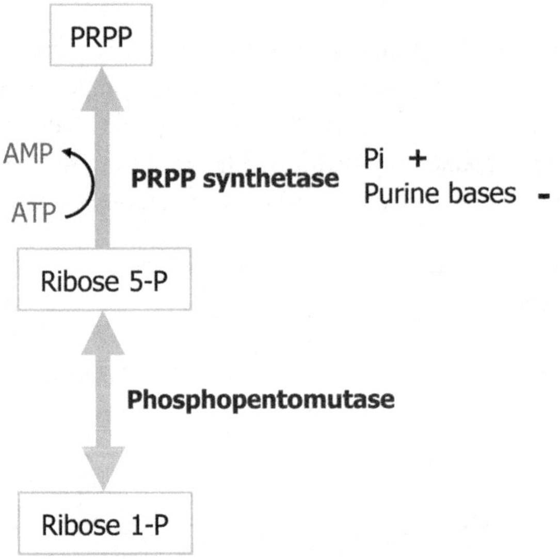

Figure 7.6: Synthesis of PRPP and regulation of PRPP synthetase.

Regulation of PRPP synthase

The enzyme, PRPP synthetase, is activated by Pi (inorganic phosphate) and inhibited by the purine bases adenine and guanine.

Synthesis of purines

Purines are composed of a bicyclic structure that is synthesized from carbon and nitrogen donated from various compounds such as carbon dioxide, glycine, glutamine, aspartate, and tetrahydrofolate (TH_4). The synthesis of purines starts with the synthesis of 5'phosphoribosylamine from PRPP and glutamine. The enzyme glutamine phosphoribosylpyrophate amidotransferase (GPAT) catalyzes this reaction and is the committed step in purine synthesis (figure 7.7). Synthesis continues for nine additional steps culminating in the synthesis of inosine monophosphate (IMP), which contains the base hypoxanthine. IMP is used to generate both AMP and GMP. The synthesis of both AMP and GMP requires energy in the form of the alternative base (i.e., the synthesis of GMP requires ATP while AMP synthesis requires energy in the form of GTP). The synthesis of AMP and GMP is regulated by feedback inhibition (figures 7.7 and 7.8). This allows for the maintenance of nucleotides in a relative ratio that is required for cellular processes. The generated nucleotide monophosphates can be converted to the di and triphosphate forms by nucleotide specific kinases, which will transfer phosphate groups to maintain a balance of the mono, di, and triphosphate forms.

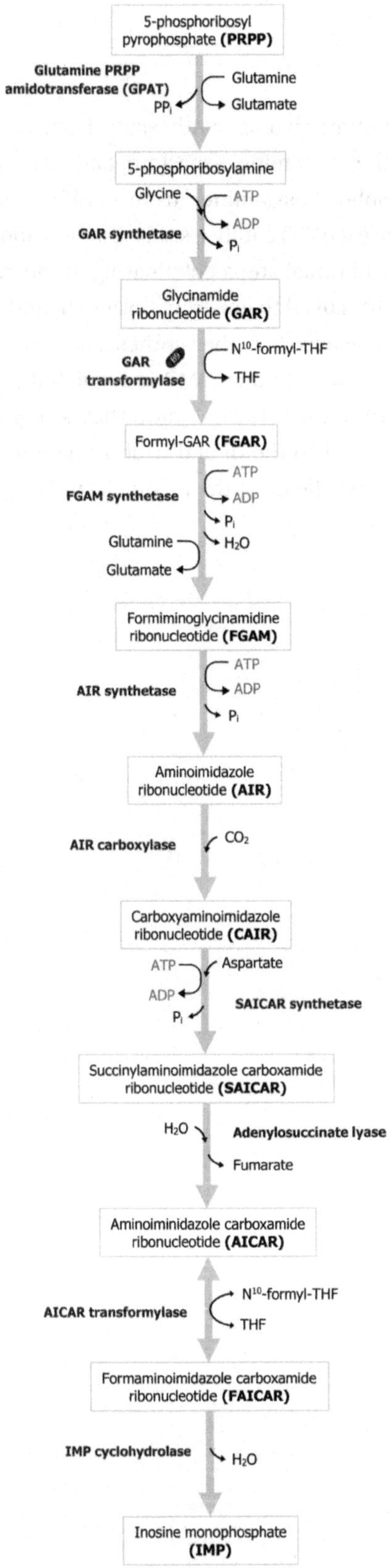

Figure 7.7: Overview of purine synthesis. The reaction catalyzed by GPAT is the regulatory enzyme of the pathway.

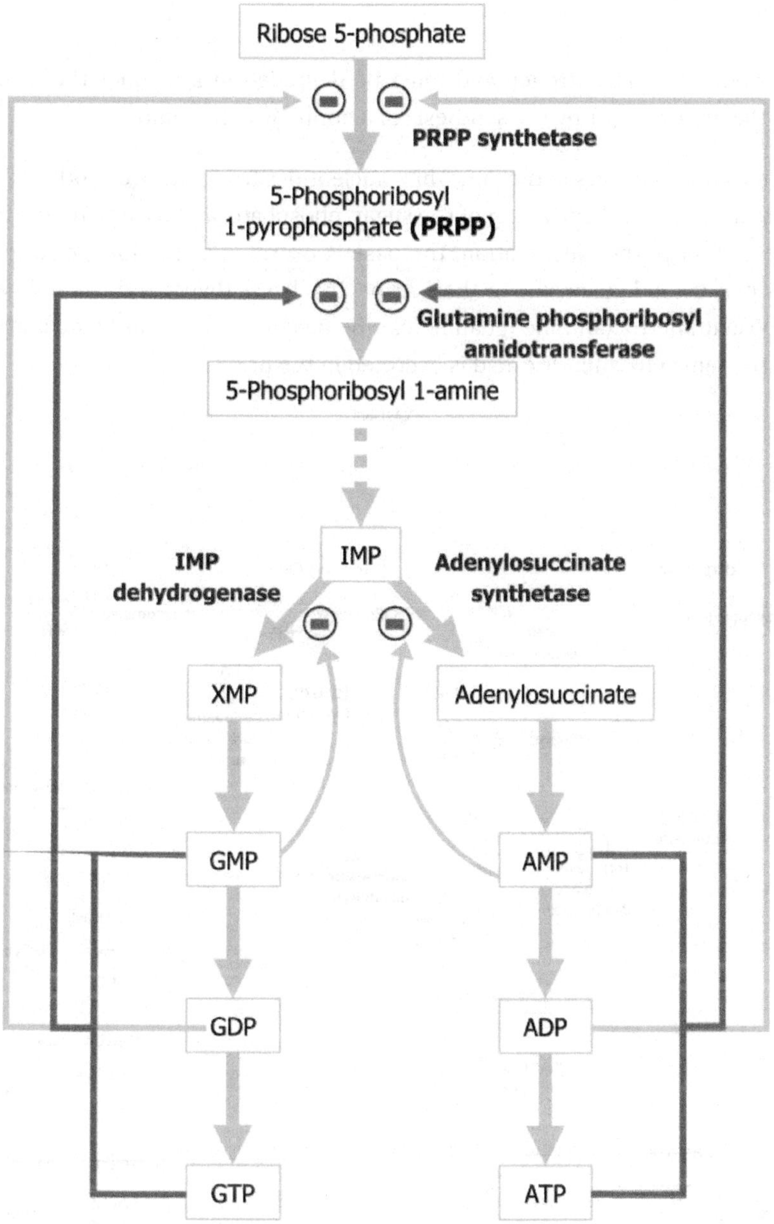

Figure 7.8: Purine synthesis and regulation of glutamine: phosphoribosylpyrophosphate amidotransferase.

Regulation of purine synthesis

The regulatory enzyme GPAT is allosterically activated by PRPP and inhibited by IMP, AMP, and GMP. All three must be present to inhibit activity of this enzyme.

Degradation of purines

Like amino acids, nucleotides contain nitrogen and must be degraded in a manner that allows for proper nitrogen disposal either through the urea cycle or by the synthesis of a nontoxic compound.

Degradation of dietary nucleotides occurs in the gut, while nucleotides from de novo synthesis are degraded in the liver. The fundamental process involves the dismantling of the sugar, phosphate, and base structure into their own respective units (figure 7.9). In the case of purine degradation, the base is excreted in the form of uric acid. Purine nucleoside phosphorylase converts inosine and guanosine to their respective bases (hypoxanthine and guanine). Finally, xanthine oxidase will oxidize hypoxanthine to xanthine (guanine can be deaminated to xanthine), and xanthine can be further oxidized to uric acid by the same enzyme. Uric acid is excreted in the urine.

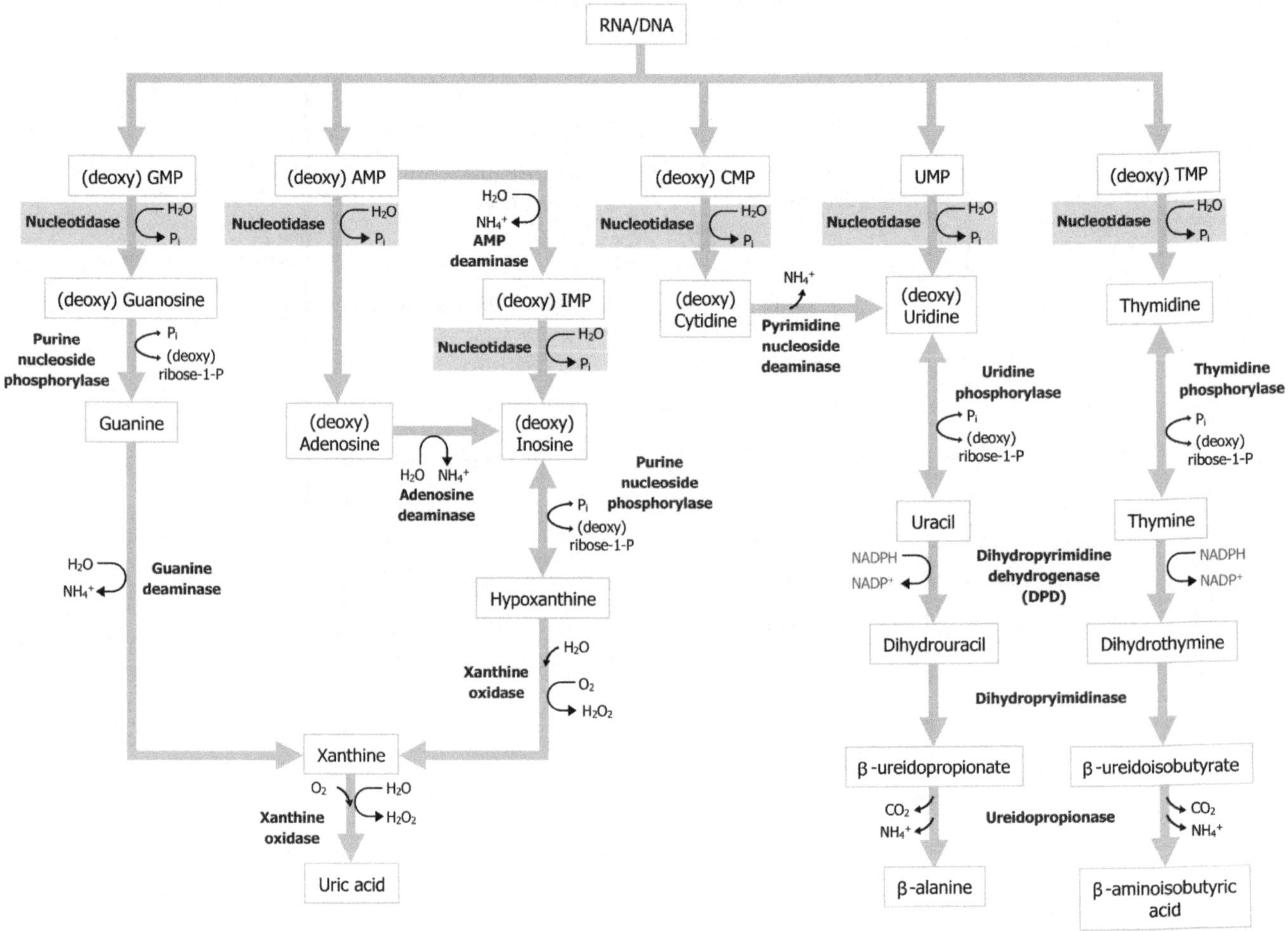

Figure 7.9: Breakdown of nucleotides.

Excess uric acid, hyperuricemia, can cause the precipitation of uric acid crystals in the joints eliciting an inflammatory reaction causing acute pain or gout. The majority of individuals diagnosed with gout present due to underexcretion of uric acid. And this can be caused by the presence of other pathologies, such as lactic acidosis or the use of diuretics. Less common presentations of gout are associated with overproduction of uric acid, which can be caused by increased activity of PRPP synthetase or deficiency in purine recycling enzyme HGPRT caused by Lesch-Nyhan syndrome (figure 7.10).

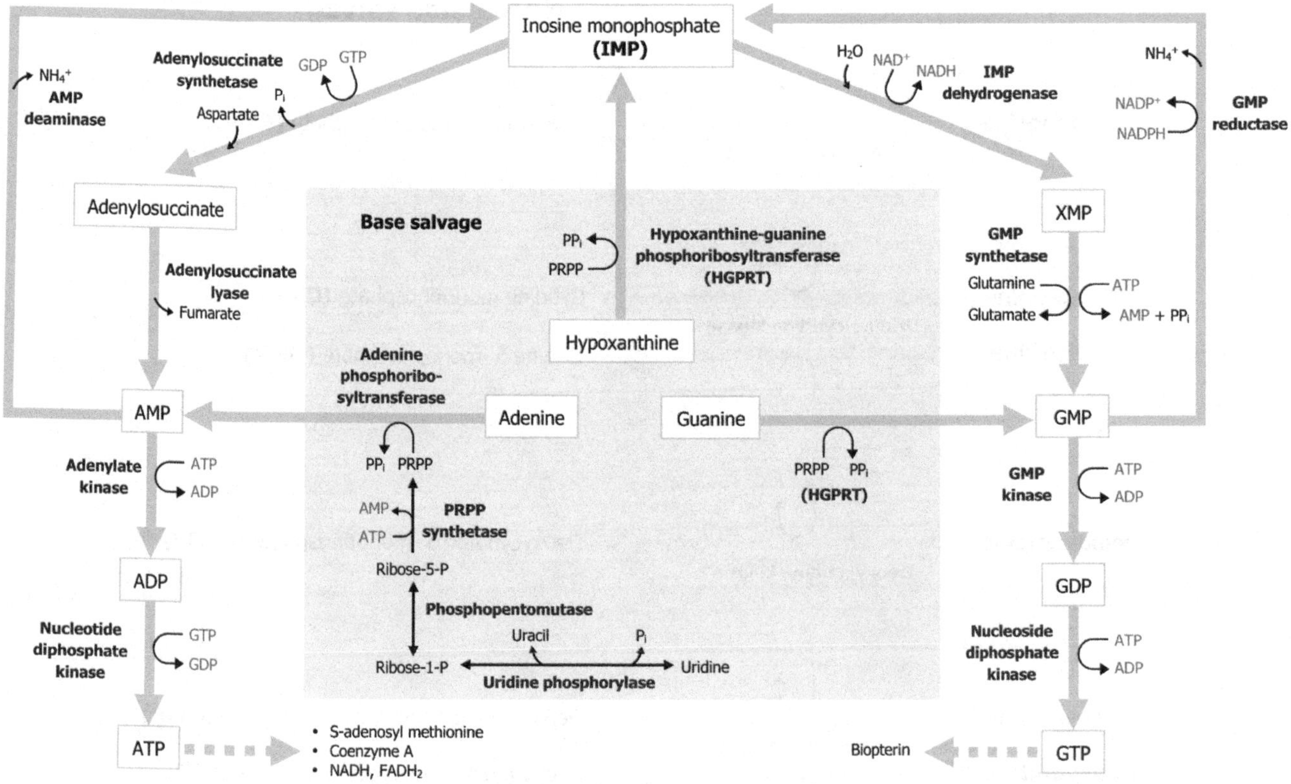

Figure 7.10: Nucleotide base salvage. Reaction catalyzed by HGPRT is clinically relevant as deficiencies can cause accumulation of uric acid.

Secondary hyperuricemia is also seen in individuals with myeloproliferative disorders undergoing therapy where there is excess cellular turnover (cell lysis leads to an accumulation of nucleotides) or in cases of Von Gierke disease or fructose intolerance, which increases substrate for PRPP synthesis. Xanthine oxidase inhibitors, such as allopurinol, are used as part of the management of gout.

Salvage of purines

The ability to recycle nucleotides is specifically important in the case of purines as de novo synthesis uses much more ATP than salvage. The degradation product of purine bases is uric acid, which is an insoluble compound, and accumulation can result in several clinical disorders as previously discussed. As such, purine bases can also undergo salvage reaction where bases are recycled and used in a new process. To reduce the amount of uric acid production, purines can be salvaged and reconverted back to their triphosphate form to be reused. There are two primary enzymes involved in the salvage pathway: adenine phosphoribosyltransferase (APRT) and xanthine-guanine phosphoribosyltransferase (HGPRT) (figure 7.10). These enzymes will recombine the base (either adenine, guanine, or hypoxanthine) with PRPP to generate AMP, GMP, or IMP respectively. Adenosine is the only nucleoside that can be rephosphorylated to its monosphosphate form using adenosine kinase (figure 7.11). All other nucleosides must be degraded to their free base before they can be salvaged.

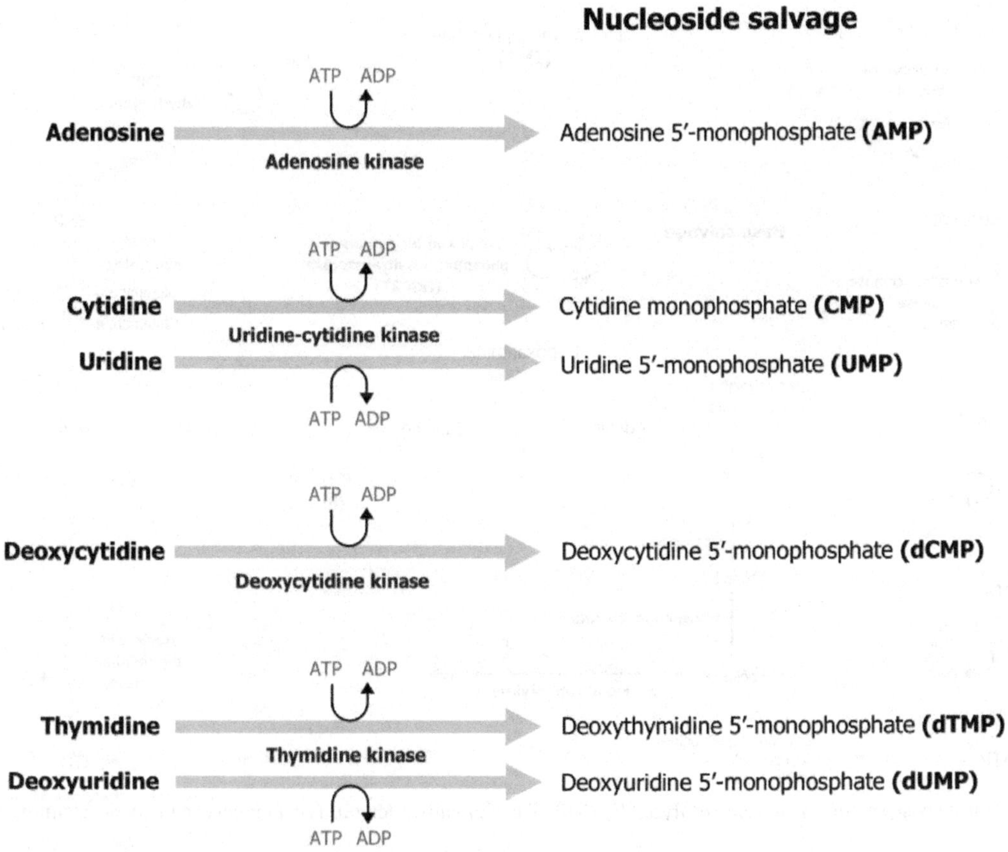

Figure 7.11: Nucleotide specific pathways for base salvage.

Synthesis of pyrimidines

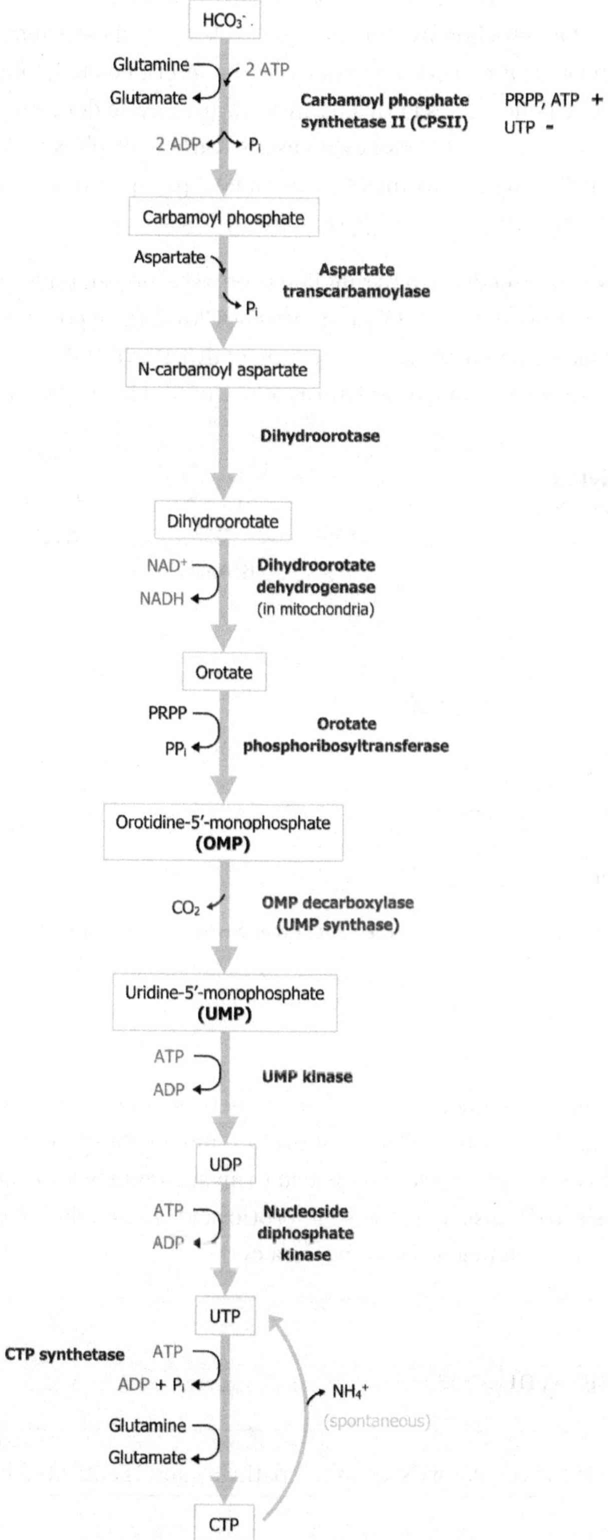

Figure 7.12: Overview of pyrimidine synthesis. The reaction catalyzed by carbamoyl phosphate synthetase I is the regulatory enzyme of the pathway.

In contrast to purine synthesis, the pyrimidine bases are synthesized before the ribose sugar and phosphate groups are added in the form of PRPP (figure 7.12). The initial step of the pathways involves the synthesis of carbamoyl phosphate from glutamine, carbon dioxide, and 2 ATP. Carbamoyl phosphate synthetase II (CSPII) catalyzes this reaction. (Note there is an analogous enzyme in the mitochondria for the urea cycle termed carbamoyl phosphate synthetase I, which also generates carbamoyl phosphate.) Of clinical importance is the intermediate orotate. Elevations of orotate (orotic acid) are consistent with enzymatic deficiencies in this pathway or urea cycle deficiencies such as a defect in ornithine transcarbamoylase. In the case of a urea cycle deficiency, an excess carbamoyl phosphate can enter pyrimidine synthesis leading to a build up of orotate. Following the synthesis of carbamoyl phosphate, a series of subsequent reactions yield uracil monosphosphate, which is the intermediate of pyrimidine synthesis.

UMP, much like IMP, serves as the intermediate to pyrimidine synthesis and can undergo sequential phosphorylation to form UTP, which can be converted to cytidine (CTP). Alternatively, UMP can be converted to a deoxy form (dUDP) to be used as substrate for the synthesis of thymidine. The conversion of dUDP to dTMP is catalyzed by thymidylate synthase, which requires folate (N5,N10 methylene tetrahydrofolate) as a methyl and hydrogen donor to complete this conversion (figure 7.13).

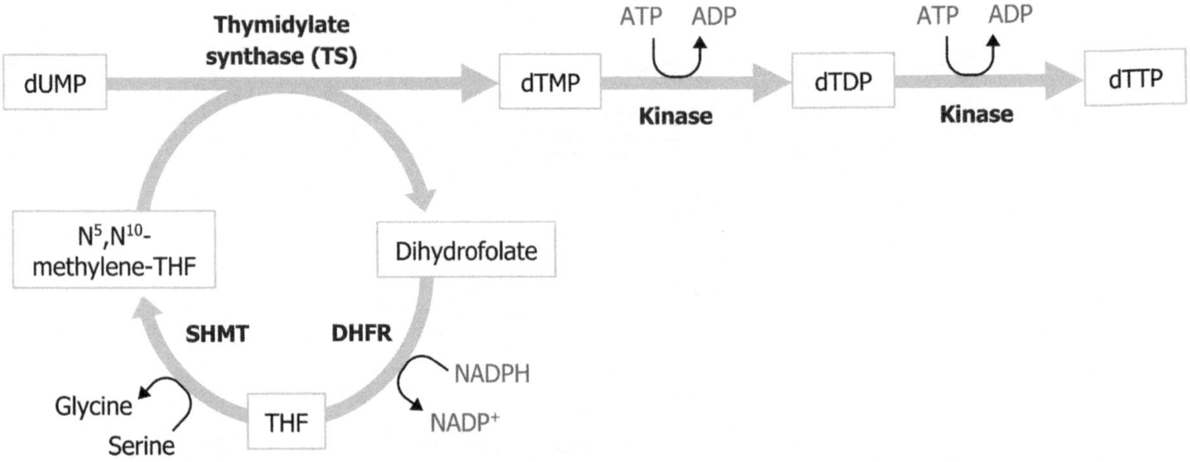

Figure 7.13: Interaction of thymidylate synthesis with the folate cycle. SHMT: serine hydroxymethyltransferase; DHFR: dihydrofolate reductase.

Defects in pyrimidine synthesis most commonly present as an increase in orotic acid in the urine. Deficiencies in the attachment of PRPP to orotate (or the decarboxylation of orotate monosphosphate) can result in the accumulation of orotic acid; similarly deficiencies of the urea cycle, which lead to an accumulation of carbamoyl phosphate, can increase flux through pyrimidine synthesis and cause an increase in orotic acid. Accumulation of orotic acid is used as a clinical indicator of pyrimidine deficiencies or deficiencies in the urea cycle.

Regulation of pyrimidine synthesis

The reaction catalyzed by CSPII is the regulatory step in the pathway and is activated by PRPP and ATP and inhibited by UTP.

Clinical importance of folate cycle inhibitors and synthesis of dTMP

Synthesis of dTMP for DNA synthesis is the rate-limiting step for the replication process, and therefore disruption of this conversion is very effective at reducing cellular proliferation. Inhibition of thymidylate synthase by 5-fluorouracil (5-FU) is a common anticancer treatment. 5-FU functions as a thymine analog and will irreversibly bind the enzyme. Similarly, methotrexate is an inhibitor of dihyrofolate reductase (DHFR), which is part of the folate cycle needed to reduce dihydrofolate to tetrahydrofolate. Inhibition of this process reduces substrate needed for the thymidylate synthase reaction and has a similar effect as inhibition of by 5-FU (figure 7.13).

Summary of pathway regulation

Metabolic pathway	Major regulatory enzyme	Allosteric effectors	Hormonal effects
Pyrimidine synthesis	CPSII	PRPP, ATP (+), UTP (-)	None
Purine synthesis	PRPP synthetase	Pi (+), Purine bases (-)	Note: PRPP synthetase is required for both purine and pyrimidine synthesis
Purine synthesis	GPAT	PRPP (+), IMP, AMP, GMP (-)	Note: PRPP synthetase is required for both purine and pyrimidine synthesis

Table 7.2: Summary of pathway regulation.

7.2 References and resources

Text

Ferrier, D. R., ed. *Lippincott Illustrated Reviews: Biochemistry*, 7th ed. Philadelphia: Wolters Kluwer Health/ Lippincott Williams & Wilkins, 2017, Chapter 13: Pentose Phosphate Pathway and NAPDH, Chapter 22: Nucleotide Metabolism.

Le, T., and V. Bhushan. *First Aid for the USMLE Step 1*, 29th ed. New York: McGraw Hill Education, 2018, 35–37, 79.

Lieberman, M., and A. Peet, eds. *Marks' Basic Medical Biochemistry: A Clinical Approach*, 5th ed. Philadelphia: Wolters Kluwer Health/Lippincott Williams & Wilkins, 2018, Chapter 27: Pentose Phosphate Pathway, Chapter 39: Purine and Pyrimidine Synthesis.

Figures

Grey, Kindred, Figure 7.5 Overview of purine and pyrimidine bases. 2021. Chemical structure by Henry Jakubowski. https://archive.org/details/7.5_20210926. CC BY 4.0.

Grey, Kindred, Figure 7.6 Synthesis of PRPP and regulation of PRPP synthetase. 2021. https://archive.org/details/7.6_20210926. CC BY 4.0.

Grey, Kindred, Figure 7.7 Overview of purine synthesis. The reaction catalyzed by GPAT is the regulatory enzyme of the pathway. 2021. https://archive.org/details/7.7_20210926. CC BY 4.0.

Grey, Kindred, Figure 7.8 Purine synthesis and regulation of glutamine:phosphoribosylpyrophosphate amidotransferase. 2021. https://archive.org/details/7.8_20210926. CC BY 4.0.

Grey, Kindred, Figure 7.9 Breakdown of nucleotides. 2021. https://archive.org/details/7.9_20210926. CC BY 4.0.

Grey, Kindred, Figure 7.10 Nucleotide base salvage. Reaction catalyzed by HGPRT is clinically relevant as deficiencies can cause accumulation of uric acid. 2021. https://archive.org/details/7.10_20210926. CC BY 4.0.

Grey, Kindred, Figure 7.11 Nucleotide specific pathways for base salvage. 2021. https://archive.org/details/7.11_20210926. CC BY 4.0.

Grey, Kindred, Figure 7.12 Overview of pyrimidine synthesis. The reaction catalyzed by carbamoyl phosphate synthetase I is the regulatory enzyme of the pathway. 2021. https://archive.org/details/7.12_20210926. CC BY 4.0.

Grey, Kindred, Figure 7.13 Interaction of thymidylate synthesis with the folate cycle. SHMT: Serine hydroxymethyltransferase; DHFR: Dihydrofolate reductase. 2021. https://archive.org/details/7.13_20210926. CC BY 4.0.

Lieberman M, Peet A. Figure 7.4 Basic structure of nucleotides. Adapted under Fair Use from Marks' Basic Medical Biochemistry. 5th Ed. pp 216. Figure 12.3 Nucleoside and nucleotide structures displayed with ribose as the sugar. 2017. Chemical structure by Henry Jakubowski.

8. Amino Acid Metabolism and Heritable Disorders of Degradation

Learning Objectives

- Define essential, conditionally essential, and nonessential amino acids, and explain how certain nonessential amino acids become essential in certain conditions.
- Integrate amino acid synthesis with specific precursors from glycolysis, citric acid cycle, and the pentose phosphate pathway.
- Identify key roles of amino acids as substrates for the synthesis of specialized products including heme, GABA, carnitine, glutathione, serotonin, histamine, ubiquinone, melanin, creatine, and dopamine.
- Review the role of transamination in the interconversion of amino acids and connection to the urea cycle; see section 5.3.
- Distinguish the following disease states associated with inborn errors of metabolism, including (A) deficient enzyme, (B) inheritance pattern of the disease, and (C) relation of the deficiency to the buildup of secondary metabolites.
- The following is a list of diseases to focus on:
    - Phenylketonuria (phenylalanine metabolism),
    - Homocystinuria (methionine metabolism),
    - Maple syrup urine disease (metabolism of branched-chain amino acids), and
    - Alkaptouria (tyrosine metabolism).

About this Chapter

There are twenty amino acids required for metabolic homeostasis. Of the twenty amino acids, eleven are considered nonessential, meaning they can be synthesized by the body. With the exceptions of tyrosine and cysteine, the others can be synthesized from glucose and a nitrogen donor. The other nine amino acids are essential and must be supplied by the diet. As mentioned previously, in addition to supplying carbon for gluconeogenesis, amino acids play important roles in the synthesis of essential cellular components. Disruptions of many of these pathways can lead to clinical disorders, many of which are identified during newborn screenings. The synthesis of all amino acids will not be addressed in this section; rather the most clinically relevant pathways will be focused on.

8.1 Amino Acid Metabolism and Specialized Products

Cofactors essential for amino acid metabolism

The metabolism of many amino acids largely relies on the availability of the cofactors pyridoxal phosphate (vitamin B_6 or PLP), tetrahydrobiopterin (BH_4), and tetrahydrofolate (TH_4). It is important to recognize that deficiencies in these cofactors could present in a similar manner as enzymatic deficiencies of specific pathways. Refer to chapter 2 for more information regarding vitamin B_6 and folate.

Pyridoxal phosphate (B_6 or PLP)

All transamination reactions require PLP as a cofactor. These reactions are essential for moving (or donating) a nitrogen from an amino acid to a keto-acid to generate a different amino acid.

Tetrahydrobiopterin (BH_4)

This is a cofactor synthesized from GTP. It is oxidized during hydroxylation reactions, most notably the conversion of phenylalanine to tyrosine. Enzymatic deficiencies leading to decreased synthesis of BH_4 can present similar to deficiencies in phenylalanine metabolism.

Tetrahydrofolate (FH_4)

Folate can exist in many forms and is often referred to as tetrahydrofolate. FH_4 is often found in various forms with a one-carbon group attached. These one-carbon groups, which make up the one-carbon pool, can be oxidized or reduced. One-carbon groups can be transferred to other compounds and play essential roles in the synthesis of glycine from serine, the synthesis of the base thymine (required for DNA synthesis), the purine bases required for both DNA and RNA synthesis, and the transfer of methyl groups to vitamin B_{12}.

Synthesis of specialized products

The following highlights some of the key aspects of amino acid metabolism.

Phenylalanine and tyrosine

Phenylalanine is an essential amino acid, and hydroxylation of Phe by phenylalanine hydroxylase (PAH) generates tyrosine (figure 8.1). This conversion requires BH_4, and deficiencies in either the cofactor or the enzyme PAH can result in phenylketonuria. Additionally, the inability to synthesize tyrosine will make this a conditionally essential amino acid and potentially negatively impact the synthesis of downstream compounds illustrated in figure 8.1.

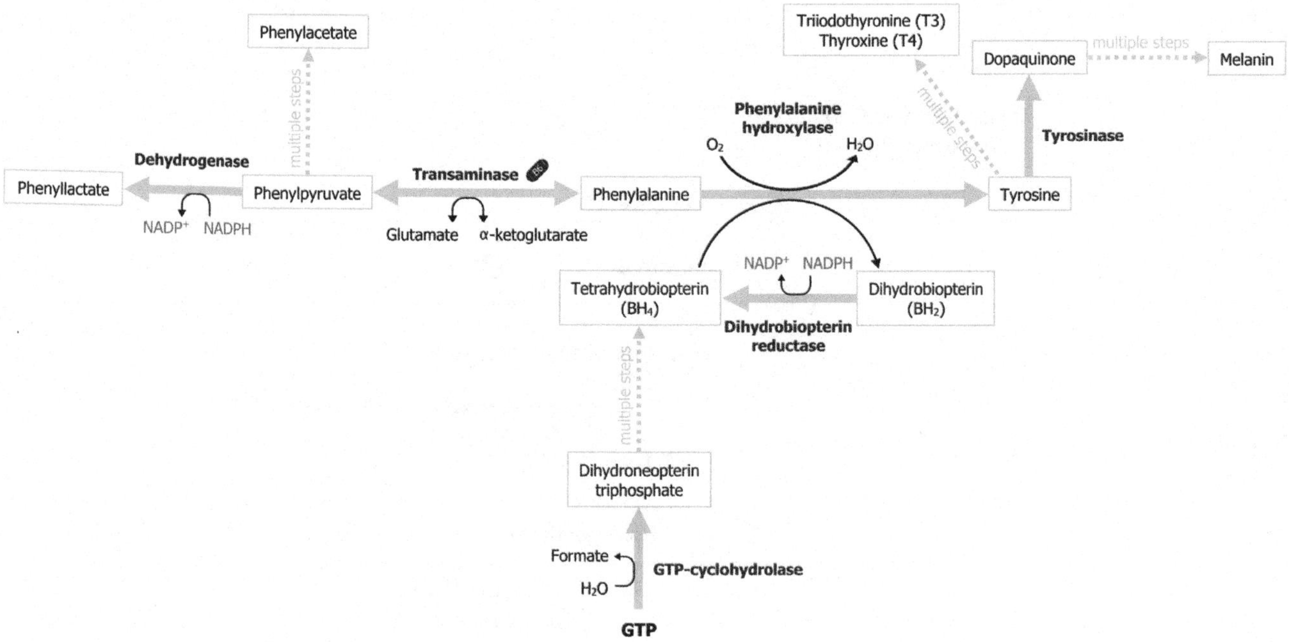

Figure 8.1: Metabolism of phenylalanine requires BH4 and also produces tyrosine. Deficiencies in cofactor or phenylalanine hydroxylase can result in phenylketonuria.

Tyrosine can be produced from phenylalanine metabolism and is required for the production of melanin and the catecholamines. Deficiencies can occur at several different locations in the pathway and result in albinism (tyrosinase), alkaptonuria (homogentisate oxidase), or tyrosinemia, which can manifest due to deficiencies in several enzymes along the pathway (figure 8.2).

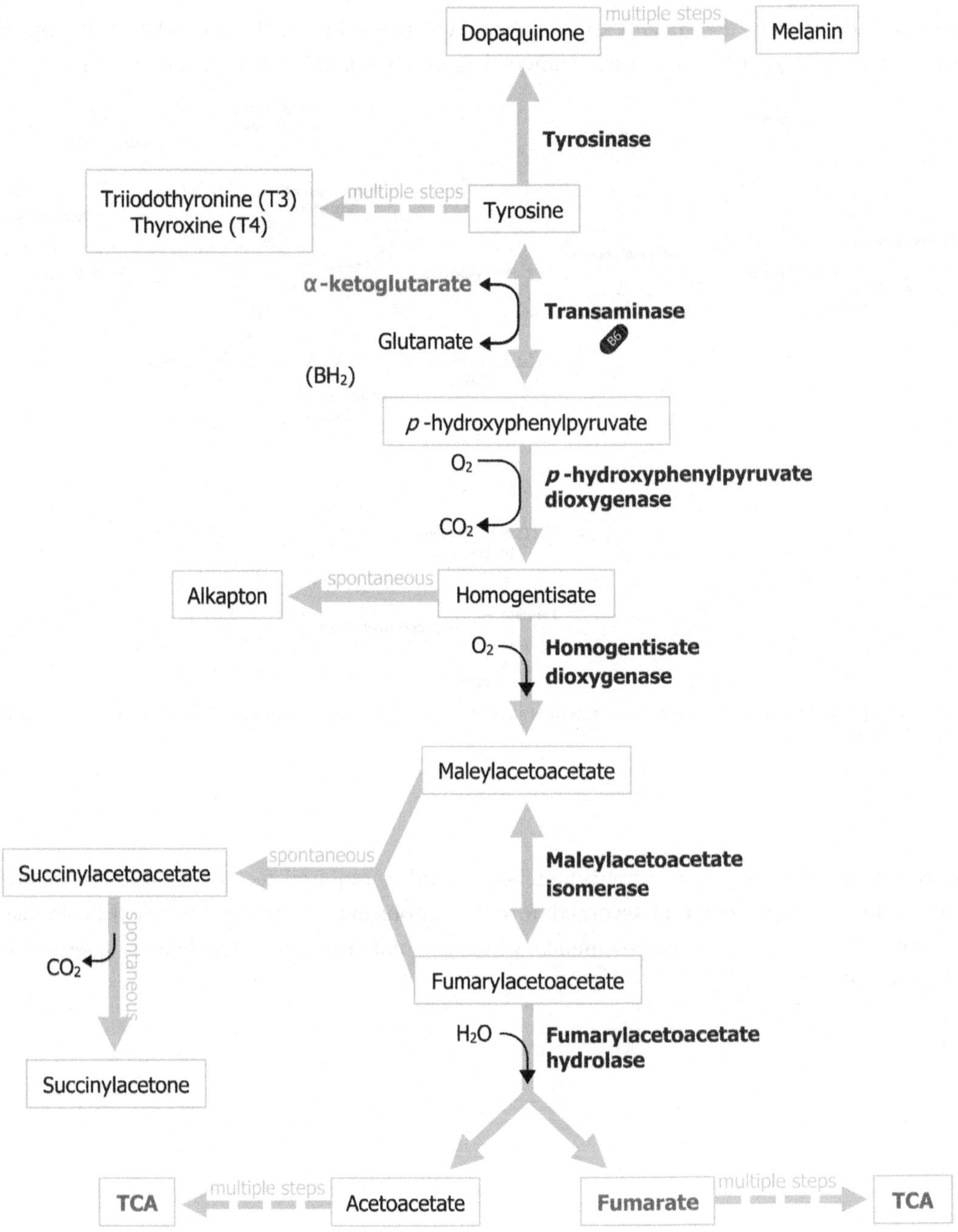

Figure 8.2: Tyrosine can be produced from phenylalanine metabolism and is required for the production of melanin and the catecholamines. Deficiencies can occur at several different locations in the pathway and result in albinism, alkaptonuria, or tyrosinemia.

Phenylketonuria

Phenylketonuria (PKU) is one of the more common amino acid metabolic disorders and is inherited in an autosomal recessive fashion. There are no symptoms of untreated phenylketonuria in the first months of life, therefore newborn screening is essential for diagnosis and initiation of treatment, which prevents the devastating effects of infantile hyperphenylalaninemia. The screening method detects elevated titers of the amino acid phenylalanine (Phe) in the blood. A positive test result (Phe greater than 150 μmol/L) prompts the physician to begin a phenylalaninerestricted formula and requires a confirmatory quantitative Phe level.

Glycine

Glycine is a key compound that functions as an essential substrate for various pathways including the folate cycle, nucleotide synthesis, and synthesis of porphyrins (heme), glutathione, and creatine. Glycine can be synthesized at the cellular level from 3-phosphoglycerate, an intermediate of glycolysis.

Arginine

Arginine is a nonessential amino acid as it can be produced in the urea cycle. Deficiencies in the urea cycle can cause arginine to become conditionally essential. In these cases, management and supplementation are needed.

Tryptophan

Tryptophan is an essential amino acid that is both ketogenic and glucogenic as it can be oxidized to produce alanine and acetyl-CoA. The ring structure can also be used to synthesize niacin, reducing the dietary requirement for this vitamin. Tryptophan metabolism to serotonin (and subsequently melatonin) requires BH_4. Deficiencies here can lead to imbalances in these neurotransmitters (figure 8.3).

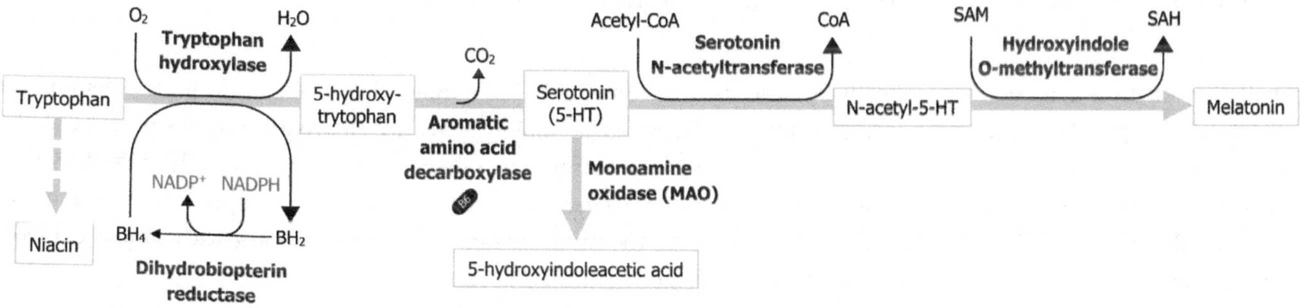

Figure 8.3: Metabolism of tryptophan to melatonin.

Glutamate

Glutamate plays many key roles in amino acid metabolism and provides substrates for GABA and glutathione synthesis (figure 8.4). Additionally, glutamate plays a key role in nitrogen movement within the body. Glutamate can be deaminated by glutamate dehydrogenase to yield α-ketoglutarate. This can enter directly into the TCA cycle or be transaminated (figure 8.4). Additionally, glutamate can be used to fix or free ammonium to generate glutamine – one of the essential, nontoxic carriers of ammonia.

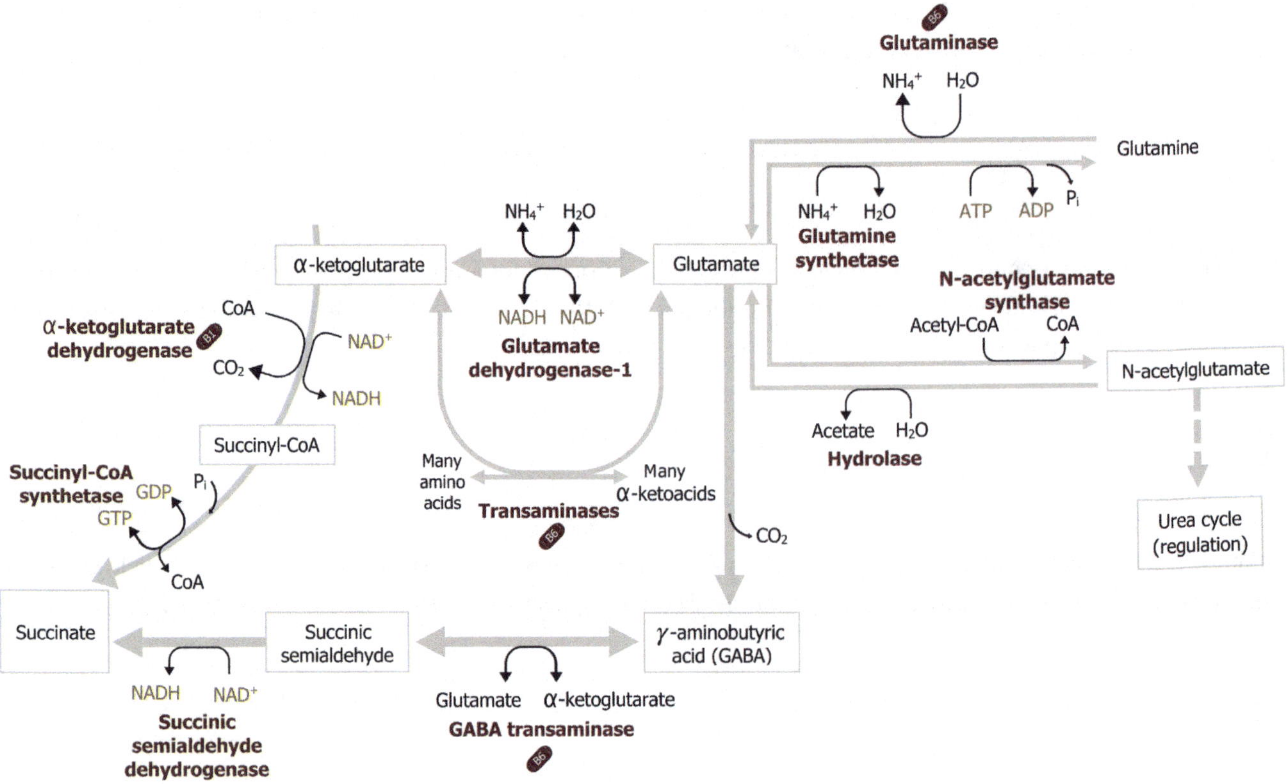

Figure 8.4: Glutamate metabolism as it interfaces with nitrogen transport and synthesis of GABA.

Isoleucine, leucine, and valine (branched-chain amino acids)

Oxidation of these amino acids, collectively described as branched-chain amino acids, occurs in all tissues (except the liver) and is a key fuel source for skeletal muscle. As these amino acids are approximately 25 percent of the amino acid pool, they provide both energy and available substrate to replenish the TCA cycle. The initial step in their metabolism, like all amino acids, is the transamination to generate a keto-acid. These compounds then undergo oxidative decarboxylation by a multiunit enzyme similar to the pyruvate dehydrogenase complex with similar cofactor requirements (section 4.1), and the remaining carbons can enter the TCA cycle.

Maple syrup urine disease

Deficiencies in metabolism of branched-chain amino acids can result in the diagnosis of maple syrup urine disease (MSUD). With an incidence of 1 in 100,000, MSUD is rare even among the inborn errors of metabolism. However, the distinct sweet odor, similar to that of maple syrup, distinguishes this condition as one of the more recognizable metabolic disorders. It is caused by deficient oxidative decarboxylation of α-keto-acid metabolites of leucine, isoleucine, and valine. Affected infants can become symptomatic during the first days of life, with poor feeding, lethargy, seizures, and occasionally coma. Milder forms of MSUD may present later in life, with developmental delays and intellectual disability. Maple syrup urine disease is primarily treated by diet but also by avoiding circumstances that increase catabolism such as high fever and dehydration. If a metabolic crisis occurs, emergency treatment in a hospital is necessary to stabilize the patient.

Methionine

Methionine is an essential amino acid with a complex metabolism of clinical importance. Its metabolism interfaces with the folate cycle, cobalamin remethylation, and the synthesis of S-adenosylmethionine (SAM). Enzymatic or cofactor deficiencies can result in elevated homocysteine levels (hyperhomocysteinemia), which can have negative impacts systemically. Methionine, required for the synthesis of SAM, can be obtained from the diet or produced from remethylation of homocysteine using vitamin B_{12}.

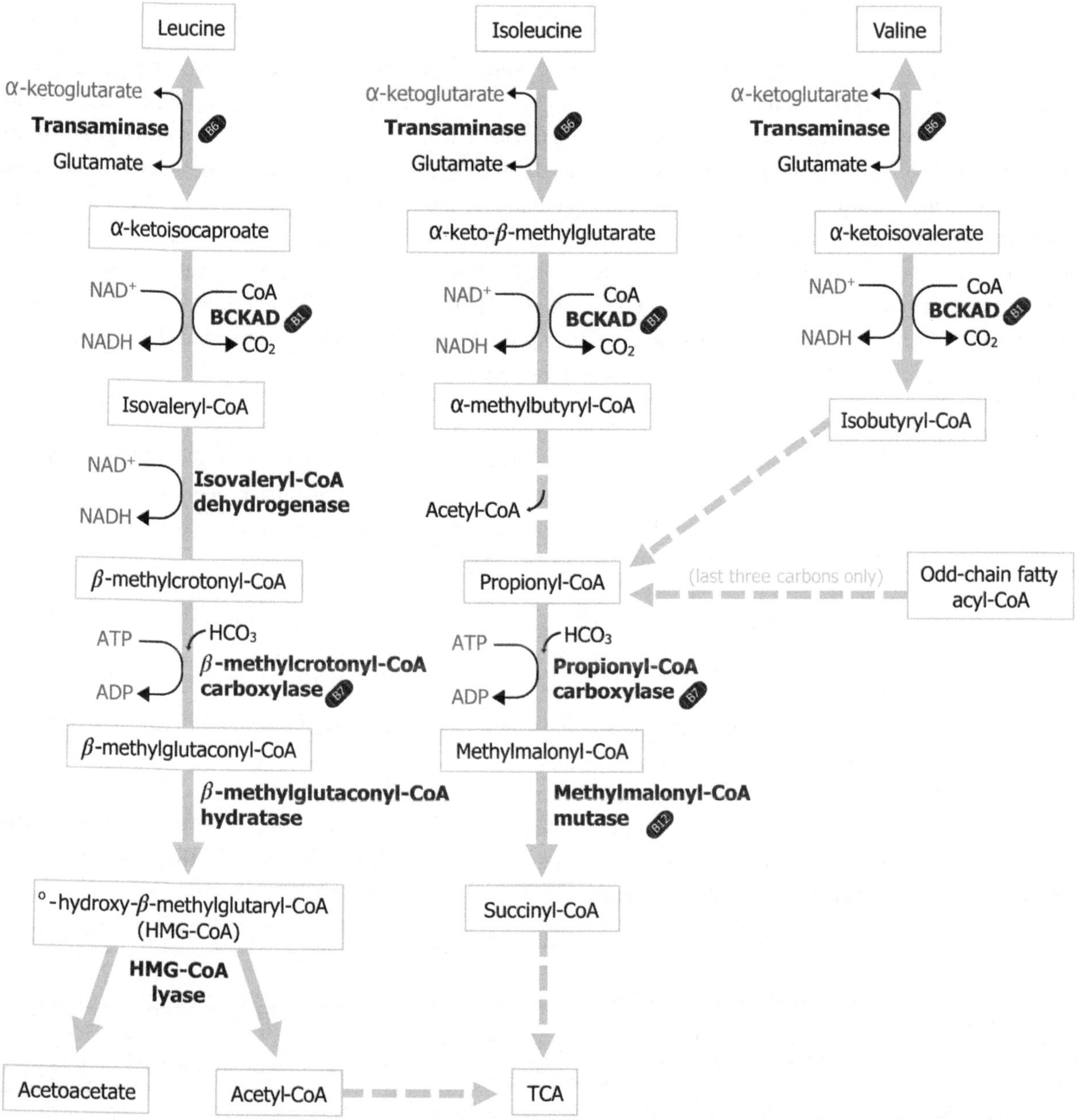

Figure 8.5: Metabolism of branched-chain amino acids. Deficiencies in branched-chain keto acid dehydrogenase (BCKAD) can result in the presentation of maple syrup urine disease.

Initially, methionine will condense with ATP to form SAM. SAM has a charged methyl group, which can be transferred to many different acceptor molecules; this step is considered irreversible as the amount of energy released is substantial.

SAM is used by many biological pathways to donate methyl groups, and it is in consistent demand. After SAM loses its methyl group, the resulting compound, S-adenosylhomocysteine (SAH), is hydrolyzed to homocysteine and adenosine.

Homocysteine, generated from this reaction, can either be remethylated in a reaction using both folate and cobalamin to resynthesize methionine or can be used for the synthesis or cysteine (figure 8.6).

Remethylation of homocysteine

Homocysteine can be converted back into methionine by using both methyl-FH_4 and vitamin B_{12}. (This is the only reaction in which methyl-FH_4 can donate the methyl group.) In this reaction, the methyl group from FH_4 is transferred to cobalamin associated with homocysteine methyltransferase. Homocysteine receives the methyl group from this charged cobalamin cofactor, and methionine is regenerated. If homocysteine methyltransferase is defective, or if vitamin B_{12} or FH_4 levels are insufficient, homocysteine will accumulate. Elevated homocysteine levels have been linked to cardiovascular and neurological diseases. A consequence of vitamin B_{12} deficiency is the accumulation of methyl-FH_4 and a decrease in other folate derivatives. This is known as the methyl-trap hypothesis; because of the B_{12} deficiency, most of the carbons in the FH_4 pool are trapped in the methyl-FH_4 form, which is the most stable. The carbons cannot be released from the folate because the one reaction in which they participate cannot occur because of the B_{12} deficiency. This leads to a functional folate deficiency, even though total levels of folate are normal.

A folate deficiency (whether functional or actual) leads to megaloblastic anemia caused by an inability of blood cell precursors to synthesize DNA and, therefore, to divide. This leads to large, partially replicated cells being released into the blood to attempt to replenish the cells that have died. Folate deficiencies also have been linked to an increased incidence of neural tube defects, such as spina bifida, in mothers who become pregnant while folate deficient.

Transsulfuration pathway

Further metabolism of homocysteine provides the sulfur atom for the synthesis of cysteine. In this two-step process, homocysteine first reacts with serine to form cystathionine. This is followed by cleavage of cystathionine, which yields cysteine and α-ketobutyrate. The first reaction in this sequence, catalyzed by cystathionine β-synthase, is inhibited by cysteine. Thus, methionine, via homocysteine, is not used for cysteine synthesis unless the levels of cysteine in the body are lower than required for its metabolic functions. An adequate dietary supply of cysteine, therefore, can "spare" (or reduce) the dietary requirement for methionine (figure 8.6).

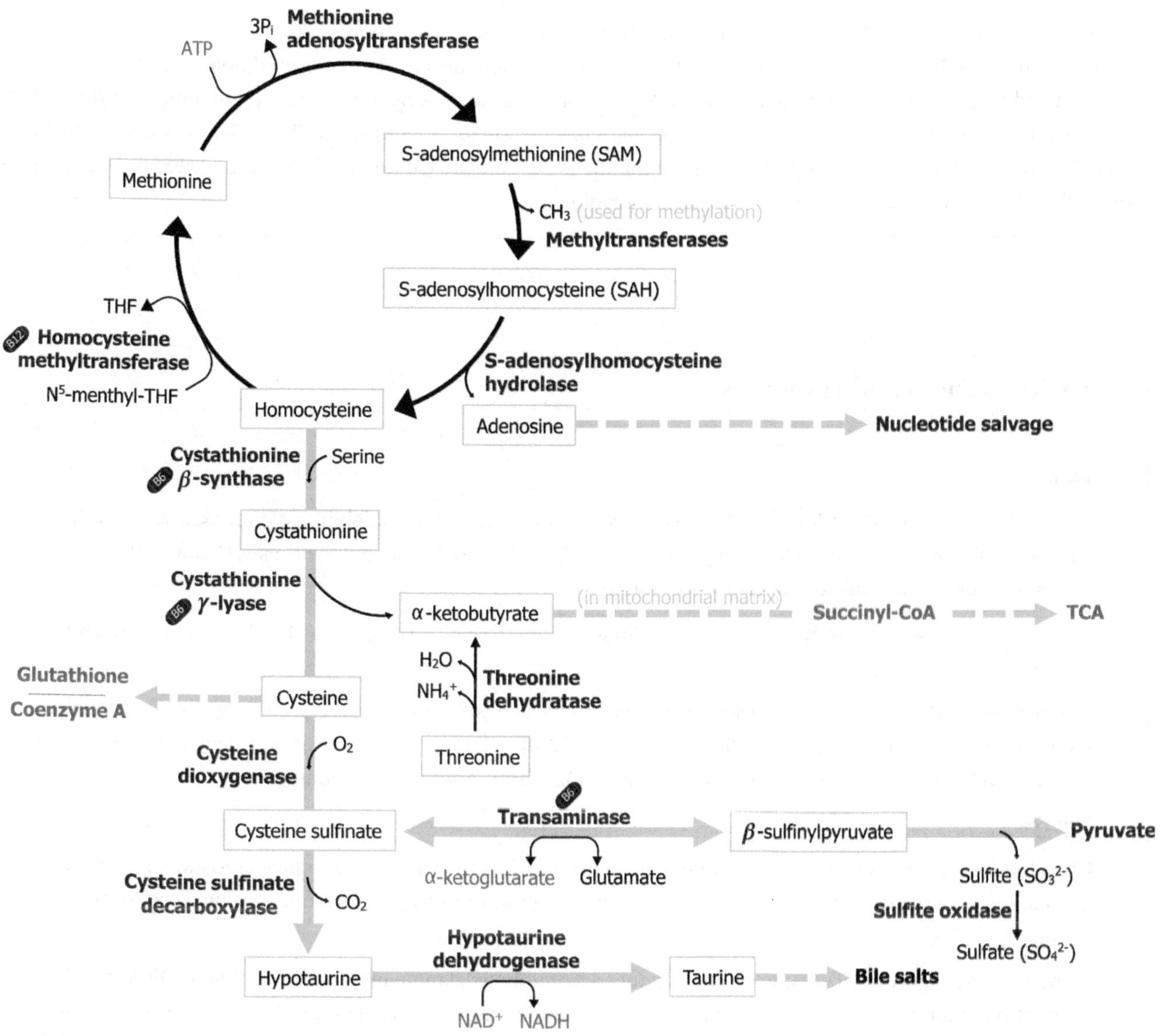

Figure 8.6: Metabolism of methionine. Remethylation and transsulfuration of homocysteine are illustrated. Cofactor or enzymatic deficiencies can result in an elevation of homocysteine.

Consequences of elevated homocysteine

Homocysteine levels can accumulate in several ways, which are related to both folic acid and vitamin B_{12} metabolism. As SAM is constantly being used as a methyl donor, this results in a consistent production of SAH. Consequently, this leads to constant production of homocysteine. The homocysteine produced can be either remethylated to methionine or condensed with serine to form cystathionine. The major pathway of homocysteine metabolism is remethylation by N5-methyl-FH4, which requires vitamin B_{12}. The liver also contains a second pathway in which betaine (a degradation product of choline) can donate a methyl group to homocysteine to form methionine, but this is a minor pathway. The conversion of homocysteine to cystathionine requires pyridoxal phosphate (PLP). Thus, if an individual is deficient in vitamin B_{12}, the conversion of homocysteine to methionine by the major route is inhibited. This directs homocysteine to produce cystathionine, which eventually produces cysteine. Homocysteine also accumulates in the blood if a mutation is present in the enzyme that converts N5,N10-methylene-FH4 to N5-methyl-FH4. When this occurs, the levels of

N5-methyl-FH4 are too low to allow homocysteine to be converted to methionine. The loss of this pathway, coupled with the feedback inhibition by cysteine on cystathionine formation, also leads to elevated homocysteine levels in the blood. A third way in which serum homocysteine levels can be elevated is by a mutated cystathionine β-synthase or a deficiency in vitamin B_6, the required cofactor for that enzyme. These defects block the ability of homocysteine to be converted to cystathionine, and the homocysteine that does accumulate cannot all be accommodated by conversion to methionine. Thus, an accumulation of homocysteine results.

8.1 References and resources

Text

Ferrier, D. R., ed. *Lippincott Illustrated Reviews: Biochemistry*, 7th ed. Philadelphia: Wolters Kluwer Health/Lippincott Williams & Wilkins, 2017, Chapter 20: Amino Acid Degradation and Synthesis, Chapter 21: Conversion of Amino Acids to Specialized Products.

Le, T., and V. Bhushan. *First Aid for the USMLE Step* 1, 29th ed. New York: McGraw Hill Education, 2018, 69, 83–85.

Lieberman, M., and A. Peet, eds. *Marks' Basic Medical Biochemistry: A Clinical Approach*, 5th ed. Philadelphia: Wolters Kluwer Health/Lippincott Williams & Wilkins, 2018, Chapter 37: Synthesis and Degradation of Amino Acids, Chapter 39: Tetrahydrofolate, Vitamin B12, and S-Adenosylmethionine.

Figures

Grey, Kindred, Figure 8.1 Metabolism of phenylalanine requires BH4 and also produces tyrosine. Deficiencies in cofactor or phenylalanine hydroxylase can result in phenylketonuria. 2021. https://archive.org/details/8.1-new. CC BY 4.0.

Grey, Kindred, Figure 8.2 Tyrosine can be produced from phenylalanine metabolism and is required for the production of melanin and the catecholamines. Deficiencies can occur at several different locations in the pathway and result in albinism, alkaptonuria or tyrosinemia. 2021. https://archive.org/details/8.2_20210926. CC BY 4.0.

Grey, Kindred, Figure 8.3 Metabolism of tryptophan to melatonin. 2021. https://archive.org/details/8.3_20210926. CC BY 4.0.

Grey, Kindred, Figure 8.4 Glutamate metabolism as it interfaces with nitrogen transport and synthesis of GABA. 2021. https://archive.org/details/8.4_20210926. CC BY 4.0.

Grey, Kindred, Figure 8.5 Metabolism of branched chain amino acids. Deficiencies in BCKAD can result in the presentation of Maple Syrup Urine Disease. 2021. https://archive.org/details/8.5_20210926. CC BY 4.0.

Grey, Kindred, Figure 8.6 Metabolism of methionine. Remethylation and transsulfuration of homocysteine are illustrated. Cofactor or enzymatic deficiencies can result in an elevation of homocysteine. 2021. https://archive.org/details/8.6_20210926. CC BY 4.0.

9. Disorders of Monosaccharide Metabolism and Other Metabolic Conditions

Learning Objectives

Monosaccharide metabolism

- Describe fructose and galactose metabolism, including the location of the pathway, substrate, and regulatory enzymes.
- Apply knowledge of metabolic regulation to determine how deficiencies in monosaccharide metabolism lead to hypoglycemia.

Alcohol metabolism

- Determine clinical consequences of increased NADH on the metabolic pathways of β-oxidation and gluconeogenesis.
- Describe the two-step process of alcohol metabolism by ADH and ALDH.

About this Chapter

Metabolism to this point has focused on the oxidation of carbohydrates (primarily glucose), lipids, and amino acids. We have addressed these processes under normal conditions without much consideration for potential interactions of other metabolites or pathologies. This section will address how some additional situations can impact the metabolism of these macromolecules. First, metabolism of both galactose and fructose is important and will be addressed. Heritable deficiencies in either of these pathways can potentially cause severe symptoms, and learning how to identify key symptoms is essential. Metabolism of alcohol is also a process to be aware of, as excess flux through this pathway has the potential to interfere with normal glucose and lipid metabolism.

9.1 Monosaccharide Metabolism

Fructose metabolism

Fructose is a dietary component of sucrose in fruit, as a free sugar in honey, and in high-fructose corn syrup. It is taken up by cells through facilitated diffusion through the GLUT5 transporter. Fructose is metabolized principally in the liver, and the initial step involves phosphorylation at the 1-position to form fructose 1-phosphate (figure 9.1). Fructokinase, the major kinase involved, phosphorylates fructose in the 1-position. Fructokinase has a high V_{max} and rapidly phosphorylates fructose as it enters the cell. Aldolase B cleaves fructose 1-phosphate into glyceraldehyde 3-phosphate and dihydroxyacetone-phosphate, which can enter directly into glycolysis.

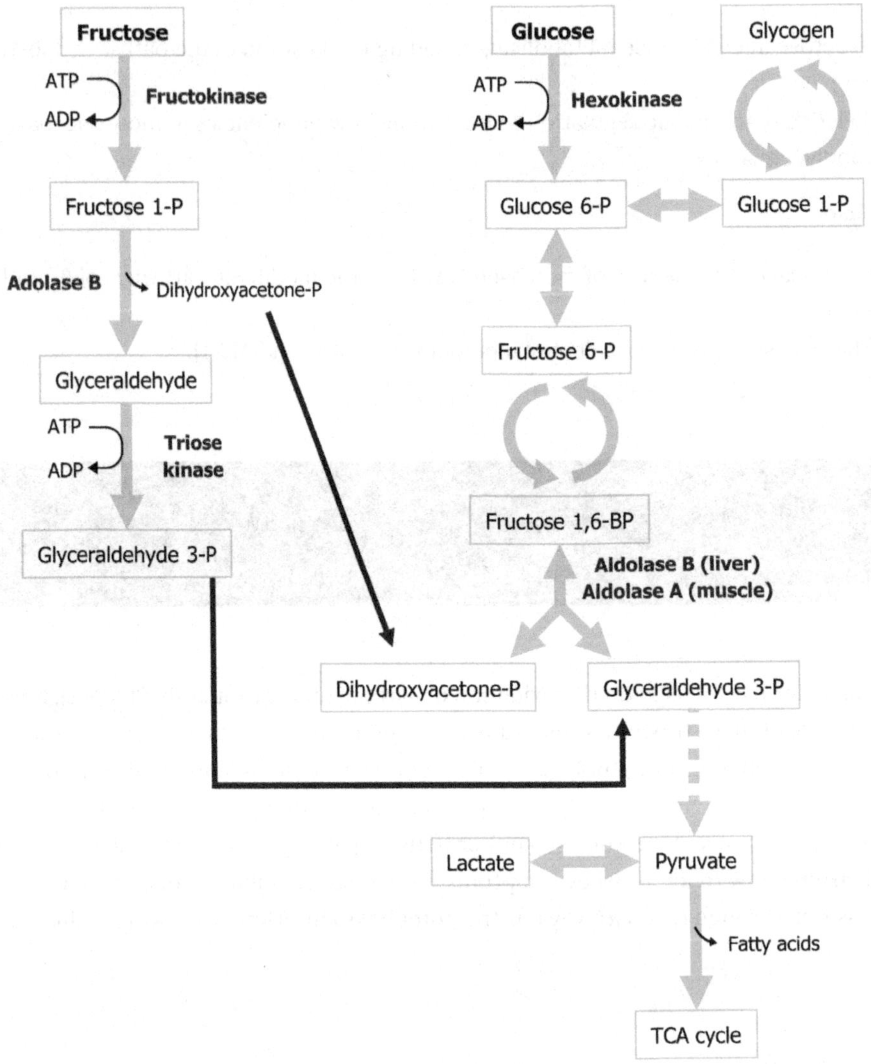

Figure 9.1: Convergence of fructose and glucose metabolism.

Aldolase B is the rate-limiting enzyme of fructose metabolism, although it is not a rate-limiting enzyme of glycolysis. Aldolase B's affinity for fructose 1-phosphate is lower than fructose 1,6-bisphosphate and is very slow at physiological levels of fructose 1-phosphate. Consequently, after high fructose consumption, fructose 1-phosphate will accumulate in the liver, and it is slowly converted to glycolytic intermediates over time (figures 9.1 and 9.2).

Deficiencies in fructose metabolism

Essential fructosuria (fructokinase deficiency) and hereditary fructose intolerance (HFI) (a deficiency of the fructose 1-phosphate cleavage by aldolase B) are inherited disorders of fructose metabolism. A deficiency in fructokinase is a benign genetic disorder. In this case, an individual will have fructosuria; fructose is not phosphorylated and trapped in the cell. Consequently, any ingested fructose is shed in the urine. Hereditary fructose intolerance is caused by a deficiency in aldolase B and results in an accumulation of fructose 1-phosphate in the hepatocytes. Inability to metabolize fructose 1-phosphate can cause significant clinical symptoms, most notably hepatomegaly and fasting hypoglyemia. The accumulation of fructose 1-phosphate eventually inhibits both glycogenolysis and gluconeogenesis (due to a lack of free phosphate), leading to bouts of fasting hypoglycemia.

Galactose metabolism

Galactose is consumed principally as lactose, which is cleaved to galactose and glucose in the intestine. Galactose is subsequently phosphorylated to galactose 1-phosphate by galactokinase (primarily in the liver). Following phosphorylation, galactose 1-phosphate is activated to a uridine diphosphate (UDP)-sugar by galactosyl uridylyltransferase (GALT). The metabolic pathway subsequently generates glucose 1-phosphate, which enters into the glycolytic pathway (figure 9.2)

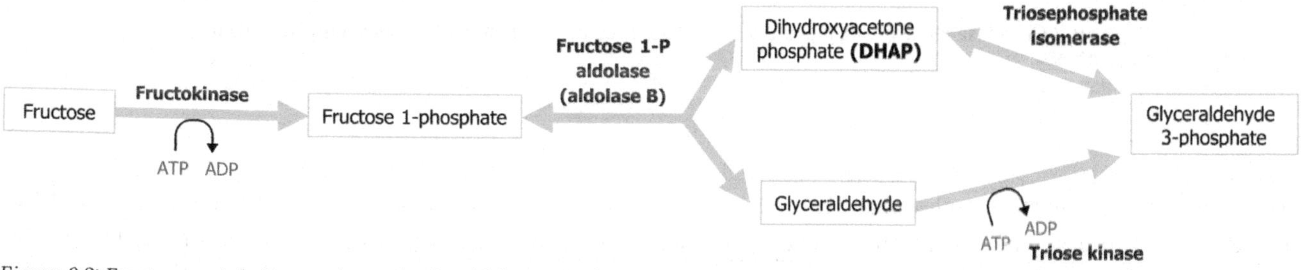

Figure 9.2: Fructose metabolism and reaction by aldolase B. Deficiencies in aldolase B can result in hereditary fructose intolerance, while deficiencies in frutokinase can result in essential fructosuria.

Deficiencies in galactose metabolism

Classical galactosemia, a deficiency of galactosyl uridylyltransferase (GALT), results in the accumulation of galactose 1-phosphate in the liver and the inhibition of hepatic glycogen metabolism and other pathways that require UDP-sugars. Cataracts can occur from the accumulation of galactose in the blood, which is converted to galactitol (the sugar alcohol of galactose) in the lens of the eye.

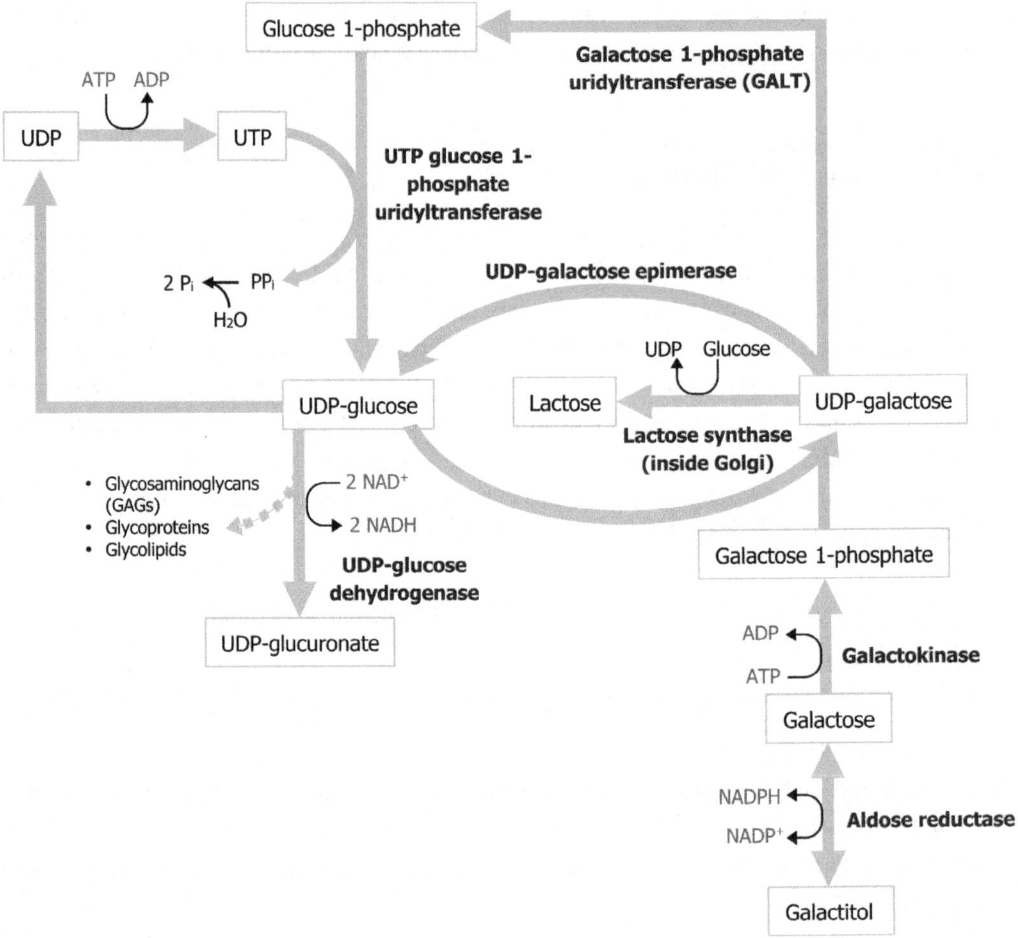

Figure 9.3: Galactose metabolism; glucose 6-phosphate is converted to glucose 1-phosphate, which enters the pathway.

The accumulating galactose 1-phosphate is especially toxic for the liver, kidneys, and central nervous system. If left untreated, the disease is fatal due to complications such as gram-negative sepsis or hepatic and renal failure. The absence of GALT activity can be detected any time after birth and screened for as part of newborn screening. It is essential to obtain results promptly, because children with classic galactosemia can have a life-threatening crisis within the first few days after birth. Infants with a positive result are placed on a lactose-free formula, and confirmatory testing is accomplished by measuring specific metabolite concentrations and enzyme activity in erythrocytes.

Nonclassical galactosemia causes fewer medical complications and presents with a different pattern of symptoms. Presentations can involve cataracts, delayed development, and kidney problems.

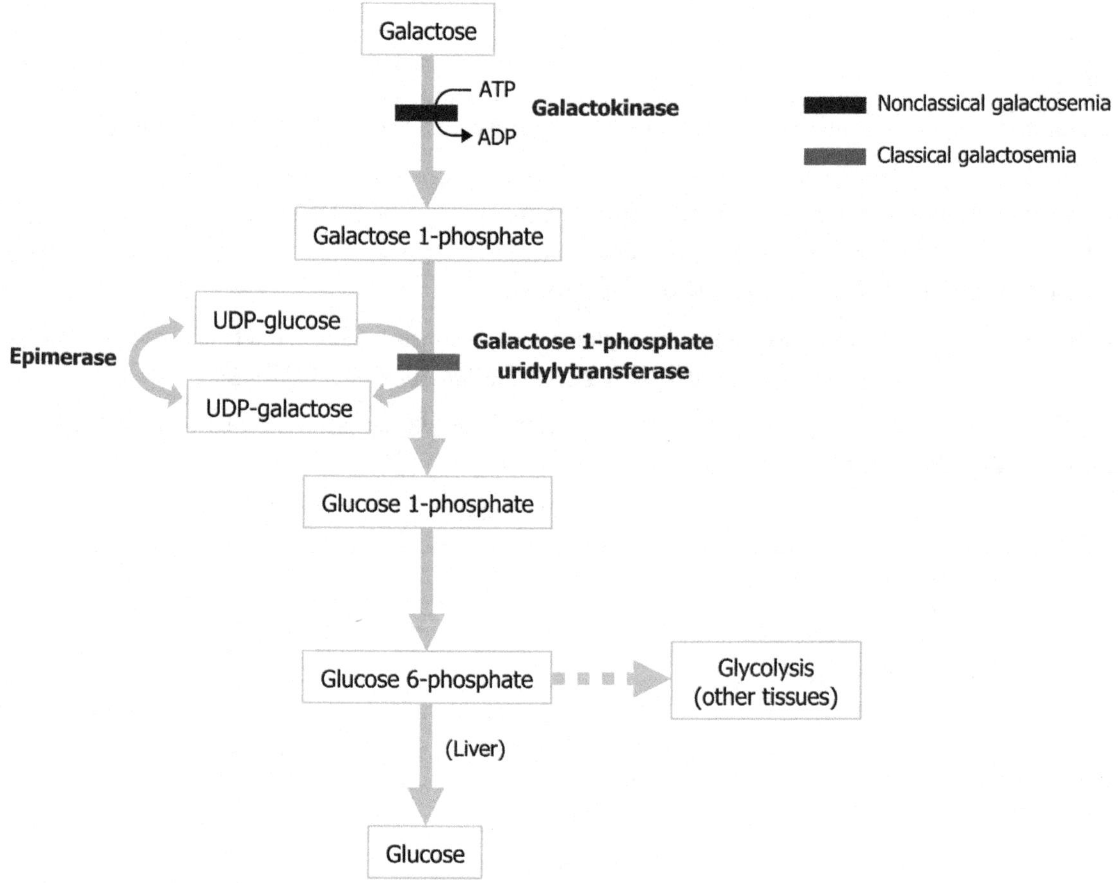

Figure 9.4: Comparison of classical and nonclassical galatosemia.

9.1 References and resources

Text

Ferrier, D. R., ed. *Lippincott Illustrated Reviews: Biochemistry*, 7th ed. Philadelphia: Wolters Kluwer Health/ Lippincott Williams & Wilkins, 2017, Chapter 12: Metabolism of Monosaccharides and Disaccharides, Chapter 23: Effects of Insulin and Glucagon: Section IV.

Le, T., and V. Bhushan. *First Aid for the USMLE Step 1*, 29th ed. New York: McGraw Hill Education, 2018, 72, 80–81.

Lieberman, M., and A. Peet, eds. *Marks' Basic Medical Biochemistry: A Clinical Approach*, 5th ed. Philadelphia: Wolters Kluwer Health/Lippincott Williams & Wilkins, 2018, Chapter 22: Generation of ATP from Glucose, Fructose and Galactose, Chapter 33: Ethanol Metabolism.

Figures

Grey, Kindred, Figure 9.1 Convergence of fructose and glucose metabolism. 2021. https://archive.org/details/9.1_20210926. CC BY 4.0.

Grey, Kindred, Figure 9.2 Fructose metabolism and reaction by Aldolase B. Deficiencies in aldolase B can result in hereditary fructose intolerance while deficiencies in frutokinase can result in essential fructosuria. 2021. https://archive.org/details/9.2_20210926. CC BY 4.0.

Grey, Kindred, Figure 9.3 Galactose metabolism; glucose 6-phosphate is converted to glucose 1-phosphate which enters the pathway. 2021. https://archive.org/details/9.3_20210926. CC BY 4.0.

Grey, Kindred, Figure 9.4 Comparison of Classical and Nonclassical galatosemia. 2021. https://archive.org/details/9.4_20210926. CC BY 4.0.

9.2 Alcohol Metabolism

Metabolism of alcohol occurs primarily in the liver through two different oxidative pathways. The activity of each pathway depends on the ethanol concentration and the frequency of ethanol consumption.

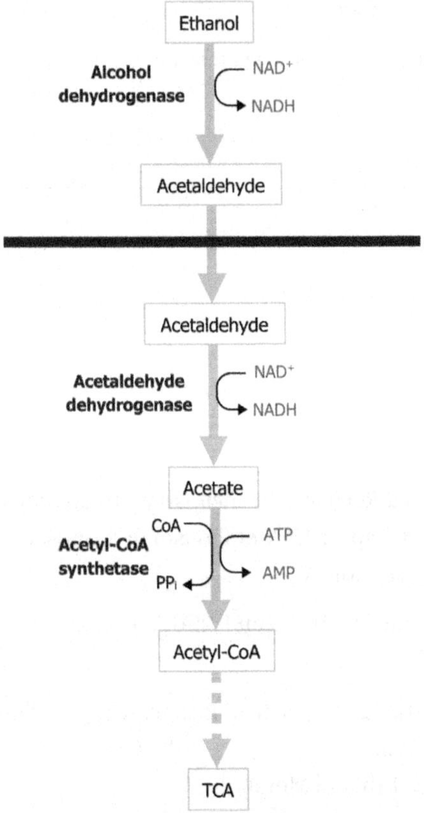

Figure 9.5: Overview of ethanol metabolism. The pathway spans the cytosol and the mitochondria, and NADH is produced in both steps of the pathway.

At low concentrations, oxidation of ethanol is a two-step process that occurs in both the cytosol and the mitochondria (figure 9.5). The first step of the reaction by alcohol dehydrogenase (ADH) occurs in the cytosol and produces acetaldehyde. Acetaldehyde is converted into acetate in the mitochondria by acetaldehyde dehydrogenase (ALDH) and can be transported in the blood to be used as an energy source for peripheral tissues (figure 9.5). The acetate can be converted to acetyl-CoA by acetyl-CoA synthetase (figure 9.6), and this will be oxidized in the TCA cycle. Each step in the oxidation of ethanol produces NADH, which increases the ratio of $NADH/NAD^+$. The increase in this ratio can alter metabolism of other substrates and cause metabolic dysfunction, which will be discussed below.

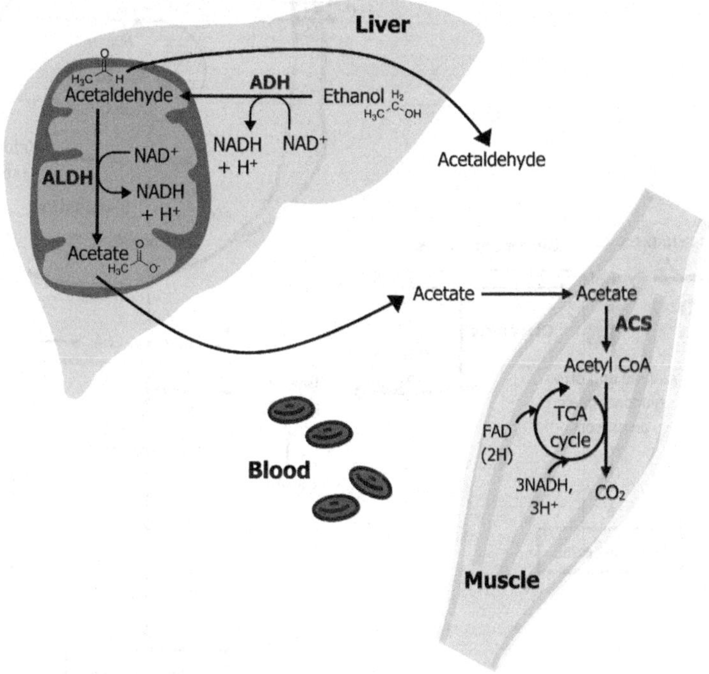

Figure 9.6: Overview of alcohol metabolism.

Consequences of ethanol metabolism in the liver

At each step in ethanol oxidation, NADH is generated in both the mitochondrial and cytosolic compartments (figure 9.5). This can have major metabolic ramifications depending on the underlying metabolic environment (figure 9.7).

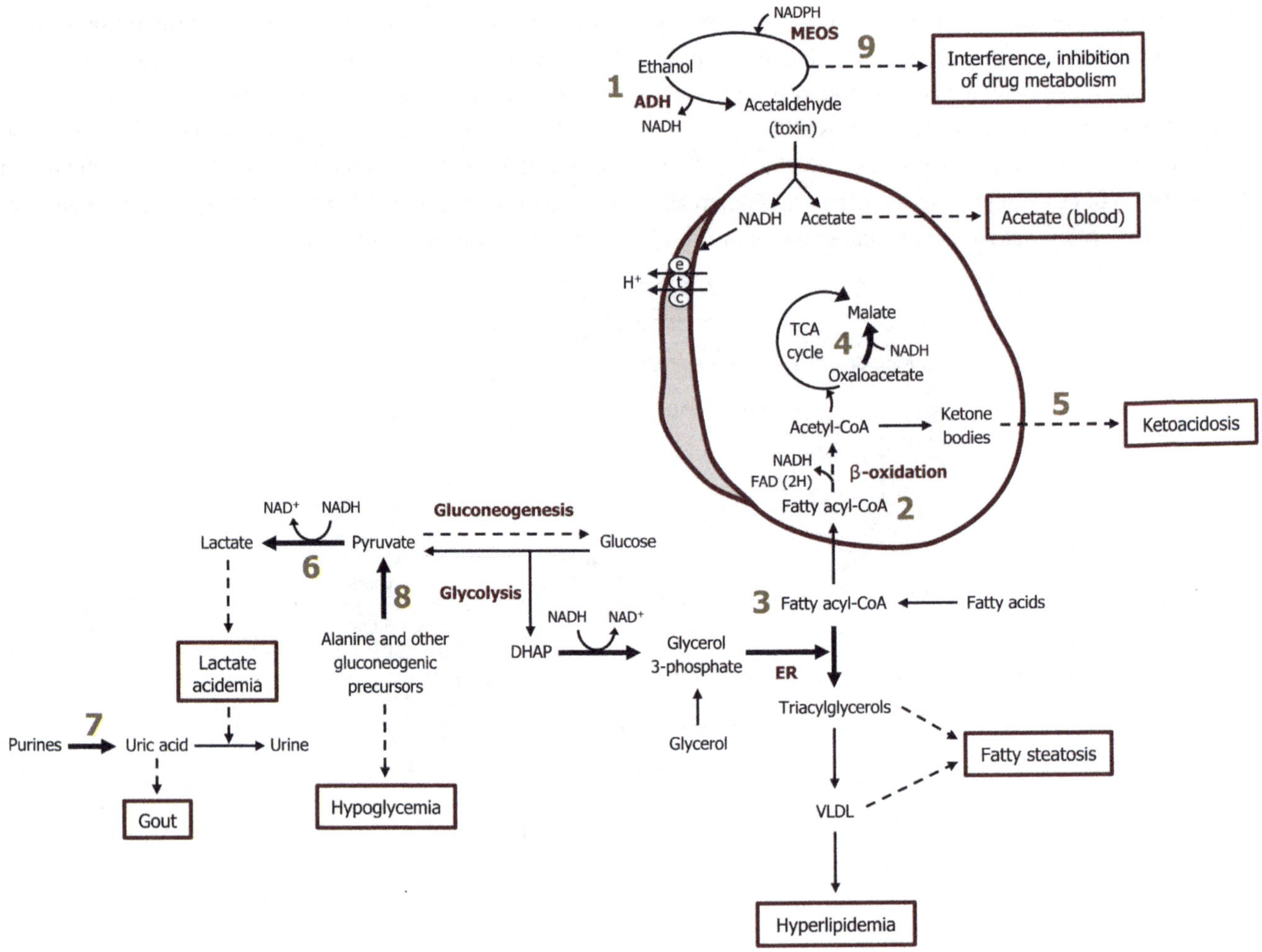

Figure 9.7: Clinical consequences of alcoholism.

1. Hypoglycemia: High NADH produced by alcohol metabolism (figure 9.7; label 1) contributes to the diversion of the gluconeogenic substrates OAA and pyruvate. The higher $NADH/NAD^+$ ratio drives the reactions toward malate and lactate, respectively. This can lead to the presentation of fasting hypoglycemia (figure 9.7; labels 4, 6, and 8).
2. Fatty steatosis: High $NADH/NAD^+$ ratio also increases the conversion of dihydroxyacetone phosphate to glycerol 3-phosphate, contributing to increased synthesis of triacylglycerol. Additionally, increases in reactive oxygen species, which can impair protein synthesis, prevent the assembly and secretion of VLDLs. This can ultimately contribute to fatty liver disease (figure 9.7; label 3).
3. Acidosis: Increases in alternative substrates for peripheral tissues (acetate from alcohol oxidation) can cause an elevation of ketones leading to ketoacidosis (figure 9.7; label 5).
4. Hyperlipidemia: The elevated NADH will negatively impact flux through the TCA by reducing the activity of the two key regulatory enzymes. This can lead to an increased shunting of citrate for fatty acid synthesis (figure 9.7; labels 2 and 3).
5. Acetaldehyde is a toxic compound that forms adducts with other proteins reducing their ability to function.

Excessive alcohol consumption

At higher concentrations of ethanol, the microsomal ethanol oxidizing system (MEOS) becomes activated (figure 9.7; label 9). This pathway consists of a series of cytochrome P450 enzymes, which have a relatively high K_m for ethanol and are located in the hepatic smooth endoplasmic reticulum (SER). This microsomal-ethanol oxidizing system also detoxifies drugs such as barbiturates (figure 9.8).

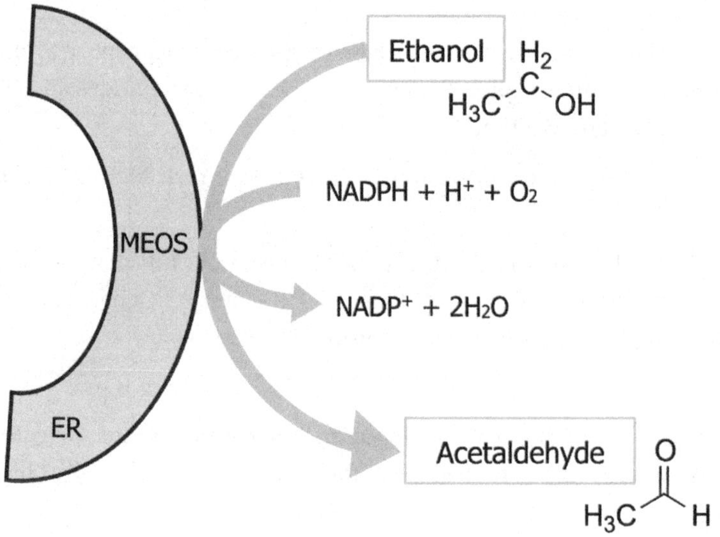

Figure 9.8: Ethanol detoxification by MEOS.

1. Chronic consumption of alcohol will increase the expression of the MEOS and proliferation of hepatic SER. Increases in expression of both CYP2E1 (P450 enzyme) and γ-glutamyltransferase (GGT), an enzyme located in the SER, are excellent markers of alcohol ingestion.
2. Ethanol oxidation by MEOS does not affect the $NADH/NAD^+$ ratio substantially, therefore, it does not have the metabolic effects described for low concentrations of ethanol.

Although the MEOS system does not impact the $NADH/NAD^+$ ratio, that is not to suggest that induction of this system is without metabolic consequences. Induction of the P450 system can negatively impact the metabolism of other drugs causing serious side effects. One example of this is altered metabolism of acetaminophen (Tylenol). Acetaminophen can be glucuronylated or sulfated in the liver for safe excretion by the kidney. However, the cytochrome P450 system can metabolize acetaminophen to the toxic intermediate N-acetyl-p-benzoquinone imine (NAPQI), which requires conjugation with glutathione prior to excretion. The enzyme that produces NAPQI, CYP2E1, is induced by alcohol through the MEOS. Thus, individuals who chronically abuse alcohol have increased sensitivity to acetaminophen toxicity because a higher percentage of acetaminophen metabolism is directed toward NAPQI, compared with an individual with low levels of CYP2E1.

Ethanol is also an inhibitor of the phenobarbital-oxidizing P450 system. When large amounts of ethanol are consumed, the inactivation of phenobarbital is directly or indirectly inhibited. Therefore, when high doses of phenobarbital and ethanol are consumed at the same time, toxic levels of the barbiturate can accumulate in the blood.

9.2 References and resources

Text

Ferrier, D. R., ed. *Lippincott Illustrated Reviews: Biochemistry*, 7th ed. Philadelphia: Wolters Kluwer Health/ Lippincott Williams & Wilkins, 2017, Chapter 12: Metabolism of Monosaccharides and Disaccharides, Chapter 23: Effects of Insulin and Glucagon: Section IV.

Le, T., and V. Bhushan. *First Aid for the USMLE Step 1*, 29th ed. New York: McGraw Hill Education, 2018, 72, 80–81.

Lieberman, M., and A. Peet, eds. *Marks' Basic Medical Biochemistry: A Clinical Approach*, 5th ed. Philadelphia: Wolters Kluwer Health/Lippincott Williams & Wilkins, 2018, Chapter 22: Generation of ATP from Glucose, Fructose and Galactose, Chapter 33: Ethanol Metabolism.

Figures

Grey, Kindred, Figure 9.5 Overview of ethanol metabolism. The pathway spans the cytosol and the mitochondria and NADH is produced in both steps of the pathway. 2021. https://archive.org/details/9.5_20210926. CC BY 4.0.

Grey, Kindred, Figure 9.6 Overview of alcohol metabolism. 2021. Chemical structure by Henry Jakubowski. https://archive.org/details/9.6_20210926. CC BY 4.0. Added Liver by Liam Mitchell from the Noun Project, Muscle by Laymik from the Noun Project, and red blood cells by Lucas Helle from the Noun Project.

Lieberman M, Peet A. Figure 9.7 Clinical consequences of alcoholism. Adapted under Fair Use from Marks' Basic Medical Biochemistry. 5th Ed. pp 709. Figure 33.6 Acute effects of ethanol metabolism on lipid metabolism in the liver. 2017.

Lieberman M, Peet A. Figure 9.8 Ethanol detoxification by MEOS. Adapted under Fair Use from Marks' Basic Medical Biochemistry. 5th Ed. pp 704. Figure 33.3 The reaction catalyzed by the microsomal ethanol-oxidizing system (MEOS; which includes CYP2E1) in the endoplasmic reticulum (ER). 2017. Chemical structure by Henry Jakubowski.

10. Genes, Genomes, and DNA

Learning Objectives

- Define the word genome, and describe what composes the eukaryotic genome.
- Describe the chemical structure and physical properties of DNA.
- Outline the levels of structure of chromatin and chromosomes.
- Define the types of chromatin (heterochromatin, euchromatin, and facultative and constitutive chromatin).
- Describe the characteristics of nonrepetitive DNA, highly repetitive DNA, and moderately repetitive DNA and its relative abundance and significance throughout the genome.
- Describe sources and types of genetic polymorphism.
- Describe the mechanisms and implications of different classes of genetic mutation (genome mutation, chromosome mutation, and gene mutation).
- Emphasize the bidirectional and semidiscontinuous nature of DNA replication and the reasons for it.
- Outline the different types of DNA damage caused by various environmental conditions.
- Outline what is known about the different types of DNA repair mechanisms.

About this Chapter

The cell is the most fundamental unit of all eukaryotic organisms. Its components and their cellular interactions are essential to the inner workings of the cell as well as influencing the surrounding environment through cell interactions. Starting at the level of DNA, we will address how individual nucleotide changes can alter cellular process leading to the change of a cell (and therefore organismal) phenotype.

10.1 DNA Structure

Nucleotides and basic DNA structure

The building blocks of DNA are nucleotides. The important components of the nucleotide are a nitrogenous (nitrogen-bearing) base, a five-carbon sugar (pentose), and a phosphate group. The nucleotide is named depending on the nitrogenous base. The nitrogenous base can be a purine, such as adenine (A) and guanine (G), or a pyrimidine, such as cytosine (C) and thymine (T). The purines have a double-ring structure with a six-membered ring fused to a five-membered ring. Pyrimidines are smaller in size; they have a single six-membered ring structure. The sugar is deoxyribose in DNA and ribose in RNA. The carbon atoms of the five-carbon sugar are numbered 1′, 2′, 3′, 4′, and 5′ (1′ is read as "one prime"). The phosphate, which makes DNA and RNA acidic, is connected to the 5′ carbon of the sugar by the formation of an ester linkage between phosphoric acid and the 5′-OH group (an ester is an acid + an alcohol). In DNA nucleotides, the 3′ carbon of the sugar deoxyribose is attached to a hydroxyl (OH) group (figures 10.1 and 10.2).

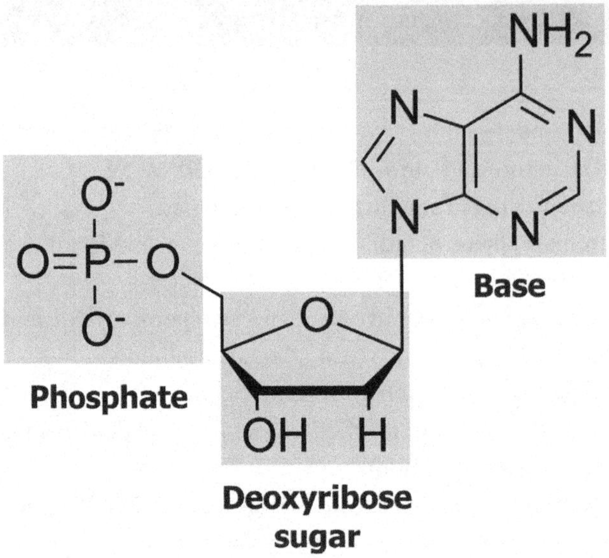

Figure 10.1: Basic structure of nucleotides including the sugar (ribose or deoxyribose), base (pyrimidine or purine), and phosphate groups.

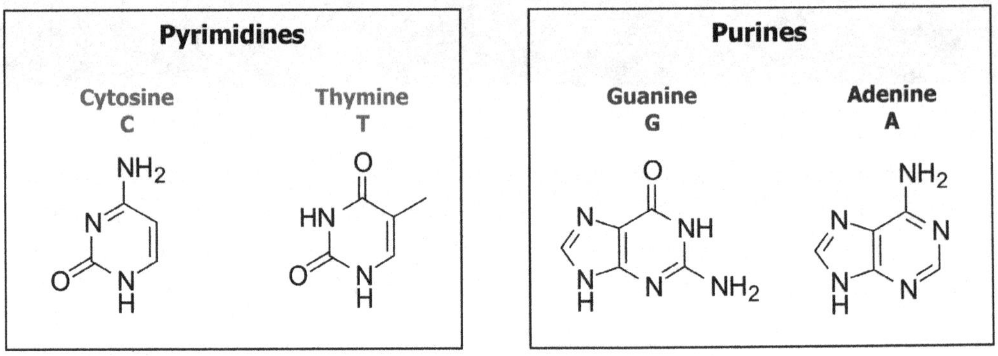

Figure 10.2: Structure of pyrimidine and purine bases.

The nucleotides combine with each other to produce phosphodiester bonds. The phosphate residue attached to the 5′ carbon of the sugar of one nucleotide forms a second ester linkage with the hydroxyl group of the 3′ carbon of the sugar of the next nucleotide, thereby forming a 5′-3′ phosphodiester bond. In a polynucleotide, one end of the chain has a free 5′ phosphate, and the other end has a free 3′-OH. These are called the 5′ and 3′ ends of the chain.

Base-pairing takes place between a purine and pyrimidine on opposite strands, so that adenine and thymine are complementary base pairs, and cytosine and guanine are also complementary base pairs. The base pairs are stabilized by hydrogen bonds: adenine and thymine form two hydrogen bonds, and cytosine and guanine form three hydrogen bonds.

The two strands are anti-parallel in nature; that is, the 3′ end of one strand faces the 5′ end of the other strand. The sugar and phosphate of the nucleotides form the backbone of the structure, whereas the nitrogenous bases are stacked inside, like the rungs of a ladder. The twisting of the two strands around each other results in the formation of uniformly spaced major and minor grooves.

DNA has a double helix structure and phosphodiester bonds; the dotted lines between thymine and adenine and guanine and cytosine represent hydrogen bonds. The major and minor grooves are binding sites for DNA-binding proteins during processes such as transcription (the copying of RNA from DNA) and replication (figure 10.3).

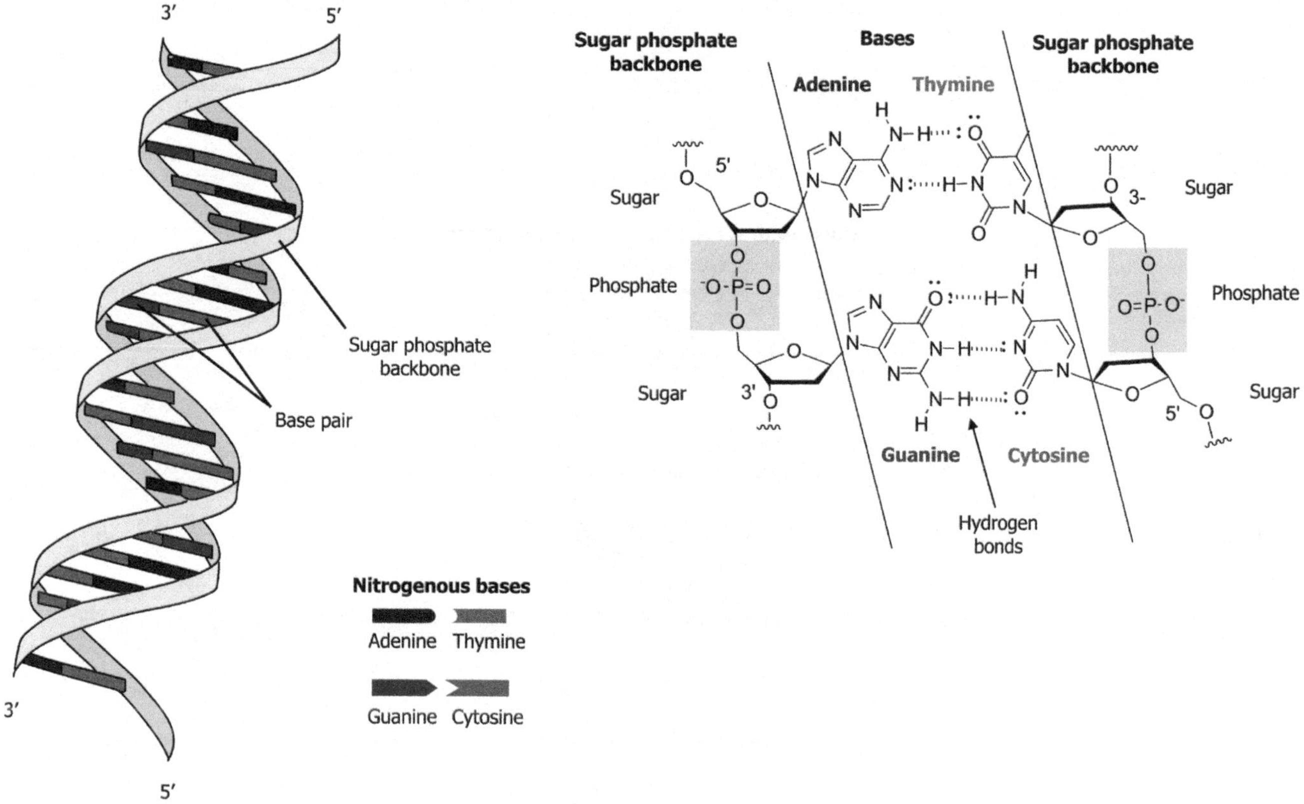

Figure 10.3: General structure and hydrogen bonding pattern of DNA.

DNA packaging and organization

Eukaryotic chromosomes consist of a linear DNA molecule complexed with protein (histones); this complex is called chromatin. Histones are evolutionarily conserved proteins that are rich in basic amino acids and form an octamer composed of two molecules of each of four different histones.

The DNA (remember, it is negatively charged because of the phosphate groups) is wrapped tightly around the histone core. This interaction is facilitated through electrostatic interactions. The negatively charged phosphate groups on the DNA backbone are attracted to a positively charged lysine on the exposed surface of histones. This nucleosome is linked to the next one with the help of a linker DNA. This is also known as the “beads on a string” structure. With the help of a fifth histone, a string of nucleosomes is further compacted into a 30 nm fiber, which is the diameter of the structure. Metaphase chromosomes are even further condensed by association with scaffolding proteins. At the metaphase stage, the chromosomes are at their most compact, approximately 700 nm in width (figure 10.4).

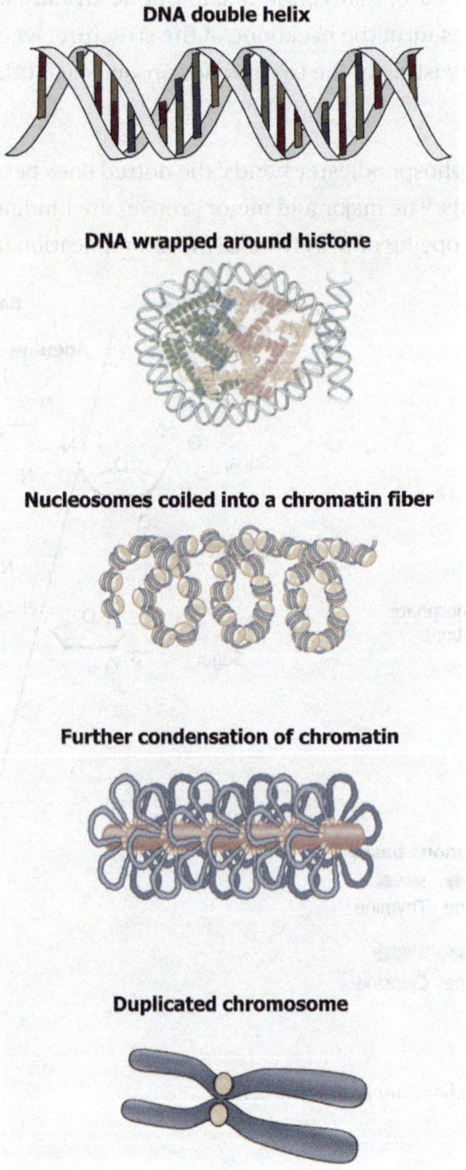

Figure 10.4: Organizational structure of DNA illustrating condensation and supercoiling into chromosomes.

In interphase, eukaryotic chromosomes have two distinct regions that can be distinguished by staining. The tightly packaged region is known as heterochromatin, and the less dense region is known as euchromatin.

Heterochromatin usually contains genes that are not expressed and is found in the regions of the centromere and telomeres.

The euchromatin usually contains genes that are transcribed, with DNA packaged around nucleosomes but not further compacted.

Histone tails can be modified through both methylation and acetylation, which will alter the histone:DNA interaction.

Histone methylation can have variable impacts on a given gene locus leading to a change in transcription. Histone acetylation relaxes the interactions of histones and DNA by removing the positive charge on lysine residues allowing the DNA to be transcriptionally accessible (euchromatin). DNA methylation, specifically to CpG islands, globally represses transcription. These modifications on histones and DNA can result in epigenetic influences that have an impact on many biological processes.

Across the three billion base pair genome, genes are organized into clusters with only a fraction of the DNA coding for translated products. The remaining DNA was historically considered "junk," however, more recently there is a new appreciation for the roles of noncoding DNA regions. Only half of the genome is unique DNA sequence, and only 1.5 percent codes for mRNA (~20,000 protein-coding genes). The remaining sequence can be categorized as:

- Moderately repetitive: DNA containing ribosomal RNA (rRNA), tandem and nontandem repeats, and short and long interspersed nuclear elements (SINE and LINE).
- Transposable elements: These are movable elements, transposons or retrotransposons, that can result in disease-causing mutations if inserted into important genomic loci.
- Highly repetitive sequence: Satellites and mini satellites are regions of high sequence repetition (trinucleotide repeats) and are difficult to replicate. This can lead to expansions of these areas as well as mutations resulting in frame shifts or loss of translational starts.

10.1 References and resources

Text

Clark, M. A. *Biology*, 2nd ed. Houston, TX: OpenStax College, Rice University, 2018, Chapter 14: DNA Structure and Function.

Karp, G., and J. G. Patton. *Cell and Molecular Biology: Concepts and Experiments*, 7th ed. Hoboken, NJ: John Wiley, 2013, Chapter 10: The Nature of the Gene and the Genome, Chapter 12: The Cell Nucleus and the Control of Gene Expression, Chapter 13: DNA Replication.

Le, T., and V. Bhushan. *First Aid for the USMLE Step 1*, 29th ed. New York: McGraw Hill Education, 2018, 34, 38–40.

Nussbaum, R. L., R. R. McInnes, H. F. Willard, A. Hamosh, and M. W. Thompson. *Thompson & Thompson Genetics in Medicine*, 8th ed. Philadelphia: Saunders/Elsevier, 2016, Chapter 2: The Introduction to the Human Genome.

Figures

Grey, Kindred, Figure 10.1 Basic structure of nucleosides including the sugar (ribose or deoxyribose), base (pyrimidine or purine) and phosphate groups. 2021. Chemical structure by Henry Jakubowski. https://archive.org/details/10.1_20210926. CC BY 4.0.

Grey, Kindred, Figure 10.2 Structure of pyrimidine and purine bases. 2021. Chemical structure by Henry Jakubowski. https://archive.org/details/10.2_20210926. CC BY 4.0.

Grey, Kindred, Figure 10.3 General structure and hydrogen bonding pattern of DNA. 2021. Chemical structure by Henry Jakubowski. https://archive.org/details/10.3_20210926. CC BY-SA 4.0. Added DNA double helix grooves by Biochemlife. CC BY-SA 4.0. From Wikimedia Commons.

Grey, Kindred, Figure 10.4 Organizational structure of DNA illustrating condensation and supercoiling into chromosomes. 2021. https://archive.org/details/10.4_20210926. CC BY-SA 4.0. Added DNA double helix grooves by Biochemlife. CC BY-SA 4.0. From Wikimedia Commons. And Figure 14.11. CC BY 4.0. From OpenStax.

10.2 DNA Repair

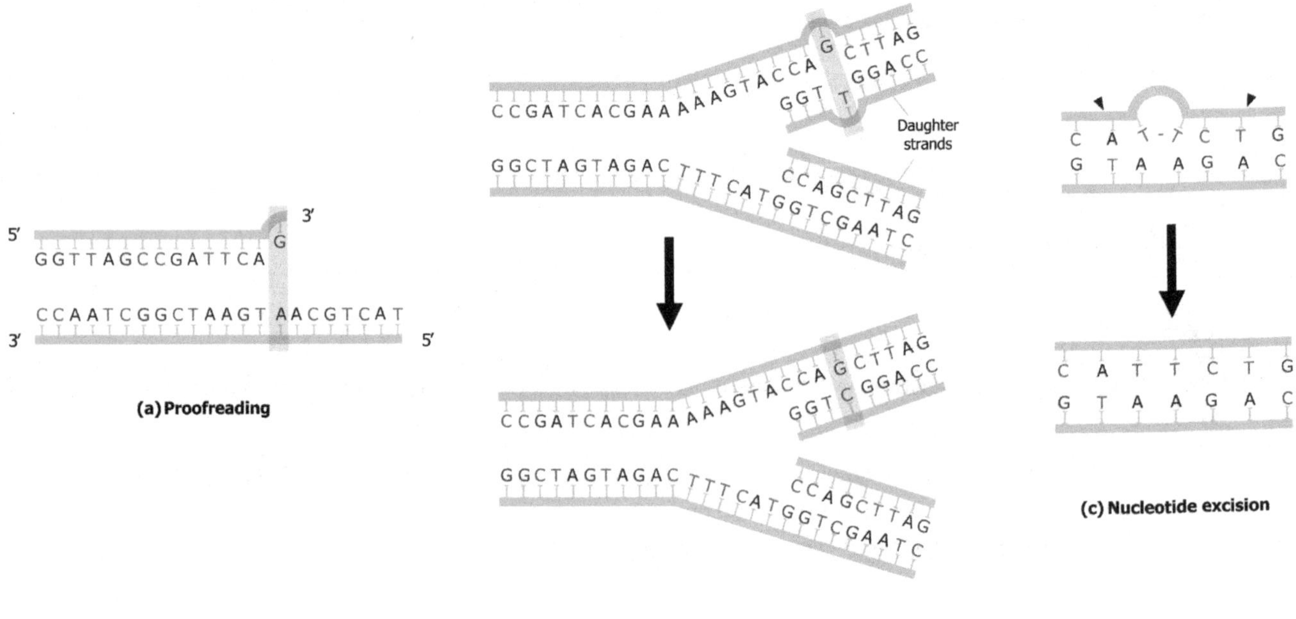

(b) Mismatch repair

Figure 10.5: Comparison on three types of repair: (A) proofreading, (B) mismatch, and (C) nucleotide excision repair.

DNA replication is a highly accurate process, but mistakes can occasionally occur, such as a DNA polymerase (DNA pol) inserting a wrong base. Uncorrected mistakes may sometimes lead to serious consequences, such as cancer. Repair mechanisms correct the mistakes. In rare cases, mistakes are not corrected, leading to mutations; in other cases, repair enzymes are themselves mutated or defective.

Most of the mistakes during DNA replication are promptly corrected by the proofreading ability of DNA polymerase itself. In proofreading, the DNA pol reads the newly added base before adding the next one, so a correction can be made. The polymerase checks whether the newly added base has paired correctly with the base in the template strand. If it is the right base, the next nucleotide is added. If an incorrect base has been added, the enzyme makes a cut at the phosphodiester bond and releases the wrong nucleotide. This is performed by the 3′ exonuclease action of DNA pol. Once the incorrect nucleotide has been removed, it can be replaced by the correct one (figure 10.5(a)).

Mismatch repair

Errors not addressed during replication are repaired through the process of mismatch repair (figure 10.5(b)). Specific repair enzymes recognize the mispaired nucleotide and excise part of the strand that contains it; the excised region is then resynthesized – typically during S phase of the cell cycle – and the enzymes involved are those used for DNA replication. If the mismatch remains uncorrected, it may lead to more permanent damage when the mismatched DNA is replicated. Deficiencies in this repair process can result in Lynch syndrome, which is characteristic of nonpolyposis colorectal cancer.

In prokaryotes, the parental strand is determined by the methyl groups on adenine bases, while the newly synthesized strand lacks them. Thus, DNA polymerase is able to remove the wrongly incorporated bases from the newly synthesized, non-methylated strand.

In eukaryotes, the mechanism is not very well understood, but it is believed to involve recognition of unsealed nicks in the new strand, as well as a short-term continuing association of some of the replication proteins with the new daughter strand after replication has completed.

Errors during DNA replication are not the only reason why mutations arise in DNA. Mutations, variations in the nucleotide sequence of a genome, can also occur because of damage to DNA. Such mutations may be of two types: induced or spontaneous. Induced mutations are those that result from an exposure to chemicals, UV rays, X-rays, or some other environmental agent. Spontaneous mutations occur without any exposure to any environmental agent; they are a result of natural reactions taking place within the body.

Nucleotide excision repair (NER)

Another type of repair mechanism, nucleotide excision repair, is similar to mismatch repair, except that it is used to remove large, bulky damaged bases rather than mismatched ones. The repair enzymes replace abnormal, bulky, bases by making a cut on both the 3′ and 5′ ends of the damaged base. The segment of DNA is removed and replaced with the correctly paired nucleotides by the action of DNA pol. Once the bases are filled in, the remaining gap is sealed with a phosphodiester linkage catalyzed by DNA ligase (figure 10.5(c)).

This repair mechanism is often employed when UV exposure causes the formation of pyrimidine dimers (thymine dimers). When exposed to UV light, thymines lying next to each other can form thymine dimers. In normal cells, they are excised and replaced. Xeroderma pigmentosa is a condition in which thymine dimerization from exposure to UV light is not repaired.

Base excision repair (BER)

The process of base excision repair (BER) is similar to NER but tends to repair small modifications to individual bases, such as deamination of cytosine to produce uracil. In this process, the aberrant base is detected by a glycosylase that will cleave the N-glycosidic bond joining the base to the deoxyribose sugar. This leaves an apurinic or apyrimidinic site (sugar phosphate backbone lacking a base), which is cleaved by an exonuclease and repaired through a similar process as mentioned above (figure 10.6).

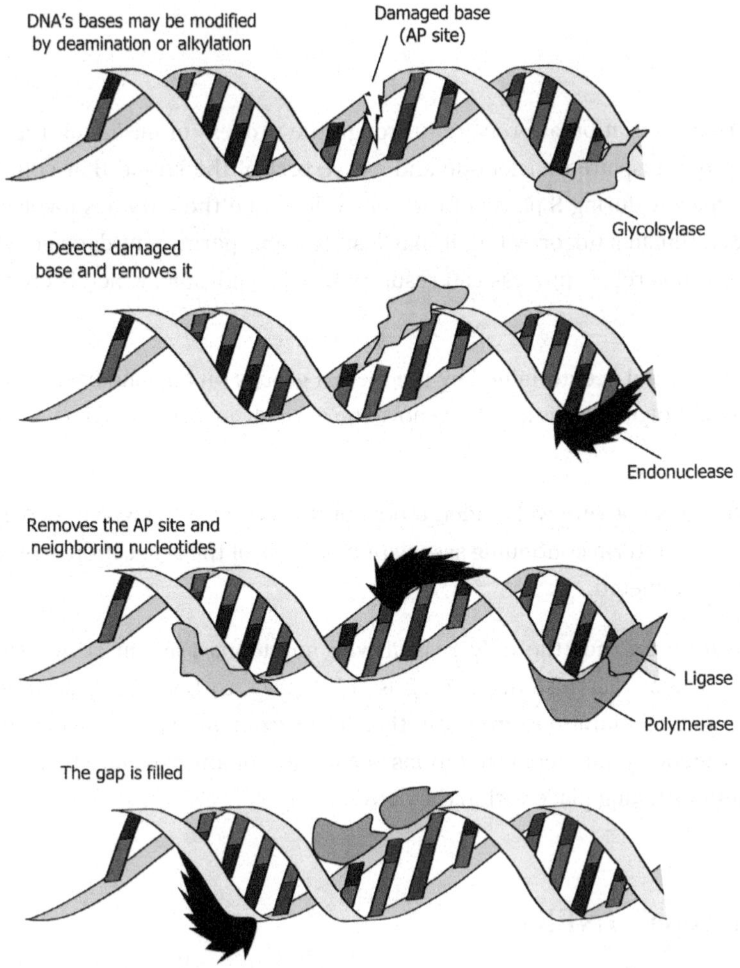

Figure 10.6: Summary of base excision repair. This is a similar process to NER but requires a glycosylase.

Double-stranded break repair

Double-stranded breaks are caused by ionizing radiation, such as X-rays or radioactive particles. This can be repaired through two processes: nonhomologous end-joining and homologous recombination. The major difference between these two processes is in nonhomologous end-joining there is direct ligation of the two ends without the need for a DNA template. This can result in some DNA being lost in the process. In contrast, homologous recombination requires a DNA template to repair the break. This allows for restoration of the duplex without a loss of nucleotides.

10.2 References and resources

Text

Clark, M. A. *Biology*, 2nd ed. Houston, TX: OpenStax College, Rice University, 2018, Chapter 14: DNA Structure and Function.

Karp, G., and J. G. Patton. *Cell and Molecular Biology: Concepts and Experiments*, 7th ed. Hoboken, NJ: John Wiley, 2013, Chapter 10: The Nature of the Gene and the Genome, Chapter 12: The Cell Nucleus and the Control of Gene Expression, Chapter 13: DNA Replication.

Le, T., and V. Bhushan. *First Aid for the USMLE Step 1*, 29th ed. New York: McGraw Hill Education, 2018, 34, 38–40.

Nussbaum, R. L., R. R. McInnes, H. F. Willard, A. Hamosh, and M. W. Thompson. *Thompson & Thompson Genetics in Medicine*, 8th ed. Philadelphia: Saunders/Elsevier, 2016, Chapter 2: The Introduction to the Human Genome.

Figures

Grey, Kindred, Figure 10.5 Comparison on three types of repair. a) Proofreading b) Mismatch and c) Nucleotide excision repair. 2021. CC BY 4.0.

Grey, Kindred, Figure 10.6 Summary of Base excision repair. This is a similar process to NER but requires a glycosylase. 2021. https://archive.org/details/10.6_20210926. CC BY-SA 4.0. Added DNA double helix grooves by Biochemlife. CC BY SA 4.0. From Wikimedia Commons.

10.3 DNA Replication

The process of DNA replication can be summarized as follows:

1. DNA unwinds at the origin of replication.
2. Helicase opens up the DNA-forming replication forks; these are extended bidirectionally.
3. Single-strand binding proteins coat the DNA around the replication fork to prevent rewinding of the DNA.
4. Topoisomerase binds at the region ahead of the replication fork to prevent supercoiling.
5. Primase synthesizes RNA primers complementary to the DNA strand.
6. DNA polymerase III starts adding nucleotides to the 3′-OH end of the primer.
7. Elongation of both the lagging and the leading strand continues.
8. RNA primers are removed by exonuclease activity.
9. Gaps are filled by DNA pol I by adding dNTPs.
10. The gap between the two DNA fragments is sealed by DNA ligase, which helps in the formation of phosphodiester bonds.

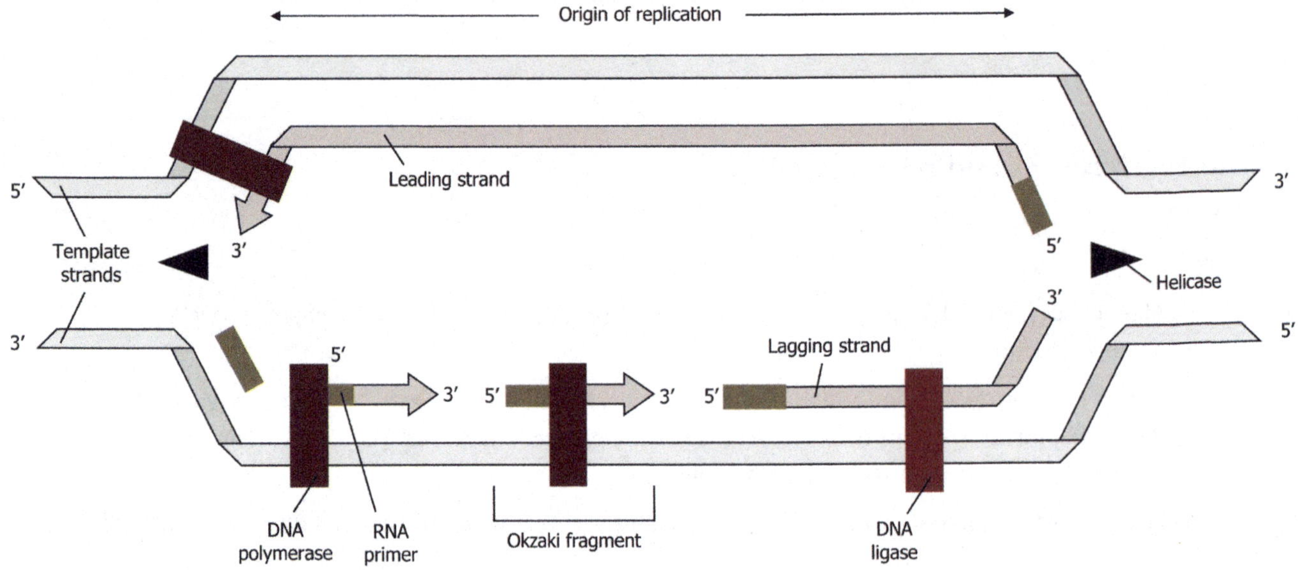

Figure 10.7: Summary of DNA replication.

DNA replication

The essential steps of replication are the same for both prokaryotes and eukaryotes. Before replication can start, the DNA has to be made available as a template. Eukaryotic DNA is bound to basic proteins known as histones to form structures called nucleosomes. Histones must be removed and then replaced during the replication process, which helps account for the lower replication rate in eukaryotes. The chromatin (the complex between DNA and proteins) may undergo some chemical modifications, so that the DNA may be able to slide off the proteins or be accessible to the enzymes of the DNA replication machinery.

One of the key players in DNA replication is the enzyme DNA polymerase, also known as DNA pol, which adds nucleotides one-by-one to the growing DNA chain that is complementary to the template strand.

In prokaryotes, three main types of polymerases are known: DNA pol I, DNA pol II, and DNA pol III.

In eukaryotes there are fourteen are known polymerases, of which five are known to have major roles during replication and have been well studied. They are known as pol α, pol β, pol γ, pol δ, and pol ε.

How does the replication machinery know where to begin?

There are specific nucleotide sequences called origins of replication where replication begins. In prokaryotes, there is typically a single origin of replication on its one chromosome, and this is in contrast to eukaryotes that have many origins of replication across the chromosomes.

The origin of replication is recognized by certain proteins that bind to this site. An enzyme called helicase unwinds the DNA by breaking the hydrogen bonds between the nitrogenous base pairs. ATP hydrolysis is required for this process. As the DNA opens up, Y-shaped structures called replication forks are formed. Two replication forks are formed at the origin of replication, and these get extended bidirectionally as replication continues. Single-strand binding proteins coat the single strands of DNA near the replication fork to prevent the single-stranded DNA from winding back into a double helix.

DNA polymerase has two important restrictions. First, it is able to add nucleotides only in the 5′ to 3′ direction (a new DNA strand can be only extended in this direction). Second, it also requires a free 3′-OH group to which it can add nucleotides by forming a phosphodiester bond between the 3′-OH end and the 5′ phosphate of the next nucleotide. This essentially means that it cannot add nucleotides if a free 3′-OH group is not available.

Then how does it add the first nucleotide? The problem is solved with the help of a primer that provides the free 3′-OH end. RNA primase synthesizes an RNA segment that is about five to ten nucleotides long and complementary to the template DNA. Because this sequence primes the DNA synthesis, it is appropriately called the primer. DNA polymerase can now extend this RNA primer, adding nucleotides one-by-one that are complementary to the template strand.

The DNA tends to become more highly coiled ahead of the replication fork. Topoisomerase breaks and reforms DNA's phosphate backbone ahead of the replication fork, thereby relieving the pressure that results from this "supercoiling." Single-strand binding proteins bind to the single-stranded DNA to prevent the helix from re-forming.

Because DNA polymerase can only extend in the 5′ to 3′ direction, and because the DNA double helix is antiparallel, there is a problem at the replication fork. The two template DNA strands have opposing orientations: one strand is in the 5′ to 3′ direction, and the other is oriented in the 3′ to 5′ direction. Only one new DNA strand, the one that is complementary to the 3′ to 5′ parental DNA strand, can be synthesized continuously toward the replication fork. This continuously synthesized strand is known as the leading strand. The other strand, complementary to the 5′ to 3′ parental DNA, is extended away from the replication fork in small fragments known as Okazaki fragments, each requiring a primer to start the synthesis. New primer segments are laid down in the direction of the replication fork, but each pointing away from it.

The overall direction of the lagging strand will be 3′ to 5′, and that of the leading strand 5′ to 3′. A protein called the sliding clamp holds the DNA polymerase in place as it continues to add nucleotides. The sliding clamp is a ring-shaped protein that binds to the DNA and holds the polymerase in place. As synthesis continues, the RNA primers are removed by the exonuclease activity of DNA pol I, which uses DNA behind the RNA as its own primer and fills in the gaps left by removal of the RNA nucleotides by the addition of DNA nucleotides. The nicks that remain between the newly synthesized DNA (that replaced the RNA primer) and the previously synthesized DNA are sealed by the enzyme DNA ligase, which catalyzes the formation of phosphodiester linkages between the 3′-OH end of one nucleotide and the 5′ phosphate end of the other fragment.

Once the chromosome has been completely replicated, the two DNA copies move into two different cells during cell division.

Telomere replication

In eukaryotes, leading strand synthesis continues until the end of the chromosome is reached. On the lagging strand, DNA is synthesized in short stretches, each of which is initiated by a separate primer. When the replication fork reaches the end of the linear chromosome, there is no way to replace the primer on the 5' end of the lagging strand.

The DNA at the ends of the chromosome thus remains unpaired, and over time these ends, called telomeres, may get progressively shorter as cells continue to divide.

Telomeres comprise repetitive sequences that code for no particular gene. In humans, a six-base-pair sequence, TTAGGG, is repeated 100 to 1,000 times in the telomere regions. In a way, these telomeres protect the genes from getting deleted as cells continue to divide. The telomeres are added to the ends of chromosomes by a separate enzyme, telomerase (figure 10.8), whose discovery helped in the understanding of how these repetitive chromosome ends are maintained. The telomerase enzyme contains a catalytic part and a built-in RNA template. It attaches to the end of the chromosome, and DNA nucleotides complementary to the RNA template are added on the 3′ end of the DNA strand. Once the 3′ end of the lagging strand template is sufficiently elongated, DNA polymerase can add the nucleotides complementary to the ends of the chromosomes. Thus, the ends of the chromosomes are replicated.

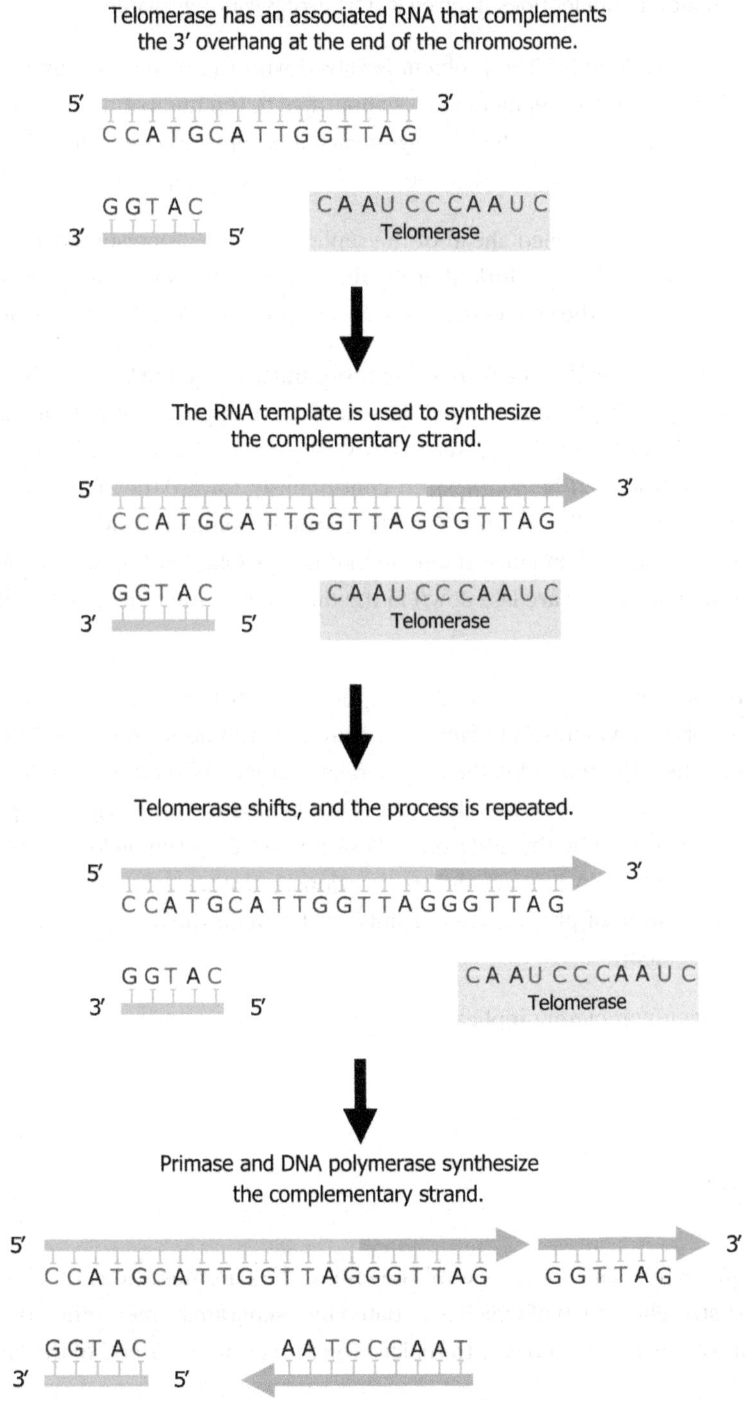

Figure 10.8: Summary of telomerase activity to fill the overhang on the lagging strand.

Prokaryotic/Eukaryotic protein	Specific function
DNA pol I	Removes RNA primer and replaces it with newly synthesized DNA
DNA pol III/Pol δ and ε	Main enzyme that adds nucleotides in the 5′-3′ direction
Helicase	Opens the DNA helix by breaking hydrogen bonds between the nitrogenous bases
Ligase	Seals the gaps between the Okazaki fragments to create one continuous DNA strand
Primase/Pol α	Synthesizes RNA primers needed to start replication
Sliding clamp	Helps to hold the DNA polymerase in place when nucleotides are being added
Topoisomerase	Helps relieve the strain on DNA when unwinding by causing breaks, and then resealing the DNA
Single-strand binding proteins (SSB)	Binds to single-stranded DNA to prevent DNA from rewinding back

Table 10.1: Prokaryotic DNA replication: enzymes and their function.

Property	Prokaryotes	Eukaryotes
Origin of replication	Single	Multiple
Rate of replication	1,000 nucleotides/s	50 to 100 nucleotides/s
DNA polymerase types	5	14
Telomerase	Not present	Present
RNA primer removal	DNA pol I	RNase H
Strand elongation	DNA pol III	Pol α, pol δ, pol ε
Sliding clamp	Sliding clamp	PCNA

Table 10.2: Difference between prokaryotic and eukaryotic replication.

10.3 References and resources

Text

Clark, M. A. *Biology*, 2nd ed. Houston, TX: OpenStax College, Rice University, 2018, Chapter 14: DNA Structure and Function.

Karp, G., and J. G. Patton. *Cell and Molecular Biology: Concepts and Experiments*, 7th ed. Hoboken, NJ: John Wiley, 2013, Chapter 10: The Nature of the Gene and the Genome, Chapter 12: The Cell Nucleus and the Control of Gene Expression, Chapter 13: DNA Replication.

Le, T., and V. Bhushan. *First Aid for the USMLE Step 1*, 29th ed. New York: McGraw Hill Education, 2018, 34, 38–40.

Nussbaum, R. L., R. R. McInnes, H. F. Willard, A. Hamosh, and M. W. Thompson. *Thompson & Thompson Genetics in Medicine*, 8th ed. Philadelphia: Saunders/Elsevier, 2016, Chapter 2: The Introduction to the Human Genome.

Figures

Grey, Kindred, Figure 10.7 Summary of DNA replication. 2021. https://archive.org/details/10.7_20210926. CC BY 4.0.

Grey, Kindred, Figure 10.8 Summary of Telomerase activity to fill the overhand on the lagging strand. 2021. CC BY 4.0.

11. Transcription and Translation

Learning Objectives

- Describe the flow of information through cells ("the central dogma") and the cell components that participate.
- Describe the structure and potential products of a gene (polypeptide, rRNA, tRNA, mRNA) and the types of proteins required for transcription (RNA polymerases, transcription factors, etc.).
- Describe the structure of mRNA, including the 5' cap and poly(A) tail.
- Summarize the processing of a pre-mRNA to mature RNA, including the splicing process (introns and exons).
- Describe the properties of the genetic code and codon assignments.
- Define the role of tRNAs in decoding the genetic code.
- Summarize the steps in all stages of translation: tRNA charging, initiation, elongation, and termination.

About this Chapter

The flow of genetic information in cells from DNA to mRNA to protein is described by the central dogma, which states that genes specify the sequence of mRNAs, which in turn specify the sequence of amino acids making up all proteins. The decoding of one molecule to another is performed by specific proteins and RNAs. Because the information stored in DNA is so central to cellular function, it makes intuitive sense that the cell would make mRNA copies of this information for protein synthesis, while keeping the DNA itself intact and protected. The copying of DNA to RNA is relatively straightforward, with one nucleotide being added to the mRNA strand for every nucleotide read in the DNA strand.

The translation to protein is a bit more complex because three mRNA nucleotides correspond to one amino acid in the polypeptide sequence. However, the translation to protein is still systematic and colinear.

11.1 Transcription

Unlike DNA synthesis, which only occurs during the S phase of the cell cycle, transcription and translation are continuous processes within the cell. The 5' to 3' strand of a DNA sequence functions as the coding (nontemplate) strand for the process of transcription such that the transcribed product will be identical to the coding strand, except for the insertion of uracil for thymidine (figure 11.1). The transcribed mRNA will serve as the template for protein translation.

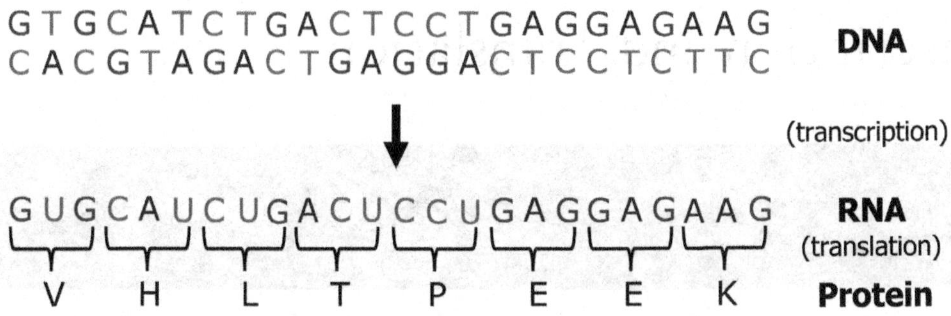

Figure 11.1: Colinearity of DNA and RNA.

Gene structure

The chromosome is organized into functional units call genes. These are specific locations on a chromosome that are composed of a transcribed region and a regulatory (or promoter) region. The transcribed region is typically (but not always) downstream of the transcriptional start and contains the following DNA elements: a 5' cap site (required for maturation of mRNA), translational start (AUG), introns and exons, and the polyadenylation site (figure 11.2).

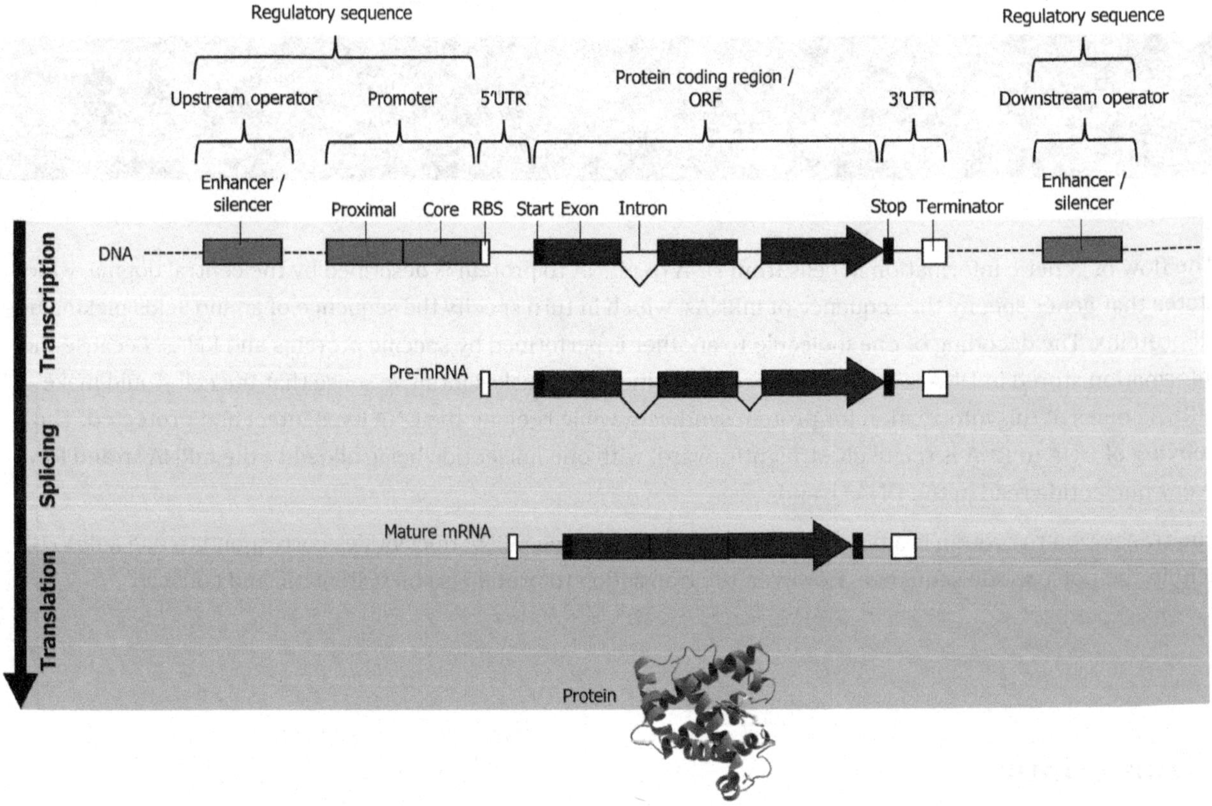

Figure 11.2: Schematic view of a eukaryotic gene structure.

The regulatory or promoter region is upstream of the transcriptional start and contains regulatory elements such as:

1. TATA box, which provides an accessible region for the DNA to begin to unwind, allowing for access by the transcriptional machinery, and
2. CAAT or GC box and enhancers or repressors (for eukaryotic transcription), which help modulate the amount of transcript produced in any given cell.

In eukaryotes, a single gene will produce one gene product as all genes are regulated independently. This is in contrast to prokaryotes, which regulate genes in an operon structure where one mRNA may be polycistronic and encode for multiple protein products.

Types of RNA polymerase

RNA polymerase I is located in the nucleolus, a specialized nuclear substructure in which ribosomal RNA (rRNA) is transcribed, processed, and assembled into ribosomes. RNA polymerase I synthesizes all the rRNAs from the tandemly duplicated set of 18S, 5.8S, and 28S ribosomal genes. (Note that the "S" designation applies to "Svedberg" units, a nonadditive value that characterizes the speed at which a particle sediments during centrifugation.)

RNA polymerase II is located in the nucleus and synthesizes all protein-coding nuclear pre-mRNAs. Eukaryotic pre-mRNAs undergo extensive processing after transcription but before translation.

RNA polymerase II is responsible for transcribing the overwhelming majority of eukaryotic genes. RNA polymerase III is also located in the nucleus. This polymerase transcribes a variety of structural RNAs that includes the 5S pre-rRNA, transfer pre-RNAs (pre-tRNAs), and small nuclear pre-RNAs. The tRNAs have a critical role in translation; they serve as the "adaptor molecules" between the mRNA template and the growing polypeptide chain. Small nuclear RNAs have a variety of functions, including "splicing" pre-mRNAs and regulating transcription factors.

Locations, products, and sensitivities of the three eukaryotic RNA polymerases

RNA polymerase	Cellular compartment	Product of transcription	α-Amanitin sensitivity
I	Nucleolus	All rRNAs except 5S rRNA	Insensitive
II	Nucleus	All protein-coding nuclear pre-mRNAs	Extremely sensitive
III	Nucleus	5S rRNA, tRNAs, and small nuclear RNAs	Moderately sensitive

Table 11.1: Locations, products, and sensitivities of the three eukaryotic RNA polymerases.

Transcription

Initiation

Eukaryotes assemble a complex of transcription factors required to recruit RNA polymerase II to a protein coding gene.

Transcription factors that bind to the promoter are called basal transcription factors. These basal factors are all called TFII (for transcription factor/polymerase II) plus an additional letter (A–J). The core complex is TFIID, which includes a TATA-binding protein (TBP). The other transcription factors systematically fall into place on the DNA template, with each one further stabilizing the pre-initiation complex and contributing to the recruitment of RNA polymerase II (figure 11.3).

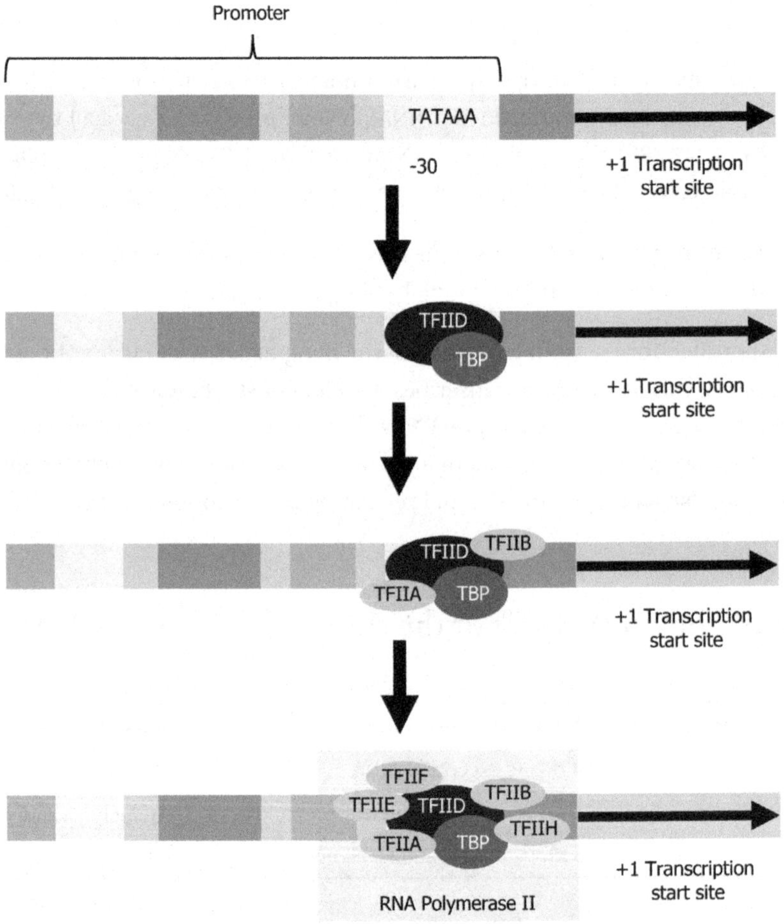

Figure 11.3: Transcription initiation.

Some eukaryotic promoters also have a conserved CAAT box (GGCCAATCT) at approximately -80. Further upstream of the TATA box, eukaryotic promoters may also contain one or more GC-rich boxes (GGCG) or octamer boxes (ATTTGCAT). These elements bind cellular factors that increase the efficiency of transcription initiation and are often identified in more "active" genes that are constantly being expressed by the cell. Other regulatory elements within the promoter region will be discussed in section 12.1.

Elongation

Following the formation of the pre-initiation complex, the polymerase is released from the other transcription factors, and elongation is allowed to proceed with the polymerase synthesizing pre-mRNA in the 5′ to 3′ direction.

Termination

The termination of transcription is different for the different polymerases. Unlike in prokaryotes, elongation by RNA polymerase II in eukaryotes takes place 1,000 to 2,000 nucleotides beyond the end of the gene being transcribed. This pre-mRNA tail is subsequently removed by cleavage during mRNA processing. Alternatively, RNA polymerases I and III require termination signals. Genes transcribed by RNA polymerase I contain a specific eighteen-nucleotide sequence that is recognized by a termination protein. The process of termination in RNA polymerase III involves an mRNA hairpin similar to rho-independent termination of transcription in prokaryotes.

Types of RNA

RNA is found in three different forms in the cell, and each is used for specific aspects of translation. Not all RNA that is transcribed is translated into a protein product; some transcribed RNA (rRNA and tRNA) is fully functional in the RNA form. mRNA (messenger RNA) is transcribed by RNA pol II.

mRNA

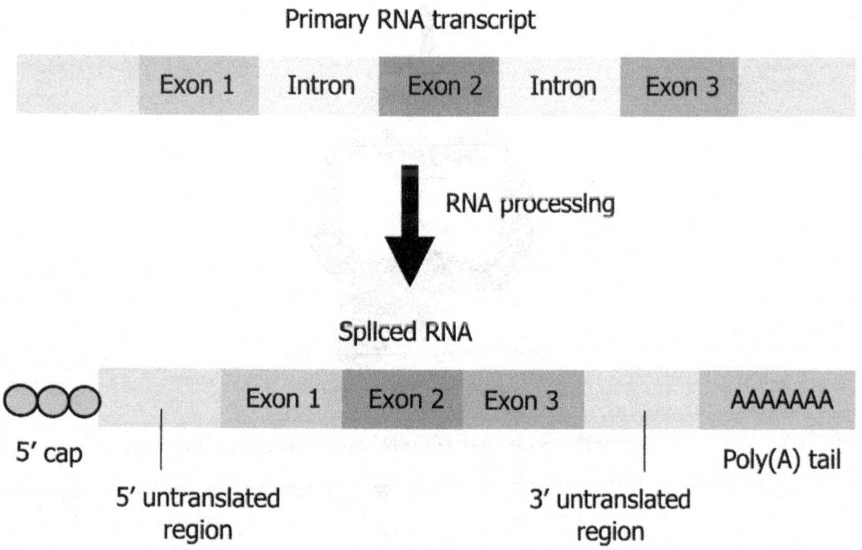

Figure 11.4: Overview of mRNA processing involving the removal of introns (splicing) and the addition of a 5' cap and 3' tail.

In eukaryotes, pre-mRNA requires maturation before use in translation including (figure 11.4):

1. 5' Capping by the addition of a 7-methylguanosine cap. Capping, resulting in the addition of two methyl groups on the 5' end, is fundamental for both mRNA stabilization and for translational initiation.
2. Addition of a poly(A) tail. The addition of the poly(A) tail also provides mRNA stability and is important for transcriptional termination. Neither the cap nor tail are part of the DNA coding regions.
3. Splicing. Splicing involves removal of introns (noncoding regions) and retention of exons (coding regions).

Splicing is a complex process mediated by a large protein RNA-associated complex called the spliceosome. The structure contains both proteins and small nuclear (sn)RNA. (Note antibodies to snRNAs are specific for systemic lupus.) Intronic sequences usually have GU at their 5′ end and AG at their 3′ end. An adenosine (A) is typically found at the branching point within the intron sequence. Small nuclear ribonucleoproteins (snRNPs) of the spliceosome recognize intron-exon junctions and splice out the intron as a "lariat" structure. Splicing starts with an autocatalytic cleavage of the 5' end of the intron leading to the formation of a circular or lariat where a 5′ UG sequence pairs with an internal adenine (A) or branch site. Finally the 3' end of the intron is cleaved, and the intron is released as a lariat, and the right side of the exon is spliced to the left side. Alternative splicing of introns and exons generates protein variation from a single mRNA (figure 11.5).

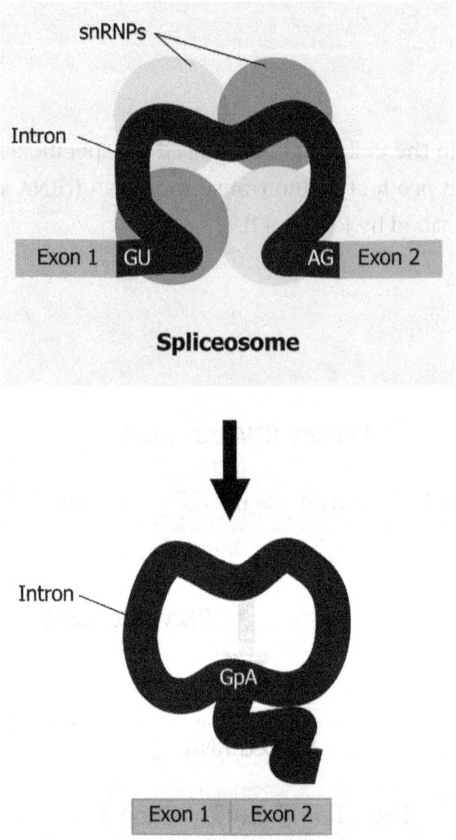

Figure 11.5: Summary of mRNA splicing.

tRNA

tRNA, transfer RNA, is transcribed by RNA pol III, and like mRNA it requires maturation including:

1. Removal of introns,
2. The addition of the 3' amino acid attachment site (CCA), and
3. Folding into a clover like structure.

tRNAs also are typical of base modifications generating nonconventional bases allowing base-pairing to several codons. This duplicity of binding is usually due to wobble in the third base pair. tRNA primarily functions to bring amino acids to the ribosome during protein translation. The anticodon on tRNA pairs with the codon on mRNA, and this determines which amino acid is added to the growing polypeptide chain.

rRNA

rRNA, ribosomal RNA, is transcribed by RNA poly I and III and requires maturation that is slightly different from mRNA and tRNA. This RNA product is not translated but rather requires methylation and is incorporated into the protein as structural support. The 18S RNA is incorporated into the 40S ribosomal subunit, and the 28S, 5.8S, and 5S is incorporated into the 60S ribosomal subunit. These combine to make the full 80S ribosome required for protein translation.

11.1 References and resources

Text

Clark, M. A. *Biology*, 2nd ed. Houston, TX: OpenStax College, Rice University, 2018, Chapter 15: Genes and Proteins.

Karp, G., and J. G. Patton. *Cell and Molecular Biology: Concepts and Experiments*, 7th ed. Hoboken, NJ: John Wiley, 2013, Chapter 11: Gene Expression: From Transcription to Translation.

Le, T., and V. Bhushan. *First Aid for the USMLE Step 1*, 29th ed. New York: McGraw Hill Education, 2018, 39, 41–45.

Nussbaum, R. L., R. R. McInnes, H. F. Willard, A. Hamosh, and M. W. Thompson. *Thompson & Thompson Genetics in Medicine*, 8th ed. Philadelphia: Saunders/Elsevier, 2016, Chapter 3: The Human Genome: Gene Structure and Function.

Figures

Grey, Kindred, Figure 11.3 Transcription initiation. 2021. https://archive.org/details/11.3_20210926. CC BY 4.0.

Grey, Kindred, Figure 11.4 Overview of mRNA processing involving the removal of introns (splicing), addition of a 5' cap and 3' tail. 2021. https://archive.org/details/11.4_20210926. CC BY 4.0.

Grey, Kindred, Figure 11.5 Summary of mRNA splicing. 2021. https://archive.org/details/11.5_20210926. CC BY 4.0.

Lieberman M, Peet A. Figure 11.1 Co-linearity of DNA and RNA. Adapted under Fair Use from Marks' Basic Medical Biochemistry. 5th Ed. pp 277. Figure 15.3 Reading frame of messenger RNA (mRNA). 2017.

Lieberman M, Peet A. Figure 11.2 Schematic view of a eukaryotic gene structure. Adapted under Fair Use from Marks' Basic Medical Biochemistry. 5th Ed. pp 255. Figure 14.4 A schematic view of a eukarytoic gene, and steps required to produce a protein product. 2017. Added Myoglobin by AzaToth. Public domain. From Wikimedia Commons.

11.2 Protein Translation

Translation is the process by which mRNAs are converted into protein products through the interactions of mRNA, tRNA, and rRNA. Even before an mRNA is translated, a cell must invest energy to build each of its ribosomes, a complex macromolecule composed of structural and catalytic rRNAs, and many distinct polypeptides. In eukaryotes, the nucleolus is completely specialized for the synthesis and assembly of rRNAs.

Ribosomes exist in the cytoplasm and rough endoplasmic reticulum of eukaryotes. Ribosomes dissociate into large and small subunits when they are not synthesizing proteins and reassociate during the initiation of translation.

- In E. *coli*, the small subunit is described as 30S, and the large subunit is 50S, for a total of 70S (recall that Svedberg units are not additive).
- Mammalian ribosomes have a small 40S subunit and a large 60S subunit, for a total of 80S. The small subunit is responsible for binding the mRNA template, whereas the large subunit sequentially binds tRNAs.

Each mRNA molecule is simultaneously translated by many ribosomes, all synthesizing protein in the same direction: reading the mRNA from 5′ to 3′ and synthesizing the polypeptide from the N terminus to the C terminus. The complete mRNA/poly-ribosome structure is called a polysome.

tRNA synthetases

Second letter

First letter	U	C	A	G	Third letter
U	UUU, UUC – Phe UUA, UUG – Leu	UCU, UCC, UCA, UCG – Ser	UAU, UAC – Tyr **UAA - STOP** **UAG - STOP**	UGU, UGC – Cys **UGA - STOP** UGG – Trp	**U C A G**
C	CUU, CUC, CUA, CUG – Leu	CCU, CCC, CCA, CCG – Pro	CAU, CAC – His CAA, CAG – Gln	CGU, CGC, CGA, CGG – Arg	**U C A G**
A	AUU, AUC, AUA – Ile **AUG** **Met**	ACU, ACC, ACA, ACG – Thr	AAU, AAC – Asn AAA, AAG – Lys	AGU, AGC – Ser AGA, AGG – Arg	**U C A G**
G	GUU, GUC, GUA, GUG – Val	GCU, GCC, GCA, GCG – Ala	GAU, GAC – Asp GAA, GAG – Glu	GGU, GGC, GGA, GGG – Gly	**U C A G**

Figure 11.6: Genetic code; each codons is three nucleotides corresponding to a specific amino acid. The code is degenerate, meaning several codes are present for the same amino acid and the codes for similar amino acids are clustered.

mRNAs are read three base pairs at a time (codon), and the reading frame will start with the first AUG (figures 11.6 and 11.7). Translation requires the formation of an aminoacyl-tRNA where tRNA is charged with the correct amino acid and brought to the translational machinery. Through the process of tRNA "charging," each tRNA molecule is linked to its correct amino acid by one of a group of enzymes called aminoacyl tRNA synthetases.

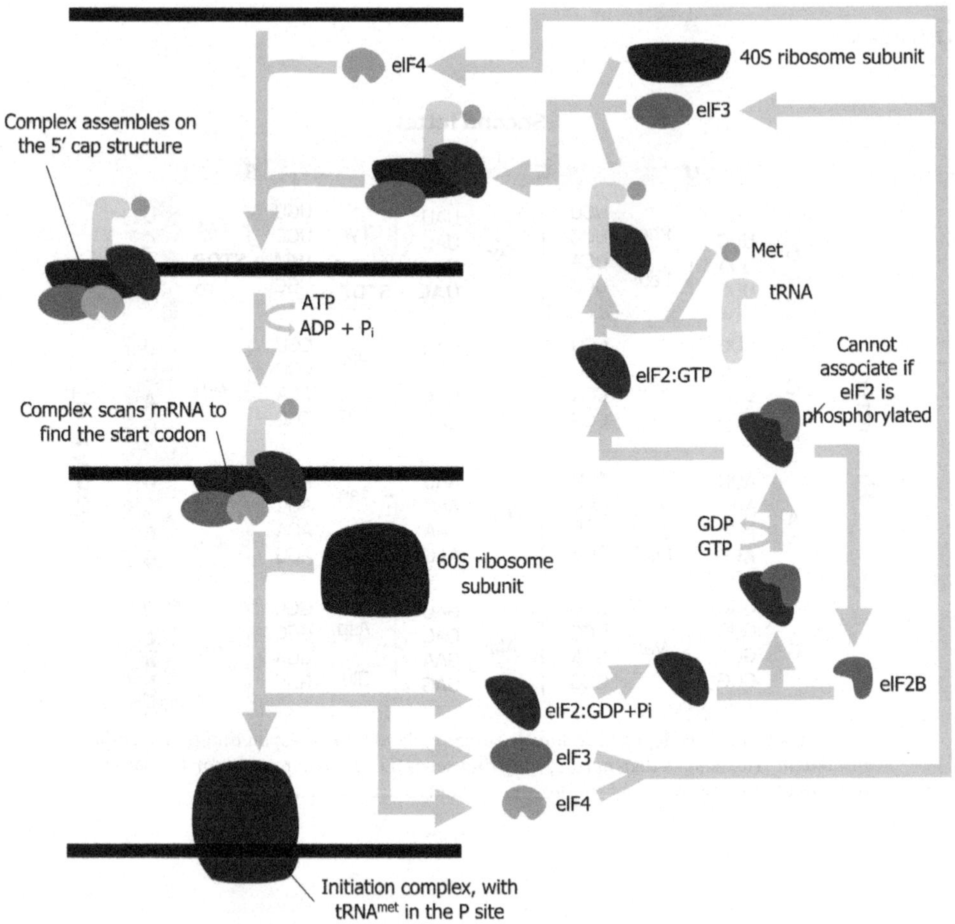

Figure 11.7: Summary of translational initiation. eIF4 recruits the small ribosomal subunit and other initiation factors to the mRNA. The charge Met-tRNA also binds the complex, and the large ribosomal subunit is recruited to the initiation complex. Once the large ribosomal subunit binds, the initiation factors can be released, and translation can proceed to elongation of the polypeptide chain.

At least one type of aminoacyl tRNA synthetase exists for each of the twenty amino acids; the exact number of aminoacyl tRNA synthetases varies by species. These enzymes first bind and hydrolyze ATP to catalyze a high-energy bond between an amino acid and adenosine monophosphate (AMP). The activated amino acid is then transferred to the tRNA, and AMP is released. The term "charging" is appropriate, since the high-energy bond that attaches an amino acid to its tRNA is later used to drive the formation of the peptide bond. Each tRNA is named for its amino acid.

Translational initiation

Translation is initiated by the assembly of the small ribosomal subunit (40S) with initiation factors (IF), which recognize the 5' cap of the mRNA. This is referred to as the cap-binding complex, and this will scan the mRNA for the initial AUG needed to start translation. Once at the cap, the initiation complex tracks along the mRNA in the 5′ to 3′ direction, searching for the AUG start codon. Many eukaryotic mRNAs are translated from the first AUG, but this is not always the case. Once the appropriate AUG is identified, the other proteins and CBP dissociate, and the 60S subunit binds to the complex of Met-tRNAi, mRNA, and the 40S subunit. This step completes the initiation of translation in eukaryotes (figure 11.8).

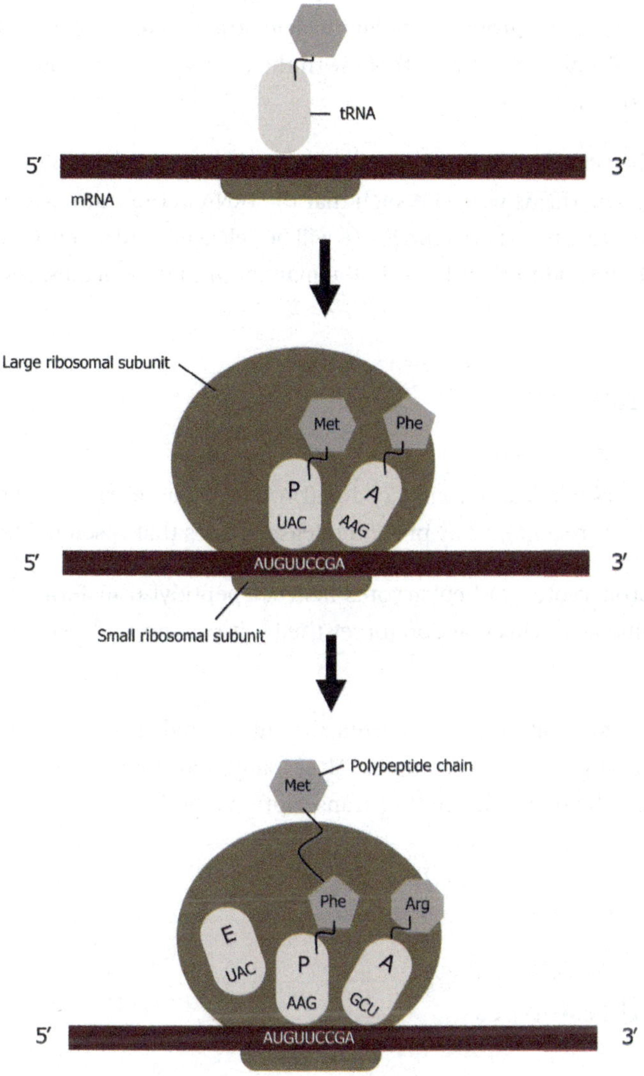

Figure 11.8: Summary of translational elongation.

Translation elongation

The ribosome has three locations for tRNA binding: A, P, and E sites.

- All tRNAs enter into the A site except for the initial methionine tRNA, which binds to the P site.
- The initial tRNA carrying methionine will attach to the ribosomal P site, and GTP is hydrolyzed, leading to the release of IF factors and recruitment of the large ribosomal subunit forming the complete ribosome.
- All tRNAs exit the ribosome through the E site.

Translation elongation requires energy in the form of GTP, and additional elongation factors (EFs) are required for this process. Elongation proceeds with charged tRNAs sequentially entering and leaving the ribosome as each new amino acid is added to the polypeptide chain. Movement of a tRNA from A to P to E sites is induced by conformational changes that advance the ribosome by three bases in the 3′ direction. GTP energy is required both for the binding of a new aminoacyl-tRNA to the A site and for its translocation to the P site after formation of the peptide bond.

Peptide bonds form between the amino group of the amino acid attached to the A-site tRNA and the carboxyl group of the amino acid attached to the P-site tRNA. A new tRNA with the corresponding amino acid coded for by the mRNA will enter into the A site of the ribosome.

The amino acid attached to the tRNA in the P site will be transferred to the tRNA in the A site; this is referred to as the peptidyl transferase react ion. The tRNAs will slide such that the tRNA in the P site will move to the E site and the tRNA in the A site will move to the P site. The tRNA in the E site will be released, and a new tRNA will enter into the A site, and the process will continue with the addition of tRNAs in the manner until the full message is transcribed (figure 11.8).

Translational termination

Termination of translation occurs when a nonsense codon (UAA, UAG, or UGA) is encountered. Upon aligning with the A site, these nonsense codons are recognized by protein release factors that resemble tRNAs.

The release factors in both prokaryotes and eukaryotes instruct peptidyl transferase to add a water molecule to the carboxyl end of the P-site amino acid. This reaction forces the P-site amino acid to detach from its tRNA, and the newly made protein is released.

The small and large ribosomal subunits dissociate from the mRNA and from each other; they are recruited almost immediately into another translation initiation complex. After many ribosomes have completed translation, the mRNA is degraded so the nucleotides can be reused in another transcription reaction.

11.2 References and resources

Text

Clark, M. A. *Biology*, 2nd ed. Houston, TX: OpenStax College, Rice University, 2018, Chapter 15: Genes and Proteins.

Karp, G., and J. G. Patton. *Cell and Molecular Biology: Concepts and Experiments*, 7th ed. Hoboken, NJ: John Wiley, 2013, Chapter 11: Gene Expression: From Transcription to Translation.

Le, T., and V. Bhushan. *First Aid for the* USMLE *Step* 1, 29th ed. New York: McGraw Hill Education, 2018, 39, 41–45.

Nussbaum, R. L., R. R. McInnes, H. F. Willard, A. Hamosh, and M. W. Thompson. *Thompson & Thompson Genetics in Medicine*, 8th ed. Philadelphia: Saunders/Elsevier, 2016, Chapter 3: The Human Genome: Gene Structure and Function.

Figures

Grey, Kindred, Figure 11.6 Genetic code, each codons is 3 nucleotides corresponding to a specific amino acid. The code is degenerate meaning several codes are present for the same amino acid and the codes for similar amino acids are clustered. 2021. https://archive.org/details/11.6_20210926. CC BY 4.0.

Grey, Kindred, Figure 11.7: Summary of translational initiation. 2021. CC BY SA 3.0. Adapted from Eukaryotic Translation Initiation by Chewie. CC BY SA 3.0. From Wikimedia Commons.

Grey, Kindred, Figure 11.8 Summary of translational elongation. 2021. CC BY 4.0.

12. Gene Regulation and the Cell Cycle

Learning Objectives

- Describe the structure of the nucleus and the nuclear envelope.
- Describe the role of transcription factors in the control of gene expression in eukaryotes.
- Describe the common features of transcription factor structure, especially DNA-binding sites.
- Describe the strategies used by eukaryotes to regulate gene expression at the level of transcription, mRNA processing, translation, and post-translation.
- Outline and define the stages in the cell cycle: M, G_1, S, G_2, and, occasionally, G_0.
- Describe the control of the cell cycle, emphasizing the participation of protein kinases and cyclins in the process.
- Emphasize the idea of checkpoints in the cell cycle and their importance to cell survival.
- Describe what is known about the mechanisms of genetic recombination during meiosis.

About this Chapter

Gene expression patterns are complex and dynamic. The expression of a gene can be regulated on many levels and will be influenced in a tissue-specific (basis for different cell types) pattern, can be developmentally controlled (temporal and spatial expression patterns), or can be environmentally influenced (induction in response to external stimuli).

Some genes (the so-called "house-keeping genes") are likely (constitutively) expressed in all cell types since certain proteins (and RNAs) are involved in the basic metabolic processes common to all cell types. Other genes are expressed in one cell type but not another (e.g., certain immune cells normally synthesize antibodies, but neurons do not). Thus, different cell types arise because of differential gene expression, and the RNA and protein content of different cell types shows considerable variation.

12.1 Eukaryotic Gene Regulation

Control of gene expression can be exerted at many levels and can be broadly divided into: changes in DNA content or position and changes in gene activity (e.g., expression patterns).

Changes to DNA content and rearrangement are addressed elsewhere. Briefly, DNA of different cell types does not vary in either amount or type. However, highly specialized cases are known to exist where DNA loss, rearrangement, and amplification profoundly influence gene expression in isolated situations.

This section will focus on changes in gene expression.

Regulation is known to occur at several different points of a multistep gene expression pathway. Four main levels of control include:

1. Transcriptional control: Determines if, how much, and when an mRNA is made.

2. Processing or post-transcriptional control: Determines if, how much, and when an mRNA is available for translation into a protein.

3. Translational control: Determines if, how much, and when a protein is made.

4. Post-translational control: Determines if, how much, and when a protein is functional.

Transcriptional control

Control of transcriptional initiation is a primary means used to regulate gene expression in eukaryotic organisms. Most eukaryotic genes are controlled at the level of transcription by proteins (trans-acting factors) that interact with specific gene sequences (cis-acting regulatory sequences).

Transcription factors: Enhancers

Along with general transcription factors, there are additional regions that help increase or enhance transcription. These regions, called enhancers, are not necessarily close to the genes they enhance. They can be located upstream of a gene, within the coding region of the gene, downstream of a gene, or thousands of nucleotides away.

Enhancer regions are binding sequences, or sites, for specific transcription factors. When a protein transcription factor binds to its enhancer sequence, the shape of the protein changes, allowing it to interact with proteins at the promotor site. However, since the enhancer region may be distant from the promoter, the DNA must bend to allow the proteins at the two sites to come into contact. DNA-bending proteins help bend the DNA and bring the enhancer and promoter regions together (figure 12.1). This shape change allows for the interaction of the specific activator proteins bound to the enhancers with the general transcription factors bound to the promoter region and the RNA polymerase. Two different genes may have the same promoter but different distal control elements, enabling differential gene expression.

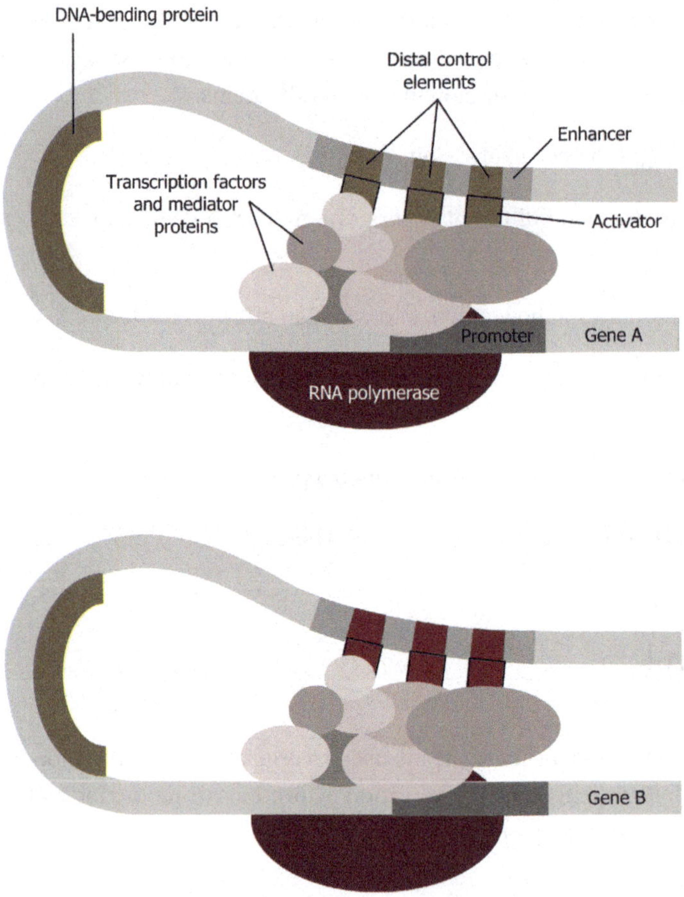

Figure 12.1: Example of transcriptional complex involving two separate genes.

Transcription factors: Repressors

Like prokaryotic cells, eukaryotic cells also have mechanisms to prevent transcription. Transcriptional repressors can bind to promoter or enhancer regions and block transcription. Like the transcriptional activators, repressors respond to external stimuli preventing the binding of activating transcription factors. This is often done by histone deacetylation, which increases the interaction of DNA and histones (figure 12.2).

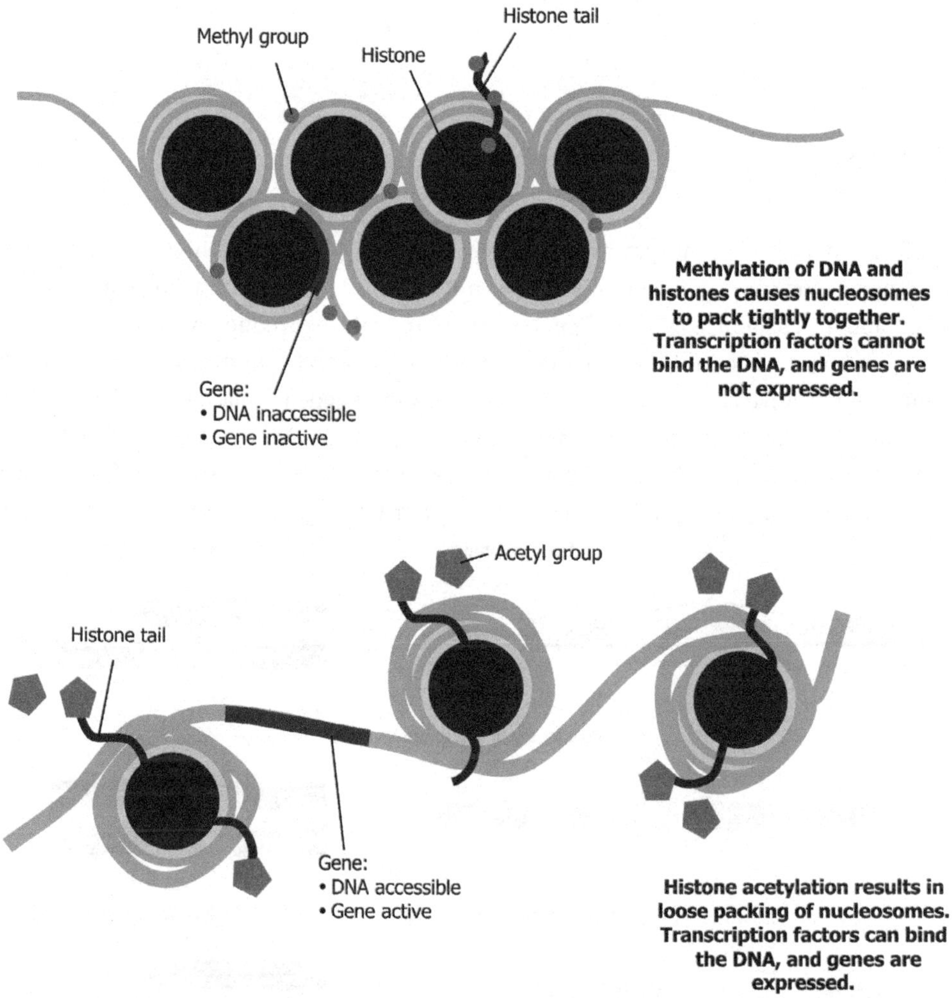

Figure 12.2: Modification of DNA and histones can alter DNA accessibility and therefore transcription.

Transcription factors: Structure and function

Structurally, transcription factors share similar characteristics but can take on very different secondary structures. Common examples of transcription factors include: Zn fingers, helix-loop-helixs, and leucine zippers. Regardless of structure, common characteristics include:

1. A positively charged DNA-binding domain,
2. Activation domain, and
3. Dimerization domain.

As noted above, one of the major roles of transcription factors is to bend or remodel the DNA in a way to allow for interactions of transcription factors and their binding sites. Chromatin remodeling by modifications of the histones (through acetylation or shifting) is common (figure 12.2).

Processing or post/cotranscription

Alternative RNA splicing

Alternative RNA splicing is a mechanism that allows different protein products to be produced from one gene when different combinations of exons are combined to form the mRNA. This alternative splicing can be haphazard, but more often it is controlled and acts as a mechanism of gene regulation, with the frequency of different splicing alternatives controlled by the cell as a way to control the production of different protein products in different cells or at different stages of development. Alternative splicing is a common mechanism of gene regulation in eukaryotes; according to one estimate, 70 percent of genes in humans are expressed as multiple proteins through alternative splicing. Although there are multiple ways to alternatively splice RNA transcripts, the original 5′-3′ order of the exons is always conserved. That is, a transcript with exons 1 2 3 4 5 6 7 might be spliced 1 2 4 5 6 7 or 1 2 3 6 7, but never 1 2 5 4 3 6 7 (figure 12.3).

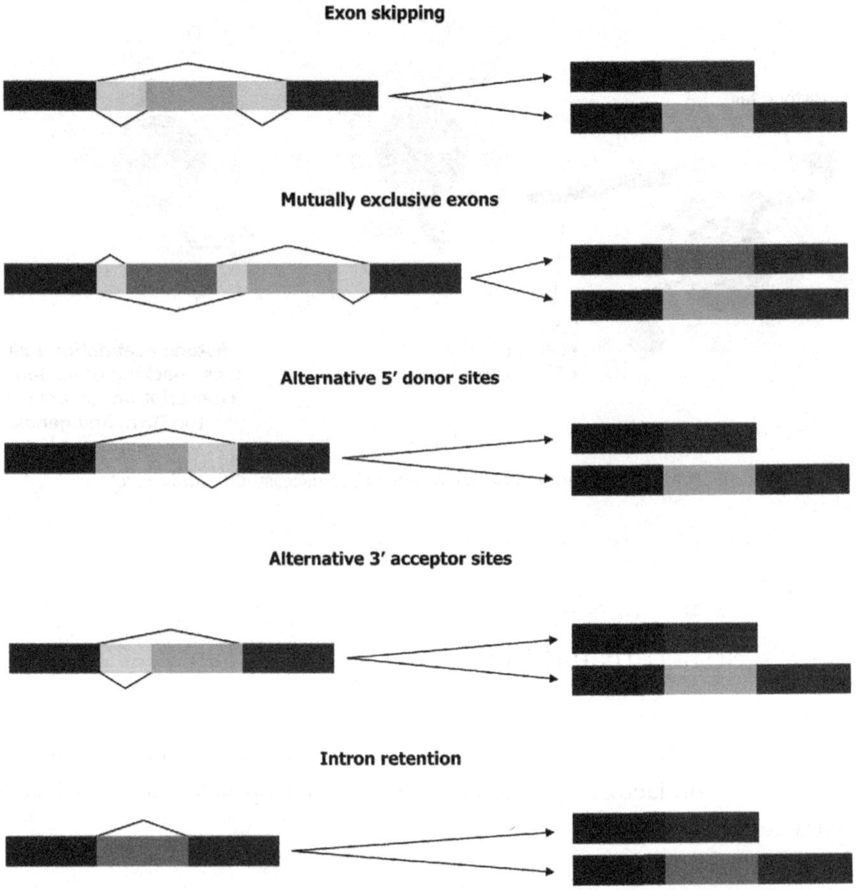

Figure 12.3: Five common modes of alternative splicing.

Translational control

Like transcription, translation is controlled by proteins that bind and initiate the process, restrict access to the mRNA, or control the localization of the transcript itself.

Localization

One fundamental way in which translation is controlled is physically by where the mRNA is located within the cell or organism. This is extremely important in development where restriction of a transcript to one side of a cell can influence the phenotype of a localized cellular region. This is largely mediated by interactions with the 5' untranslated region (UTR).

Translational initiation

In translation, the complex that assembles to start the process is referred to as the translation initiation complex, and similar to transcription, this complex can be activated or inhibited. In eukaryotes, translation is initiated by binding the initiating met-tRNAi to the 40S ribosome.

Initially the met-tRNAi is brought to the 40S ribosome by a protein initiation factor, eukaryotic initiation factor-2 (eIF-2). The eIF-2 protein binds to the high-energy molecule guanosine triphosphate (GTP), and the tRNA-eIF2-GTP complex then binds to the 40S ribosome.

The cap-binding protein eIF4F brings the mRNA complex together with the 40S ribosome complex. The ribosome then scans along the mRNA until it finds a start codon AUG. When the anticodon of the initiator tRNA and the start codon are aligned, the GTP is hydrolyzed, the initiation factors are released, and the large 60S ribosomal subunit binds to form the translation complex. Insulin increases the efficiency of formation of the cap-binding complex, therefore increasing the rate of protein synthesis.

The binding of eIF-2 to the RNA is controlled by phosphorylation. If eIF-2 is phosphorylated, it undergoes a conformational change and cannot bind to GTP. Therefore, the initiation complex cannot form properly, and translation is impeded (figure 12.4).

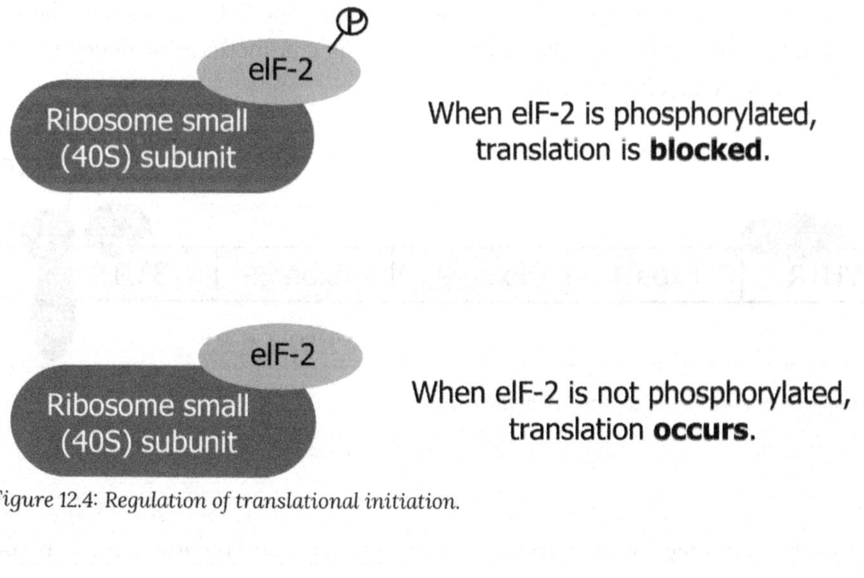

Figure 12.4: Regulation of translational initiation.

When eIF-2 remains unphosphorylated, the initiation complex can form normally, and translation can continue.

Control of RNA stability

Before the mRNA leaves the nucleus, it is given two protective "caps" that prevent the ends of the strand from degrading during its journey. These changes protect the two ends of the RNA from exonuclease attack.

1. The 5′ cap, which is placed on the 5′ end of the mRNA, is usually composed of a methylated guanosine triphosphate molecule (GTP). The GTP is placed "backward" on the 5′ end of the mRNA, so that the 5′ carbons of the GTP and the terminal nucleotide are linked through three phosphates.
2. The poly(A) tail, which is attached to the 3′ end, is usually composed of a long chain of adenine nucleotides.

Once the RNA is transported to the cytoplasm, the length of time that the RNA resides there can be controlled. Each RNA molecule has a defined lifespan and decays at a specific rate. This rate of decay can influence how much protein is in the cell.

- If the decay rate is increased, the RNA will not exist in the cytoplasm as long, shortening the time available for translation of the mRNA to occur.
- Conversely, if the rate of decay is decreased, the mRNA molecule will reside in the cytoplasm longer and more protein can be translated.

RNA-binding proteins

Binding of proteins to the RNA can also influence its stability. Proteins called RNA-binding proteins, or RBPs, can bind to the regions of the mRNA just upstream or downstream of the protein-coding region. These regions in the RNA that are not translated into protein are called the untranslated regions, or UTRs (figure 12.5). They are not introns (those have been removed in the nucleus). Rather, these are regions that regulate mRNA localization, stability, and protein translation. The region just before the protein-coding region is called the 5′ UTR, whereas the region after the coding region is called the 3′ UTR. The binding of RBPs to these regions can increase or decrease the stability of an RNA molecule, depending on the specific RBP that binds.

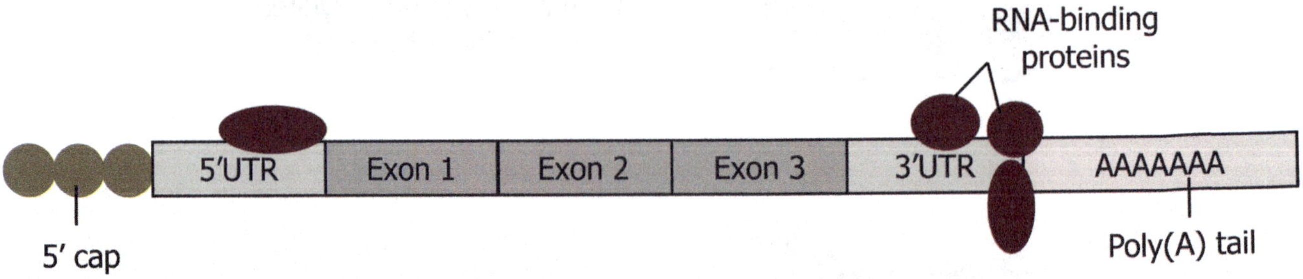

Figure 12.5: RNA-Binding proteins can increase stability of the transcript.

One classic example of this is the regulation of transferrin receptor (TR) and ferritin levels in response to iron.

- Iron is transported in the blood bound to the iron transport protein, transferrin. Transferrin receptors (TRs) are required to bring extracellular iron from the bloodstream into cells (i.e., iron uptake).
- Ferritin, a protein involved in iron storage, is also regulated post-transcriptionally. The half-life of these mRNAs is regulated by iron concentrations.

- The translation of ferritin mRNAs is regulated by the concentration of iron.
- The 5' UTR of transferrin receptor mRNA contains a single irons response element (IRE) that mediates the effect.
  - When iron is low, the iron-responsive protein (IRP) binds the IRE to block ferritin mRNA translation.
  - When iron is high, IRP cannot bind IRE, and ferritin mRNA is translated.

microRNAs

In addition to RBPs that bind to and control (increase or decrease) RNA stability, other elements called microRNAs can bind to the RNA molecule. These microRNAs, or miRNAs, are short RNA molecules that are only twenty-one to twenty-four nucleotides in length. The miRNAs are made in the nucleus as longer pre-miRNAs.

These pre-miRNAs are chopped into mature miRNAs by a protein called dicer. Like transcription factors and RBPs, mature miRNAs recognize a specific sequence and bind to the RNA; however, miRNAs also associate with a ribonucleoprotein complex called the RNA-induced silencing complex (RISC). The RNA component of the RISC base-pairs with complementary sequences on an mRNA and either impede translation of the message or lead to the degradation of the mRNA.

Post-translation regulation

Chemical modifications

Proteins can be chemically modified with the addition of groups including methyl, phosphate, acetyl, and ubiquitin groups.

The addition or removal of these groups from proteins can have many effects and can be in response to many cellular changes. For example:

- Covalent modifications can regulate protein activity.
- Sometimes these modifications can regulate where a protein is found in the cell — for example, in the nucleus, in the cytoplasm, or attached to the plasma membrane.
- Chemical modifications occur in response to external stimuli such as stress, the lack of nutrients, heat, or ultraviolet light exposure.
- These changes can alter epigenetic accessibility, transcription, mRNA stability, or translation — all resulting in changes in expression of various genes.

This is an efficient way for the cell to rapidly change the levels of specific proteins in response to the environment. Because proteins are involved in every stage of gene regulation, the phosphorylation of a protein (depending on the protein that is modified) can alter accessibility to the chromosome, can alter translation (by altering transcription factor binding or function), can change nuclear shuttling (by influencing modifications to the nuclear pore complex), can alter RNA stability (by binding or not binding to the RNA to regulate its stability), can modify translation (increase or decrease), or can change post-translational modifications (add or remove phosphates or other chemical modifications).

Protein degradation

The addition of an ubiquitin group to a protein marks that protein for degradation. Ubiquitin acts like a flag indicating that the protein lifespan is complete. These proteins are moved to the proteasome, an organelle that functions to remove proteins, to be degraded. One way to control gene expression, therefore, is to alter the longevity of the protein (figure 12.6).

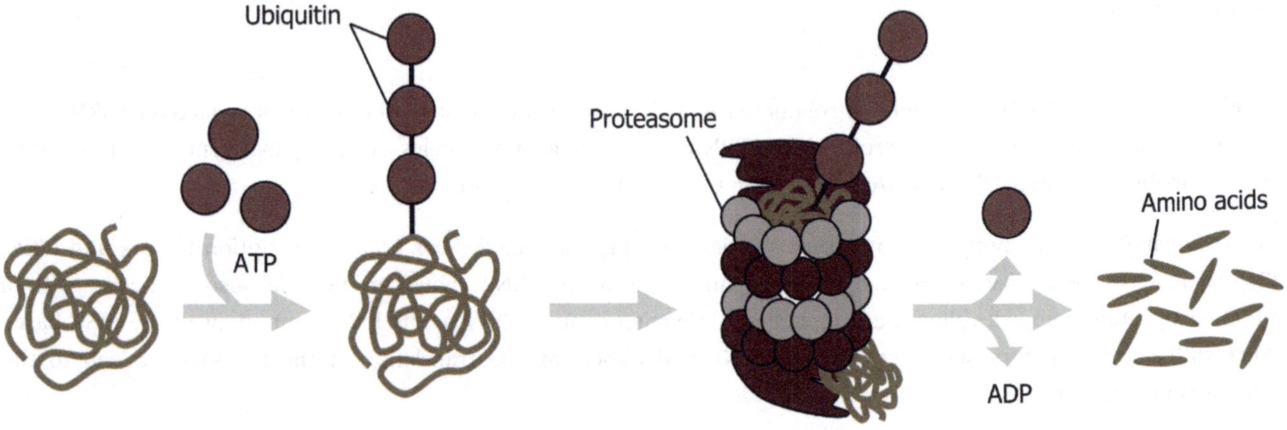

Figure 12.6: Proteasome-mediated degradation.

12.1 References and resources

Text

Clark, M. A. *Biology*, 2nd ed. Houston, TX: OpenStax College, Rice University, 2018, Chapter 10: Cell Reproduction, Chapter 11: Meiosis and Sexual Reproduction, Chapter 16: Gene Expression.

Karp, G., and J. G. Patton. *Cell and Molecular Biology: Concepts and Experiments*, 7th ed. Hoboken, NJ: John Wiley, 2013, Chapter 11: Gene Expression: From Transcription to Translation, Chapter 12: The Cell Nucleus and the Control of Gene Expression, Chapter 13: DNA Replication and Repair, Chapter 14: Cellular Reproduction.

Le, T., and V. Bhushan. *First Aid for the USMLE Step 1*, 29th ed. New York: McGraw Hill Education, 2018, 41–43, 46.

Nussbaum, R. L., R. R. McInnes, H. F. Willard, A. Hamosh, and M. W. Thompson. *Thompson & Thompson Genetics in Medicine*, 8th ed. Philadelphia: Saunders/Elsevier, 2016, Chapter 3: The Human Genome: Gene Structure and Function.

Figures

Grey, Kindred, Figure 12.1 Example of transcriptional complex involving two separate genes. 2021. CC BY 4.0. Adapted from Biology 2e Figure 16.10 Interaction between proteins at the promoter and enhancer sites. CC BY 4.0. From OpenStax.

Grey, Kindred, Figure 12.2 Modification of DNA and histones can alter DNA accessibility and therefore transcription. 2021. CC BY 4.0. Adapted from Biology 2e. Figure 16.8 Nucleosomes can slide along DNA. CC BY 4.0. From OpenStax.

Grey, Kindred, Figure 12.3 Five common modes of alternative splicing. 2021. https://archive.org/details/12.3_20210926. CC BY 4.0.

Grey, Kindred, Figure 12.4 Regulation of translational initiation. 2021. https://archive.org/details/12.4_20210926. CC BY 4.0.

Lieberman M, Peet A. Figure 12.5 RNA Binding proteins can increase stability of the transcript. Adapted under Fair Use from Marks' Basic Medical Biochemistry. 5th Ed. pp 312. Figure 16.21 Translational regulation of ferritin synthesis. 2017.

Lieberman M, Peet A. Figure 12.6 Proteasome mediated degradation. Adapted under Fair Use from Marks' Basic Medical Biochemistry. 5th Ed. pp 312. Figure 35.6 The proteasome and regulatory proteins. 2017.

12.2 Cell Cycle

Note

Checkpoints are the most critical, and the full summary of mitosis is for background.

Cells on the path to cell division proceed through a series of precisely timed and carefully regulated stages of growth, DNA replication, and division that produce two genetically identical cells. The cell cycle has two major phases: interphase and the mitotic phase. During interphase, the cell grows, and DNA is replicated. During the mitotic phase, the replicated DNA and cytoplasmic contents are separated, and the cell divides.

The cycle is divided into four distinct phases, G_1, S, G_2, and M (mitosis), and for most mammalian cells in culture this process takes about twenty-four hours to complete. The majority of differentiated cells in the body are not dividing, retained in a resting state or G_0 (figure 12.7).

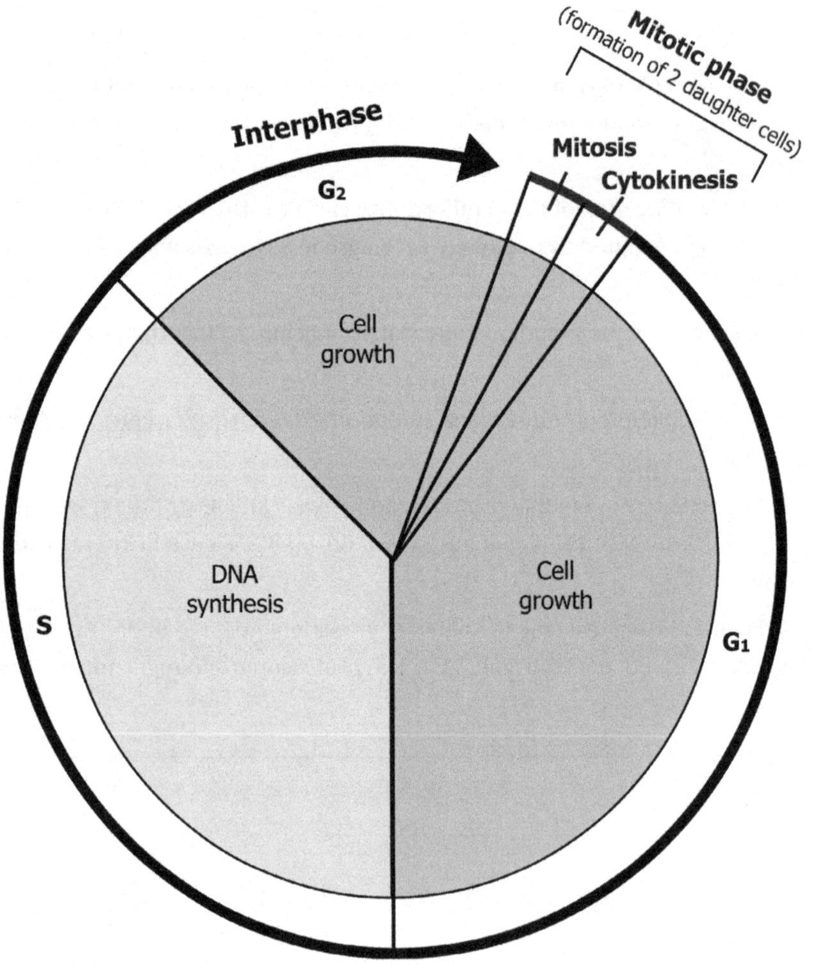

Figure 12.7: Overview of the cell cycle.

Interphase

During interphase, the cell undergoes normal processes while also preparing for cell division. For a cell to move from interphase to the mitotic phase, many internal and external conditions must be met. The three stages of interphase are called G_1, S, and G_2.

G_1 phase

The first stage of interphase is called the G_1 phase, or first gap, because little change is visible. However, during the G_1 stage, the cell is quite active at the biochemical level. The cell is accumulating the building blocks of chromosomal DNA and the associated proteins, as well as accumulating enough energy reserves to complete the task of replicating each chromosome in the nucleus.

S phase

Throughout interphase, nuclear DNA remains in a semicondensed chromatin configuration. In the S phase (synthesis phase), DNA replication results in the formation of two identical copies of each chromosome (sister chromatids) that are firmly attached at the centromere region. At this stage, each chromosome is made of two sister chromatids and is a duplicated chromosome. The centrosome is duplicated during the S phase. The two centrosomes will give rise to the mitotic spindle, the apparatus that orchestrates the movement of chromosomes during mitosis. The centrosome consists of a pair of rod-like centrioles at right angles to each other. Centrioles help organize cell division.

G_2 phase

In the G_2 phase, or second gap, the cell replenishes its energy stores and synthesizes the proteins necessary for chromosome manipulation. Some cell organelles are duplicated, and the cytoskeleton is dismantled to provide resources for the mitotic spindle. The final preparations for the mitotic phase must be completed before the cell is able to enter the first stage of mitosis.

The mitotic phase

To make two daughter cells, the contents of the nucleus and the cytoplasm must be divided. The mitotic phase is a multistep process during which the duplicated chromosomes are aligned, separated, and moved to opposite poles of the cell, and then the cell is divided into two new identical daughter cells. The first portion of the mitotic phase, mitosis, is composed of five stages, which accomplish nuclear division. The second portion of the mitotic phase, called cytokinesis, is the physical separation of the cytoplasmic components into two daughter cells (figure 12.8).

Mitosis

Mitosis is divided into a series of phases — prophase, prometaphase, metaphase, anaphase, and telophase — that result in the division of the cell nucleus (figure 12.8).

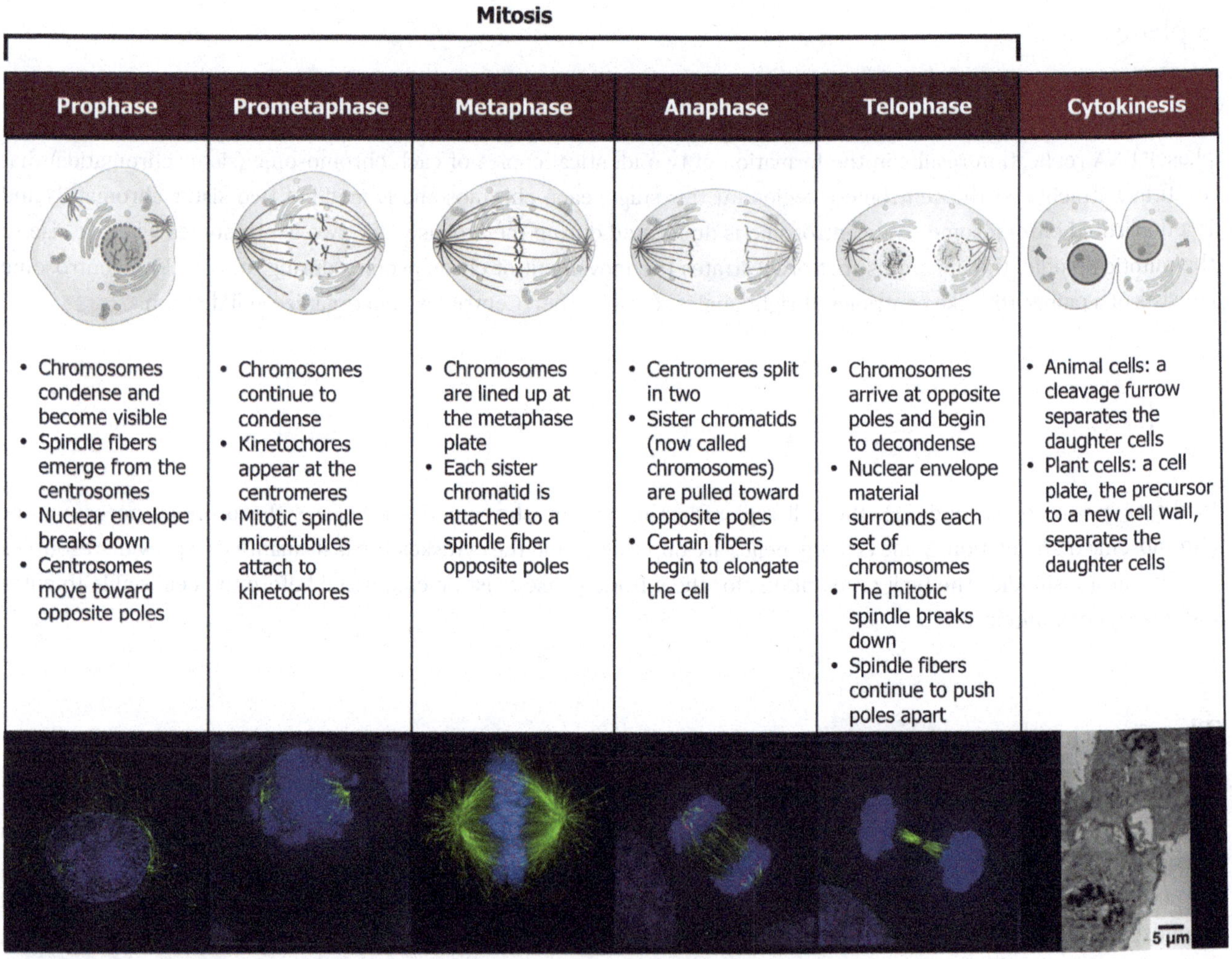

Figure 12.8: Summary of the mitotic phase.

During **prophase**, the "first phase," several events must occur to provide access to the chromosomes in the nucleus. The nuclear envelope starts to break into small vesicles, and the Golgi apparatus and endoplasmic reticulum fragment and disperse to the periphery of the cell. The nucleolus disappears. The centrosomes begin to move to opposite poles of the cell. The microtubules that form the basis of the mitotic spindle extend between the centrosomes, pushing them farther apart as the microtubule fibers lengthen. The sister chromatids begin to coil more tightly and become visible under a light microscope.

During **prometaphase**, many processes that were begun in prophase continue to advance and culminate in the formation of a connection between the chromosomes and cytoskeleton. The remnants of the nuclear envelope disappear. The mitotic spindle continues to develop as more microtubules assemble and stretch across the length of the former nuclear area. Chromosomes become more condensed and visually discrete. Each sister chromatid attaches to spindle microtubules at the centromere via a protein complex called the kinetochore.

During **metaphase**, all the chromosomes are aligned in a plane called the metaphase plate, or the equatorial plane, midway between the two poles of the cell. The sister chromatids are still tightly attached to each other. At this time, the chromosomes are maximally condensed.

During **anaphase**, the sister chromatids at the equatorial plane are split apart at the centromere. Each chromatid, now called a chromosome, is pulled rapidly toward the centrosome to which its microtubule was attached. The cell becomes visibly elongated as the nonkinetochore microtubules slide against each other at the metaphase plate where they overlap.

During **telophase**, all the events that set up the duplicated chromosomes for mitosis during the first three phases are reversed. The chromosomes reach the opposite poles and begin to decondense (unravel). The mitotic spindles are broken down into monomers that will be used to assemble cytoskeleton components for each daughter cell. Nuclear envelopes form around chromosomes.

Control of the cell cycle

There are three key checkpoints in the cell cycle that provide regulation oversight:

- G_1 checkpoint,
- G_2/M checkpoint, and
- Metaphase checkpoint.

Progress through these checkpoints is regulated by a family of cyclin dependent kinases (CDKs). These proteins are constitutive (always present) and inactive. CDKs bind specific cyclin activators, which are required for activity of the kinase. CDKs are present throughout the cell cycle, but expression of the cyclins is restricted to certain times in the cycle, and they are rapidly degraded as the cells progress through the checkpoints. Through binding of cyclins and negative regulation by phosphorylation by CDK inhibitors (CKIs), the cycle is tightly regulated in a restricted manner.

The cyclin and CDK complex can be produced from a combination of different cyclins (A-D) and different CDKs (1-6).

Rb-protein

Rb-protein (pRb, retinoblastoma protein) is an important substrate of the G_1/S-CDK complexes. During the G_0 and G_1 phases, Rb is present in an unphosphorylated (hypophosphorylationed) form, which binds to the transcription factor E2F and thereby blocks it from initiating transcription. When the cycle moves into the S1 phase, pRb becomes phosphorylated (by the CyclinD/CDK4/6 active complex), which allows for the release of E2F.

DNA damage

During the process of DNA replication, DNA damage will halt the process until it can be repaired. Likewise, extrinsic damaging factors can trigger a DNA repair process. Protein p53 is commonly known for its role in DNA repair mechanisms. Under nonstressful conditions it is bound to mdm2 within the cytosol. In response to stress and DNA damage, it is activated, through ATM- or ATR-mediated phosphorylation. Once active, it functions as a transcription factor and induces the synthesis of protein p21.

p21 will then act as a CDK inhibitor (Cip/Kip family) and blocks the action of the G_1-CDK complex. This will halt the cell cycle at the transition to the S1 phase, and the DNA can be repaired at leisure (figure 12.9). When this has been successfully completed, p53 is dephosphorylated, ubiquitinylated, and passed on to the proteasome. Thus, p53 does not accumulate in normal cells.

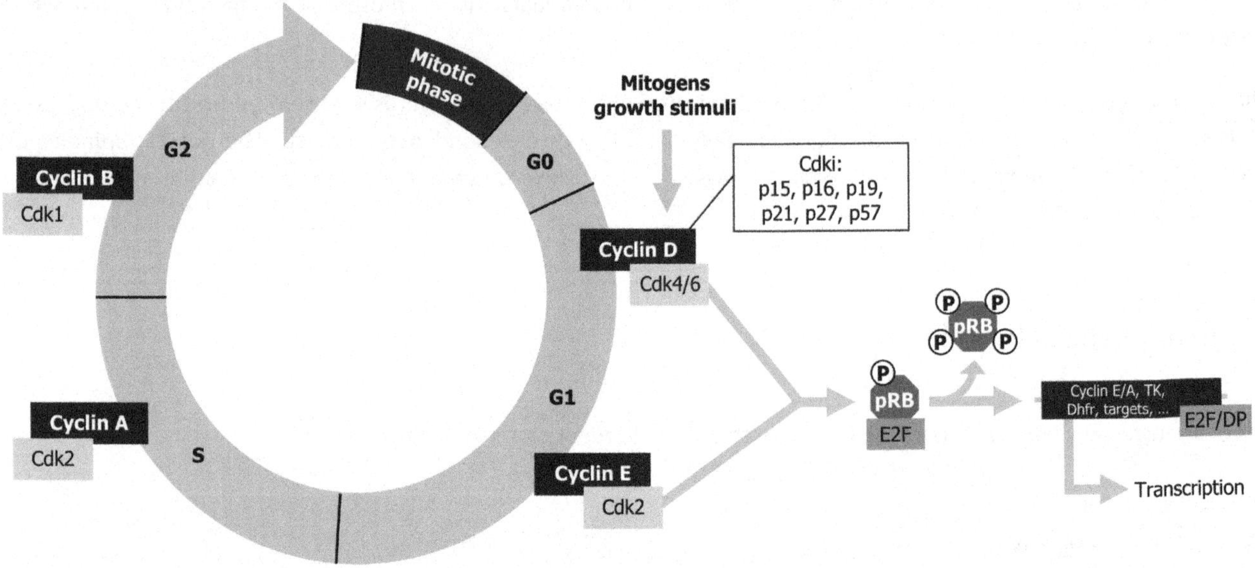

Figure 12.9: Summary of cell cycle checkpoints and the role of CDK inhibitors in halting cell cycle progress.

If the DNA repair systems do not succeed in eliminating the DNA damage, a steady increase in the concentration of phosphorylated p53 finally drives the cell into apoptosis. Proteins pRb and p53 are products of tumor suppressor genes. Complete absence of them, due to mutations, leads to accelerated cell division, a typical feature of tumors. In fact, somatic mutations in pRb and p53 have been found in more than half of all human tumors (figure 12.9).

12.2 References and resources

Text

Clark, M. A. *Biology*, 2nd ed. Houston, TX: OpenStax College, Rice University, 2018, Chapter 10: Cell Reproduction, Chapter 11: Meiosis and Sexual Reproduction, Chapter 16: Gene Expression.

Karp, G., and J. G. Patton. *Cell and Molecular Biology: Concepts and Experiments*, 7th ed. Hoboken, NJ: John Wiley, 2013, Chapter 11: Gene Expression: From Transcription to Translation, Chapter 12: The Cell Nucleus and the Control of Gene Expression, Chapter 13: DNA Replication and Repair, Chapter 14: Cellular Reproduction.

Le, T., and V. Bhushan. *First Aid for the USMLE Step 1*, 29th ed. New York: McGraw Hill Education, 2018, 41–43, 46.

Nussbaum, R. L., R. R. McInnes, H. F. Willard, A. Hamosh, and M. W. Thompson. *Thompson & Thompson Genetics in Medicine*, 8th ed. Philadelphia: Saunders/Elsevier, 2016, Chapter 3: The Human Genome: Gene Structure and Function.

Figures

Grey, Kindred, Figure 12.7 Overview of the cell cycle. 2021. https://archive.org/details/12.7_20210926. CC BY 4.0.

Grey, Kindred, Figure 12.8 Summary of the mitotic phase. 2021. https://archive.org/details/12.8_20210926. CC BY 4.0. Added Mitosis cells sequence by LadyofHats. Public domain. From Wikimedia Commons. And Figure 2. CC BY 4.0. From Lumen.

Grey, Kindred, Figure 12.9 Summary of cell cycle checkpoints and role of CDK inhibitors in halting cell cycle progress. 2021. https://archive.org/details/12.9_20210926. CC BY 4.0.

12.3 Meiosis

The twenty-three chromosome pairs in humans accounts for all the genetic information needed to survive. For most of the components within the cell, only an approximation of division is needed during cell replication, however, with respect to division of DNA, this duplication and segregation must be exact. The integrity of the genetic information within the cell is critical for the well-being of the organisms and its offspring, so these processes are clearly controlled.

Within the cell cycle, the process of mitosis is largely responsible for this intricate chromosomal division of the somatic (body) cells by which two identical diploid daughter cells are produced through deoxyribonucleic acid (DNA) replication and cytoplasmic division.

In contrast, meiosis is a specialized process of the germline (sperm and eggs) that involves one round of DNA replication followed by two cell divisions to produce four haploid germ cells. Unlike mitosis, the resulting germ cells differ in males and females.

Male meiosis results in the production of four equally sized, functional spermatozoa, while female meiosis results in a single large functional ovum and three small nonfunctional polar bodies. Abnormalities in these processes include chromosomal nondisjunction, which results in the loss or gain of one or more chromosomes, and chromosomal breakage due to unrepaired DNA damage, which results in the formation of abnormal chromosomes and an increased risk for neoplasia.

Meiosis

Meiosis is composed of two distinctive cell divisions, meiosis I and meiosis II, which are found only in the germline. Through these two divisions, haploid gametes are formed from diploid somatic cells. There is only one replication of the DNA, but there are two divisions of the chromosomes. The first division differs from the second in that there is pairing and recombination between homologous chromosomes resulting in variation in the genetic makeup of the gametes. Segregation of the homologues occurs during the first meiotic (reductional) division, reducing the forty-six chromosomes to twenty-three, one from each homologous pair. The second (equational) division is similar to mitosis with segregation of sister chromatids into daughter cells (figure 12.10).

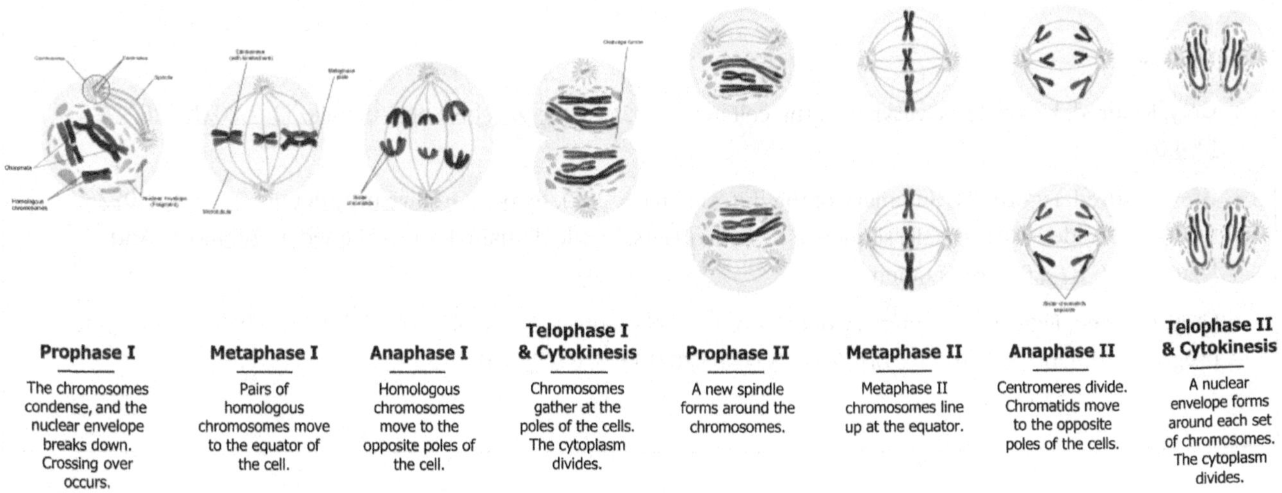

Figure 12.10: Overview of meiosis.

Meiosis I: Reductional division

Before meiosis, gametic stem cells replicate through mitosis. At the very beginning of meiosis, the last G_1 phase of the diploid stem cells is followed by chromosome replication during S phase and G_2, ending the last somatic interphase. Thus, each cell enters meiosis with two copies of the diploid genome (2n, 2c). At this point, the spermatogonium (male somatic cell) enlarges to become a primary spermatocyte, and the oogonium (female somatic cell) enlarges to become a primary oocyte.

These cells then enter prophase I, which is subdivided into five stages: leptotene, zygotene, pachytene, diplotene, and diakinesis. In female meiosis, there is an additional stage following diplotene called dictyotene in which the oocyte remains from early fetal gestation until ovulation when diakinesis occurs.

Prophase I

During prophase I, homologous chromosomes pair and undergo recombination through crossing over. This is visualized by the presence of X-shaped connections between homologues, called chiasmata, as the homologues begin to repel each other. These chiasmata will aid in the proper segregation of the chromosomes and become more prominent during diplotene. This is where the synaptoneal complex dissolves, allowing for chromosomal condensation to continue and for the repulsion of homologous chromosomes. The separation of the homologous chromosomes causes the chiasmata to appear. Individual chromatids can be visualized during this stage. (The dictyotene stage is unique to female meiosis in which there is a decondensation of chromosomal bivalents. The oocyte remains in this state for many years until follicle maturation and ovulation.)

At diakinesis, chromosomal condensation is completed. The chiasmata on each arm of the chromosomes move distally toward the telomeres. Each bivalent contains four chromatids, and pairs of sister chromatids are linked at the centromeres.

Metaphase I

The spindle forms, and the nuclear membrane disappears. Bivalents align on the metaphase plate still held together by the chiasmata. The centromeres of the two homologous chromosomes are separate, aligning on either side of the equatorial plate.

Anaphase I

Homologous chromosomes separate from each other by final terminalization of the chiasmata. They move to opposite poles, pulled by the centromere, which is attached to spindle fibers.

Telophase I

The chromosomes reach the poles, a nuclear membrane is formed, and cell division occurs. In male meiosis, the cytoplasm is divided equally, and the two resulting cells become secondary spermatocytes. In female meiosis, the division is unequal; most of the cytoplasm is retained in the secondary oocyte, while very little is retained by the first polar body. This period is very brief, and chromosomes move immediately to the second meiotic division. Each cell at this stage is haploid (1n) but with each chromosome formed of sister chromatids (2c). The sister chromatids may be unique due to recombination during the two homologues in prophase I.

Meiosis II: Equational division

This division is similar to mitosis in that individual chromosomes align on the metaphase plate, and sister chromatids separate and move to opposite poles at anaphase. The single copy (1c) of each chromosome is represented by one sister chromatid in the spermatids or mature ova.

Male meiosis

In humans, the male is the heterogametic sex, producing two kinds of normal sperm: 23,X and 23,Y. Spermatogenesis is a constant event beginning at puberty and continuing throughout life to produce four functional spermatids from each primary gametocyte. At puberty, the number of spermatogonia (diploid stem cells) increases. These develop into primary spermatocytes after several mitotic divisions. Each primary spermatocyte undergoes the first meiotic division to become two secondary spermatocytes. These cells then undergo the second meiotic division to become four spermatids of equal size with a haploid set of chromosomes. Spermiogenesis then transforms the spermatids into mature spermatozoa by elimination of the cytoplasm, elongation of the head of the sperm, and formation of a tail. The entire process from the enlargement of the spermatogonium to formation of the mature spermatozoa takes approximately sixty-four days.

Female meiosis

This is in contrast to meiosis in females, which begins before birth and produces only a single type of normal ovum: 23,X. The precursors to the germ cells are oogonia; these increase in number through mitosis, reaching a maximum number of approximately 7 million. Each individual oogonium enlarges to form a primary oocyte, which becomes surrounded by ovarian stromal cells to form a primary follicle. The vast majority of primary oocytes are formed during the third and fourth months of fetal life.

The primary oocyte begins the first meiotic division to become a secondary oocyte with the extrusion of a small polar body as the follicle matures and completes metaphase I with expulsion from the mature follicle at ovulation. The secondary oocyte does not complete the second meiotic division until fertilization, when a second polar body is extruded to form a mature ovum with a haploid set of chromosomes. Thus, each primary oocyte produces one functional gamete, the mature ovum, and three polar bodies. A nuclear membrane forms a pronucleus around the haploid set of maternal chromosomes, while a second pronucleus forms from the haploid set of chromosomes from the sperm head. These two pronuclei then fuse to begin the first mitotic division.

Meiotic pairing

Homologous pairing is unique to meiosis and plays two important roles: genetic recombination and chromosomal stabilization. While it has long been believed that the former is the most important, the latter is now accepted as the primary significance of meiotic recombination. During meiosis I, the pairing of homologues facilitates recombination, which is initiated by programed double-stranded breaks occurring at synaptic initiation sites (SISs). A subset of these breaks will resolve into the formation of the synaptonemal complex. When pairing is completed, synapsis occurs between the homologues, which completes the crossing over event. Each crossover event forms chasmata, which play an analogous role to the centromere and stabilize the maternal and paternal chromosomes. The stabilization of the metaphase chromosomes using this mechanism is key to normal chromosomal alignment and maintenance of an intact genome. Without recombination, the total number of unique gametic combinations of genes for each parent would be just over 8 million. However, crossing over greatly increases the total number of possible gene combinations such that the likelihood of either parent producing identical gametes is vanishingly small.

12.3 References and resources

Text

Clark, M. A. *Biology*, 2nd ed. Houston, TX: OpenStax College, Rice University, 2018, Chapter 10: Cell Reproduction, Chapter 11: Meiosis and Sexual Reproduction, Chapter 16: Gene Expression.

Karp, G., and J. G. Patton. *Cell and Molecular Biology: Concepts and Experiments*, 7th ed. Hoboken, NJ: John Wiley, 2013, Chapter 11: Gene Expression: From Transcription to Translation, Chapter 12: The Cell Nucleus and the Control of Gene Expression, Chapter 13: DNA Replication and Repair, Chapter 14: Cellular Reproduction.

Le, T., and V. Bhushan. *First Aid for the USMLE Step* 1, 29th ed. New York: McGraw Hill Education, 2018, 41–43, 46.

Nussbaum, R. L., R. R. McInnes, H. F. Willard, A. Hamosh, and M. W. Thompson. *Thompson & Thompson Genetics in Medicine*, 8th ed. Philadelphia: Saunders/Elsevier, 2016, Chapter 3: The Human Genome: Gene Structure and Function.

Figures

Grey, Kindred, Figure 12.10 Overview of Meiosis. 2021. https://archive.org/details/12.10_202109. CC BY 4.0. Added Meiosis Stages by Ali Zifan. CC BY 4.0. From Wikimedia Commons.

13. Human Genetics

Learning Objectives

Introduction to human genetics and genetic testing

- Understand how the following studies are performed and what kind of genetic information can/can't be obtained from each: karyotype, FISH, array CGH, Southern, Northern, and Western blots.
- Be able to select the appropriate technique (from the list above) to study chromosomes, chromosome segments containing several genes or single genes, microsatellites/copy number variants, DNA mutations/sequence alterations, RNA, and proteins.
- Understand how genes can be cloned using either a vector or PCR.
- Be able to describe both Sanger sequencing and "shotgun sequencing".
- Be able to describe the information obtained from whole exome sequencing.

Genetics methodology

- Understand how the following studies are performed and what kind of information can/can't be obtained from each: exome, Sanger sequencing, microarray, RFLP analysis, and FISH.
- Use the genetic code table to construct a protein sequence.
- Become familiar with DNA sequence variant nomenclature.

About this Chapter

The human genome project was a collaborative effort to sequence the human genome with the general idea that we would be able to identify all the genes coded for in DNA and determine how all genes functioned. This global understanding would change the way diseases are diagnosed and treated. When the project concluded in 2003, it was clear that DNA sequence was only a single piece of this equation, and just knowing what genes are present does not give a clear picture of how genes are expressed and regulated. What it has illustrated is that the modalities of inheritance and genetic influence over human phenotype is more complex that previously appreciated.

13.1 Chromosomal Structure and Cytogenetics

Chromosomes can be analyzed from living tissue and arranged in a karyotype (figure 13.1). Chromosomes can be sorted into the autosomal pairs (twenty-two) and sex chromosomes and classified to determine any abnormalities. A normal karyotype for a female is 46,XX, and a male is 46,XY. Deviations from this patterning can result in chromosomal abnormalities, which may or may not produce viable offspring.

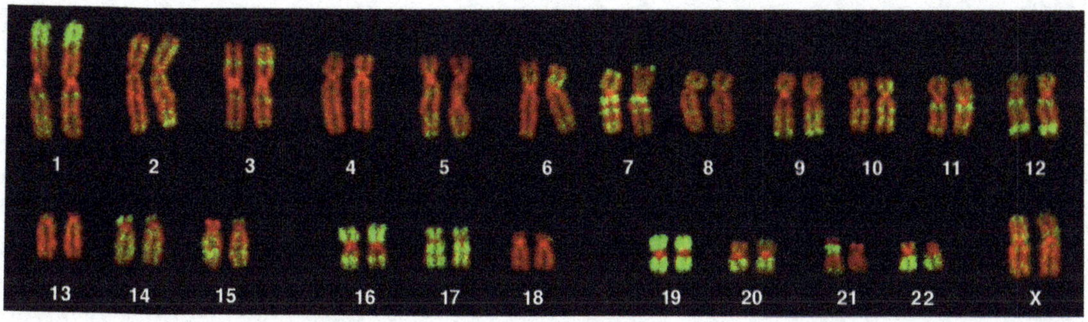

Figure 13.1: Representative karyotype illustrating twenty-two pairs of autosomes and one pair of sex chromosomes.

Chromosome structure

Each chromosome is made up of a p and q arm held together by the centromere. The position of the centromere is a distinguishing characteristic and can be classified as metacentric, submetacentric, or acrocentric. The position of the centromere plays a key role in mitotic and meiotic division as chromosomes with skewed centromeres are more likely to be involved in nondisjunction events (figure 13.2).

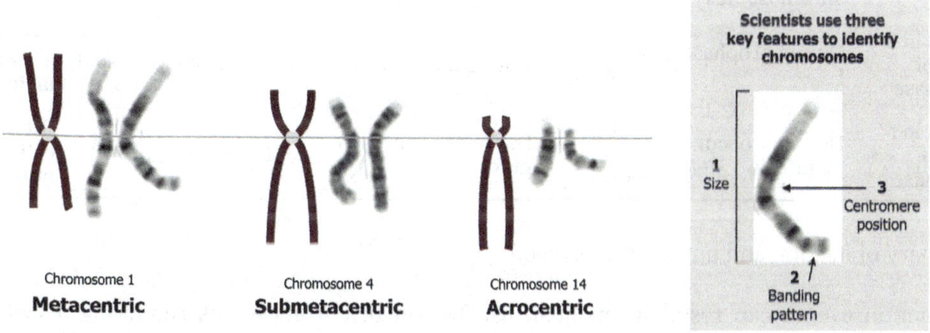

Figure 13.2: Basics of chromosome structure.

Nondisjunction

The precise pairing and segregation during the two meiotic divisions ensures the equal division of the somatic diploid set of chromosomes into the four resulting haploid cells (figure 13.3). Nondisjunction is the term used when the two homologous chromosomes in the first division or the two sister chromatids in the second do not segregate from each other at anaphase, but instead move together into the same daughter cell. This term may also be used for the same occurrence in mitotic cell divisions when the sister chromatids fail to segregate properly.

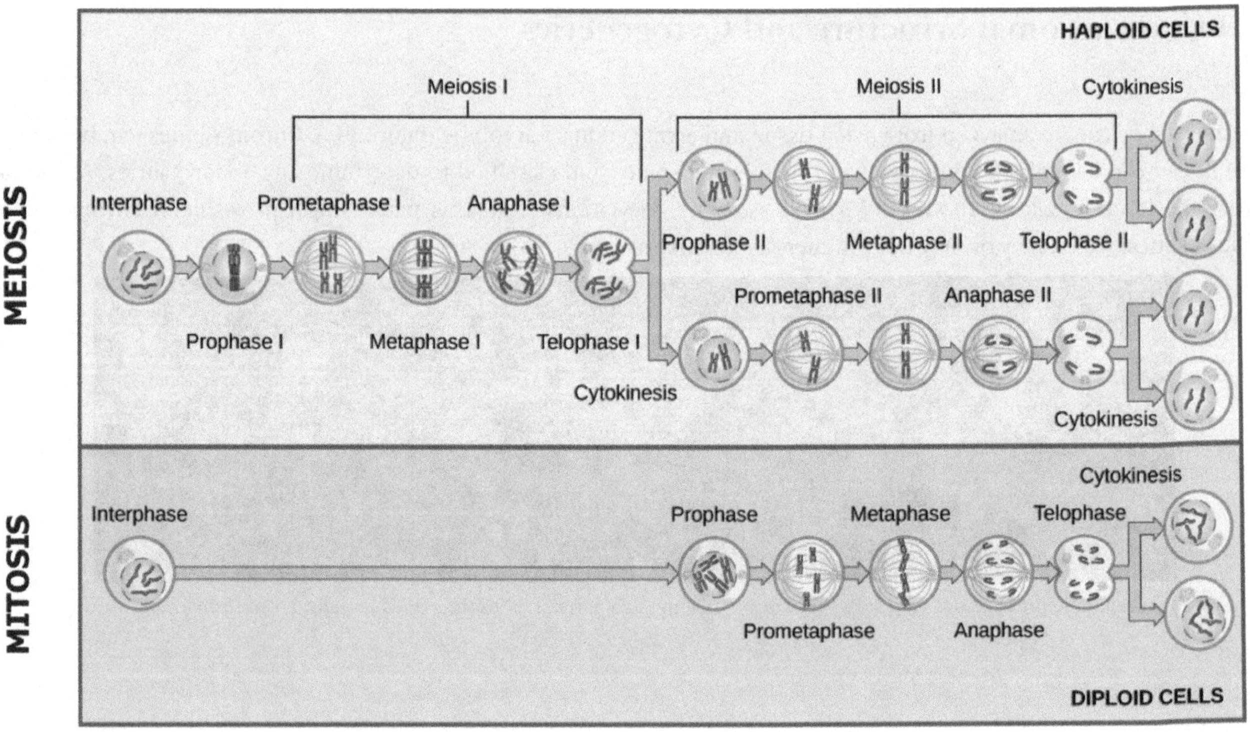

Figure 13.3: Summary of meiotic and mitotic cell divisions.

	DNA synthesis	Synapsis of homologous chromosomes	Crossover	Homologous chromosomes line up at metaphase plate	Sister chromatids line up at metaphase plate	
Meiosis	Occurs in S phase of interphase	During prophase I	During prophase I	During metaphase I	During metaphase II	**Outcome: Four haploid cells at the end of meiosis II**
Mitosis	Occurs in S phase of interphase	Does not occur in mitosis	Does not occur in mitosis	Does not occur in mitosis	During metaphase	**Outcome: Two diploid cells at the end of mitosis**

Table 13.1: Summary of meiotic and mitotic cell divisions.

These nondisjunction events can result in unequal distribution of chromosomes rendering a cell with an atypical chromosome number. A cell that is euploid would contain all twenty-three chromosomes, while polyploidy would suggest additional chromosomes within the cell. In humans, aneuploidy of autosomes are the most clinically important abnormalities to address, and the most common cause of this is a nondisjunction event.

Meiotic nondisjunction

Normally, one copy of each chromosome is inherited from each parent; however, when there is nondisjunction at either anaphase I or anaphase II, gametes will contain either two copies or no copies of the chromosome, which failed to disjoin. At fertilization, when the gamete provided by the other parent contributes one copy of each chromosome, the newly formed zygote will instead possess three copies (trisomy) or one copy (monosomy) of the chromosome, which failed to disjoin. Trisomy and monosomy are both examples of aneuploidy, a general term that denotes an abnormality in the number of copies of any given chromosome.

Chromosomal trisomies caused by nondisjunction at meiosis I can be distinguished from those occurring at meiosis II by examining the inheritance patterns of polymorphic markers near the centromere in cells obtained from the trisomic offspring (figure 13.4).

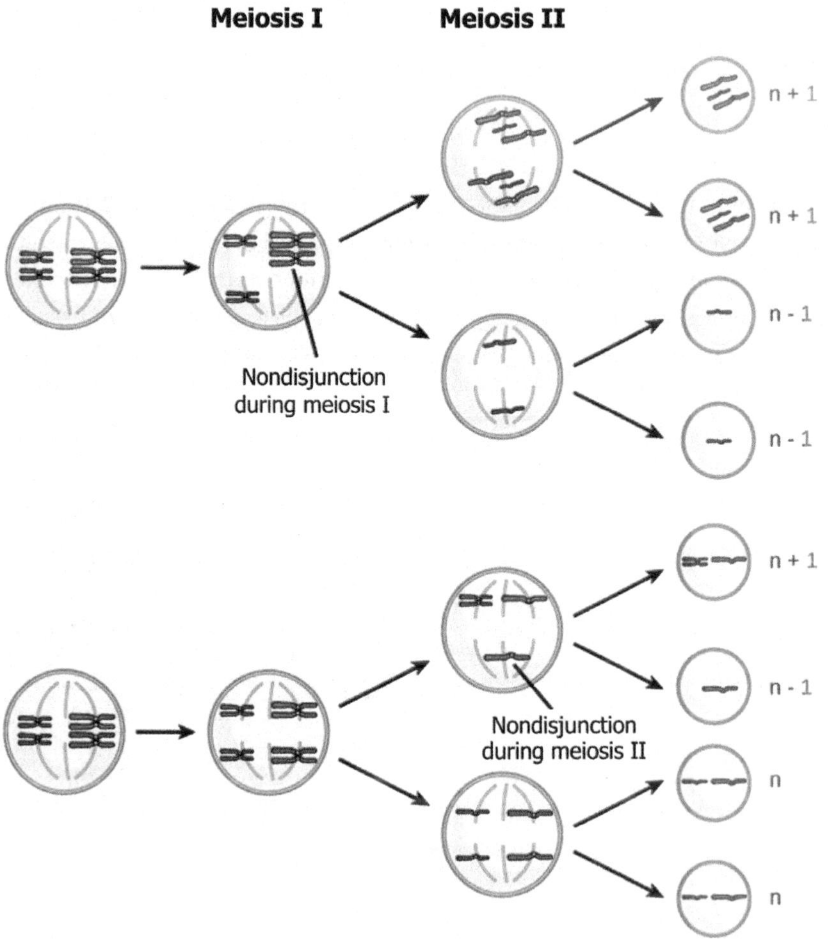

Figure 13.4: Comparison of nondisjunction in meiosis I versus meiosis II.

- Nondisjunction during the first division results in one copy of each of the two different markers being present on the two copies of the chromosome present in the abnormal gamete.
- Nondisjunction at meiosis II results in two copies of the same marker being present (figure 13.4).

Meiotic nondisjunction is the cause of the most common and clinically significant class of chromosomal abnormalities. This is true for chromosomal abnormalities found in spontaneous abortions where approximately 35 percent of miscarriages have a trisomy or monosomy, in stillbirths with approximately 4 percent being aneuploid, and also in live births with 0.3 percent being affected. Most autosomal trisomies and virtually all autosomal monosomies result in pregnancy failure or spontaneous abortion. Trisomies for chromosomes 13, 18, or 21 can result in the live birth of an infant with birth defects and intellectual disability. Extra copies of the X or Y chromosome are compatible with live birth, as is a small fraction of the conceptions with only a single X chromosome (Turner syndrome).

Increasing maternal age is considered a risk factor for increased frequency of nondisjunctional events. This maternal age effect is seen in both meiosis I and meiosis II, with the majority of these events occurring at meiosis I. Only a small proportion of chromosomal aneuploidies are due to errors in male meiosis, and these generally involve the sex chromosomes. Although there is little correlation with increasing paternal age and nondisjunctional events, there is some evidence to suggest that increased paternal age increases risk for other conditions (neurofibromatosis and achondroplasia) and should therefore not be ignored when determining risk.

Mitotic nondisjunction

Mitotic nondisjunction occurs after zygote formation and may be the result of misdivision of a cell after a normal conception with gain (or loss) of a chromosome during embryogenesis. This typically results in mosaicism (figure 13.5), the presence of multiple and genetically distinct cell populations in the same individual. The timing of mitotic nondisjunction events determines the ratio of aneuploid to normal cells and the types of tissues affected. For example, if the nondisjunction occurs early in development, the majority of cells and tissues would carry this aneuploidy, which would result in an increased clinical severity.

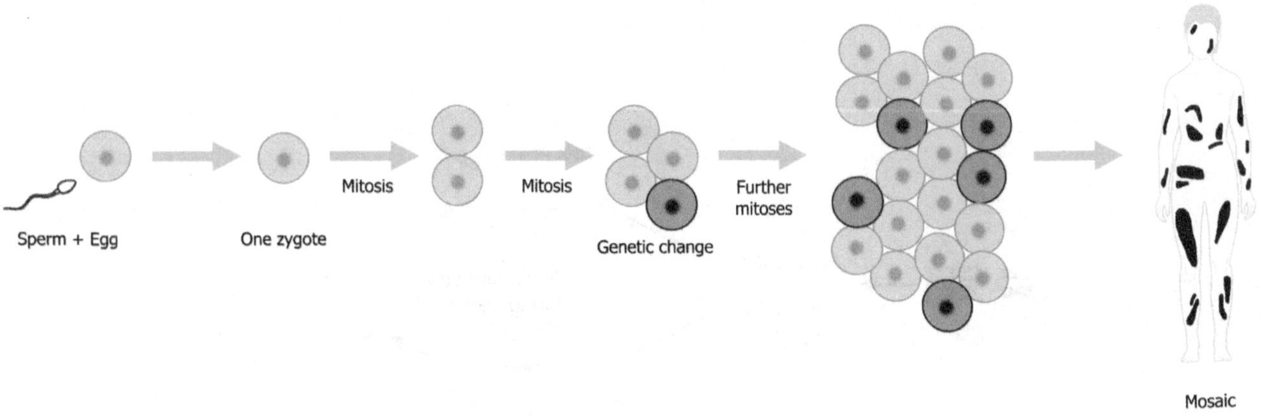

Figure 13.5: Mosaicism resulting in cells with differing genetics across the body.

Mosaicism is often found in sex chromosome abnormalities and some autosomal trisomies. Over half of mosaic trisomy 21 cases have been shown to be the result of loss of the extra 21 in subsequent mitotic divisions after a trisomic conception, while trisomy 8 mosaicism typically seems to be acquired during mitotic divisions after a normal conception.

Chimaerism is similar to mosaicism in that multiple, genetically distinct cell lines are present in the same individual. Here, however, the cell lines begin as different zygotes rather than arising through changes during mitosis. This can arise naturally from the fusion of closely implanted twins or migration of cells between embryos in multiple gestations, or it can be caused by the transplantation of tissues or organs from donors for medical treatment.

Chromosome structural defects

In addition to copy number defects, parts of the chromosome may be lost or altered. These rearrangements, regardless of the type, may be balanced or unbalanced (where the rearrangement does not produce a loss or gain).

Deletions and duplications

A deletion occurs when a chromosome breaks at two sites and the segment between them gets lost. Depending on the size and breakage site, varying numbers of genes can be lost. In rare cases the deletions are large enough to be visible under the light microscope. Smaller deletions have traditionally been identified by molecular cytogenetic (FISH) analyses, although they are now routinely detected with chromosome oligonucleotide arrays. These are called microdeletions, while the resulting pathologies are called microdeletion syndromes.

An example of this is Prader-Willi syndrome, a rare disorder due to the deletion or loss of expression from the paternal chromosome 15. This short region of genes is subject to maternal imprinting and typically only expressed from a single chromosomal loci. In these individuals, loss of expressivity from the paternal allele (either through a microdeletion or loss of chromosome 15) and imprinting of the maternal allele leads to this presentation. If both copies of the region are inherited from the paternal allele the result is the presentation of Angelman syndrome (figure 13.6).

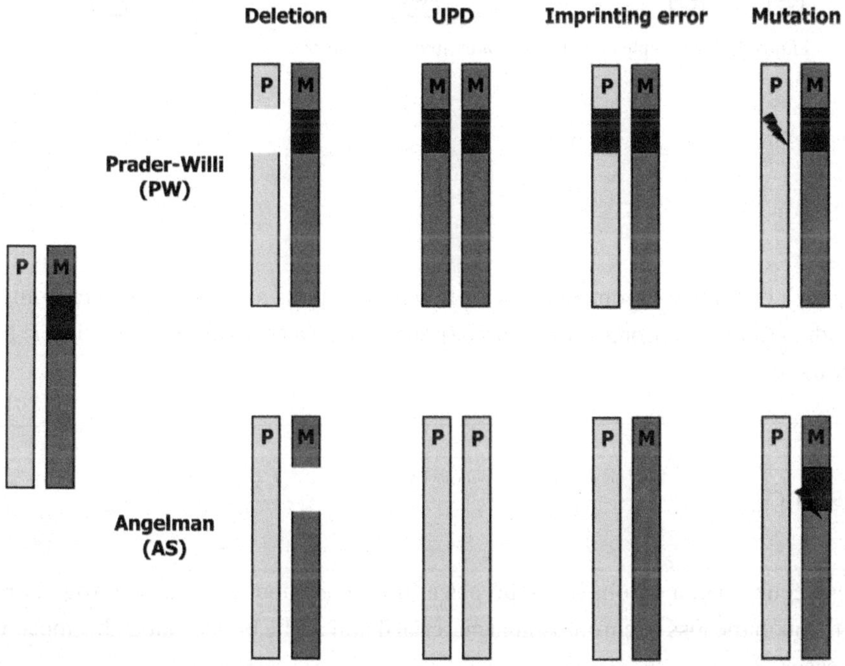

Figure 13.6: Genetic basis of Prader-Willi syndrome (PWS) and Angelman syndrome (AS). UPD: Uniparental disomy; Square: imprinting on the maternal allele.

Duplications refer to a chromosome segment appearing in two (often sequentially inserted) copies on a single homolog. Most of the time, this is caused by a nonhomologous recombination in the first meiotic division.

Inversion

Inversion occurs when a chromosome segment between two breaks is rotated 180 degrees before reinsertion. The gene copy number remains the same; clinical symptoms may arise if there is an additional deletion or duplication, if the breaks occur within the coding region of a gene, or if the regulation of a gene is altered. Like other balanced chromosomal aberrations, inversions may cause infertility, recurrent miscarriages, or an unbalanced chromosome complement in a child (figure 13.7).

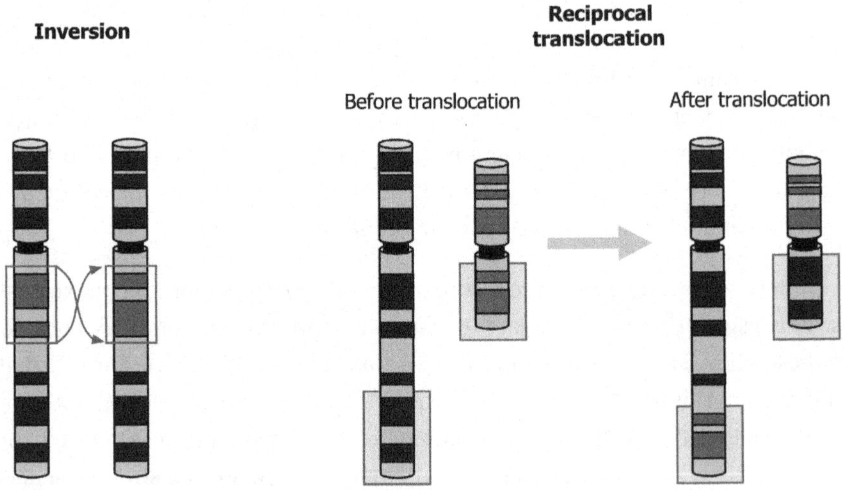

Figure 13.7: Example of a chromosome inversion and translocation.

Isochromosome

An isochromosome is a derivative chromosome with two homologous arms after the centromere divided transversely rather than longitudinally. An isochromosome can be thought of as a "mirror image" of either the short arm or the long arm of a given chromosome.

Ring chromosome

Ring chromosomes occur when a chromosome breaks at both ends and the ends join together. They typically become clinically relevant through the loss of chromosomal material distal to the breaks. Ring chromosome X causes 5 percent of Turner syndrome cases.

Translocations

Translocations occur most often during meiosis if unequal crossing over occurs. Additionally, translocations (interchange of genetic material between nonhomologous chromosomes) can be another source of chromosomal abnormality (figure 13.7).

Translocations can be classified as either reciprocal or Robertsonian.

- Reciprocal translocations occur when there is a break in two different chromosomes and the material is mutually exchanged. The newly formed "derivate chromosomes" have a full genetic complement, and the carrier is typically unaffected as no genetic information is lost.
- Robertsonian translocations occur when the short arms of two nonhomologous chromosomes are lost and the long arms (q) fuse to form a single chromosome. The acrocentric chromosomes (13, 14, 15, 21, and 22) are very susceptible to this type of translocation as they are acrocentric with very short arms. The short arms typically carry very little genetic material, so the loss of them does not usually result in a carrier phenotype. These individuals have forty-five chromosomes.

13.1 References and resources

Text

Clark, M. A. *Biology*, 2nd ed. Houston, TX: OpenStax College, Rice University, 2018, Chapter 10: Cell Reproduction, Chapter 11: Meiosis and Sexual Reproduction, Chapter 13: Modern Understandings of Inheritance, Chapter 17: Biotechnology and Genomics.

Le, T., and V. Bhushan. *First Aid for the USMLE Step* 1, 29th ed. New York: McGraw Hill Education, 2018, 52–55.

LeClair, R. J., and R. G. Best. "Chromosome Mechanics." *eLS* (2016): 1–11. https://onlinelibrary.wiley.com/doi/....a0001441.pub3.

Nussbaum, R. L., R. R. McInnes, H. F. Willard, A. Hamosh, and M. W. Thompson. *Thompson & Thompson Genetics in Medicine*, 8th ed. Philadelphia: Saunders/Elsevier, 2016, Chapter 5: Principles of Clinical Cytogenetics.

Figures

Bolzer A, Kreth G, Solovei I, et al. Figure 13.1 Representative karyotype illustrating 22 pairs of autosomes and one pair of sex chromosomes. PLoSBiol3.5.Fig7ChromosomesAluFish. CC BY 2.5. From WIkimedia Commons.

Csink AK, Henikoff S. Figure 13.6 Genetic basis of Prader-Willi (PWS) and Angelman syndrome(AS). Adapted under Fair Use from Trends in Genetics. Volume 14, Issue 5, 1 May 1998, pp 194-200. Figure 2. Prader-Willi and Angelman syndromes.

Grey, Kindred, Figure 13.2 Basics of chromosome structure. 2021. https://archive.org/details/13.2_20210926. CC BY 4.0. Added Karyotype (normal) by National Cancer Institute. Public domain. From Wikimedia Commons.

Grey, Kindred, Figure 13.3 Summary of meiotic and mitotic cell divisions. 2021. https://archive.org/details/13.3_20210926. CC BY 4.0. Adapted from Figure 1. CC BY 4.0. From Open Oregon.

Grey, Kindred, Figure 13.4 Comparison on nondisjunction in meiosis I vs. meiosis II. 2021. https://archive.org/details/13.4_20210926. CC BY 4.0. Adapted from Figure 8. CC BY 4.0. From Open Oregon.

13.2 Biotechnology

Basic techniques to manipulate genetic material (DNA and RNA)

To evaluate genetic disorders a variety of biochemical techniques can be used. The type, kind, and size of the projected genetic variation will determine what approach is taken.

Following DNA extraction there are a variety of techniques that can be employed. The lowest resolution technique for evaluating the genome is the karyotype followed by high-resolution banding. From here, smaller genomic changes can be observed using comparative genome hybridization, fluorescence in situ hybridization (FISH) analysis, or microarrays. Finally, specific nucleotide changes can be examined by whole genome sequencing.

DNA and RNA extraction

To study or manipulate nucleic acids, one must first isolate or extract the DNA or RNA from the cells. Most nucleic acid extraction techniques involve steps to break open the cell and use enzymatic reactions to destroy all macromolecules that are not desired. Enzymes such as proteases that break down proteins inactivate macromolecules, and ribonucleases (RNAses) that break down RNA are inhibited to ensure sample stability. Using alcohol precipitates the DNA. Human genomic DNA is usually visible as a gelatinous, white mass. One can store the DNA samples frozen at -80°C for several years (figure 13.8).

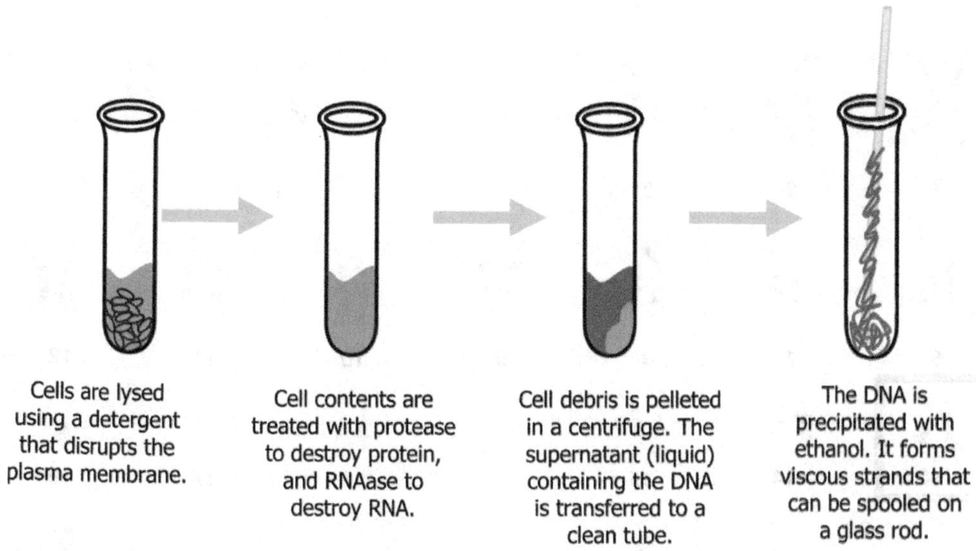

Figure 13.8: Basic process for DNA extraction.

Scientists perform RNA analysis to study gene expression patterns in cells. RNA is naturally very unstable because RNAses are commonly present in nature and very difficult to inactivate. Similar to DNA, RNA extraction involves using various buffers and enzymes to inactivate macromolecules and preserve the RNA.

Karoytype and high-resolution banding

Karyotyping can be used to look at general chromosome morphology and chromosome number. To do this, cells are harvested and arrested in metaphase allowing for the chromosomes to be fixed, spread on slides, and stained by one of several techniques. Giemsa banding (G banding) is the gold standard for the detection and characterization of structural and numerical genomic abnormalities in clinical diagnostic settings for both constitutional (postnatal or prenatal) and acquired (cancer) disorders.

The pattern of light and dark bands on each chromosome is numbered on each arm from the centromere to the telomere, and comparison of a patient sample to a standard map can be used to precisely identify changes in chromosome structure. Microdeletion syndromes can be detected with this technique (figure 13.9).

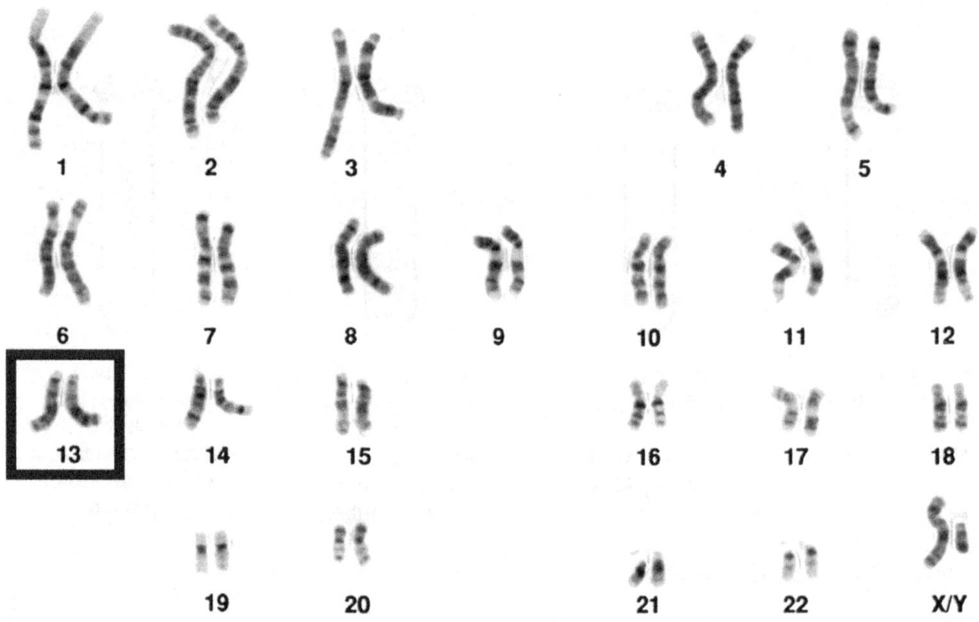

Figure 13.9: Male karyotype with G-banding patterns.

Fluorescence in situ hybridization (FISH)

FISH is a targeted approach using a sequence-specific probe to detect the presence or absence of a particular DNA sequence or for evaluating the number or organization of a chromosome or chromosomal region in situ.

This technique has several advantages and can be used to identify a varicty of different chromosomal changes:

1. DNA probes specific for chromosomal regions, or genes, can be labeled with different fluorochromes and used to identify particular chromosomal rearrangements.
2. Repetitive DNA probes allow detection of satellite DNA or other repeated DNA elements localized to specific chromosomal regions.

Microarrays

Although FISH can detect chromosome changes, microarrays can simultaneously query the whole genome to detect relative copy number variations, gains, or losses by hybridizing a control genome to one of a patient. In looking at the results, an excess of sequences from one genome would represent an overrepresentation in a gene locus within an individual (duplication). This technique can also be used to look at single nucleotide polymorphisms to determine allele frequency.

DNA sequencing techniques

Sanger sequencing is commonly referred to as the dideoxy chain termination method. The method is based on the use of chain terminators, the dideoxynucleotides (ddNTPs). The ddNTPSs differ from the deoxynucleotides by the lack of a free 3′ OH group on the five-carbon sugar. If a ddNTP is added to a growing DNA strand, the chain cannot be extended any further because the free 3′ OH group needed to add another nucleotide is not available. By using a predetermined ratio of deoxyribonucleotides to dideoxynucleotides, it is possible to generate DNA fragments of different sizes.

The DNA sample to be sequenced is denatured (separated into two strands by heating it to high temperatures). The DNA is divided into four tubes in which a primer, DNA polymerase, and all four nucleoside triphosphates (A, T, G, and C) are added. In addition, limited quantities of one of the four dideoxynucleoside triphosphates (ddCTP, ddATP, ddGTP, and ddTTP) are added to each tube respectively. The tubes are labeled as A, T, G, and C according to the ddNTP added. For detection purposes, each of the four dideoxynucleotides carries a different fluorescent label. Chain elongation continues until a fluorescent dideoxy nucleotide is incorporated, after which no further elongation takes place. After the reaction is over, electrophoresis is performed. Even a difference in length of a single base can be detected (figure 13.10).

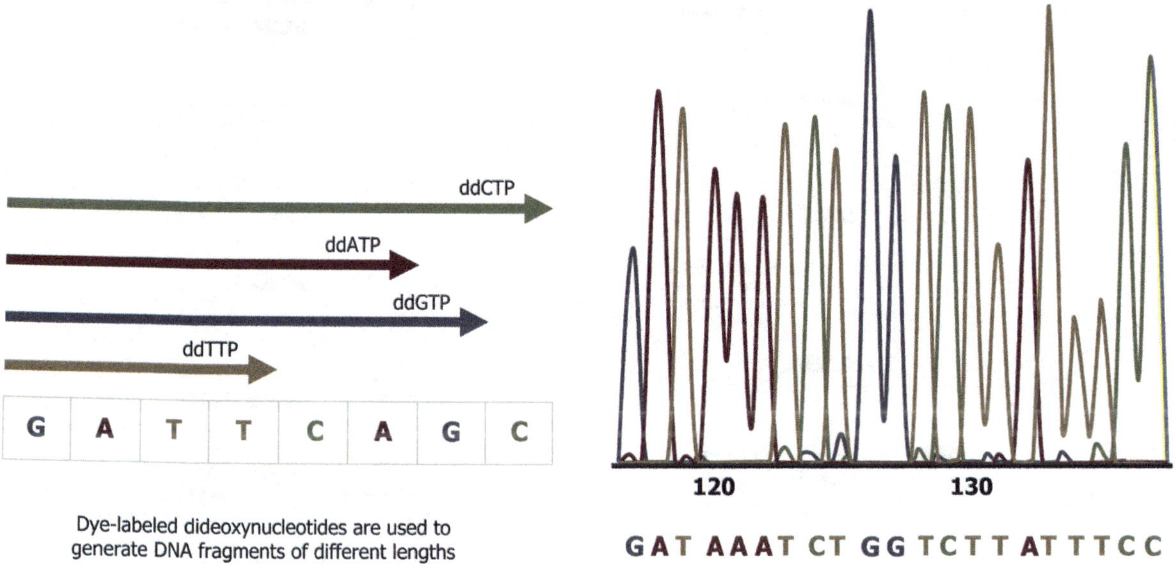

Figure 13.10: Schematic of Sanger sequencing technique.

Nucleic acid fragment amplification by polymerase chain reaction (PCR)

DNA analysis often requires focusing on one or more specific genome regions. Polymerase chain reaction (PCR) is a technique that scientists use to amplify specific DNA regions for further analysis (figure 13.11). Researchers use PCR for many purposes in laboratories, such as cloning gene fragments to analyze genetic diseases, identifying contaminant foreign DNA in a sample, and amplifying DNA for sequencing. More practical applications include determining paternity and detecting genetic diseases.

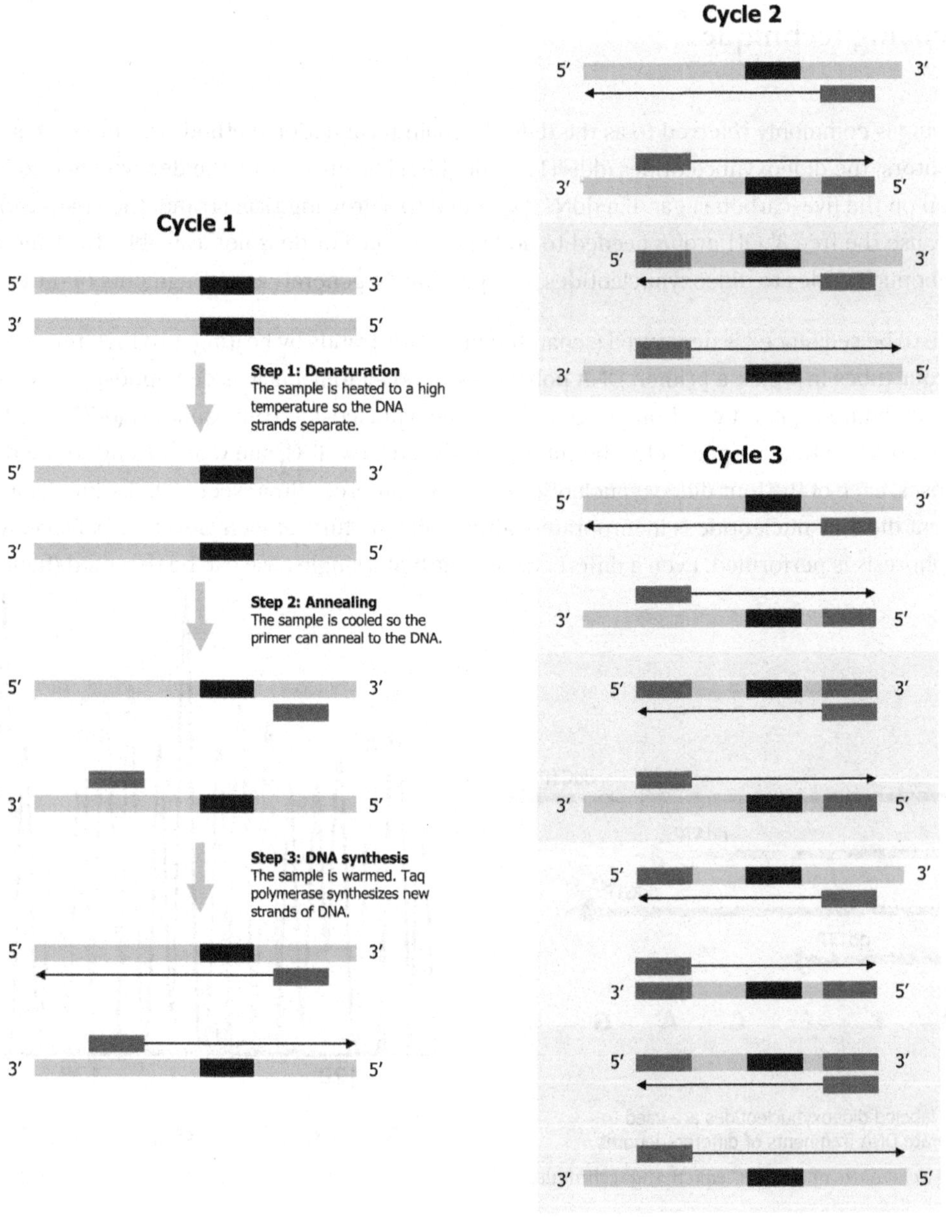

Figure 13.11: Overview of polymerase chain reaction.

Scientists use polymerase chain reaction, or PCR, to amplify a specific DNA sequence. Primers are short pieces of DNA complementary to each end of the target sequence combined with genomic DNA, Taq polymerase, and deoxynucleotides.

Reverse transcriptase PCR (RT-PCR) is similar to PCR, but cDNA is made from an RNA template before PCR begins. DNA fragments can also be amplified from an RNA template in a process called reverse transcriptase PCR (RT-PCR). The first step is to recreate the original DNA template strand (called cDNA) by applying DNA nucleotides to the mRNA. This process is called reverse transcription. This requires the presence of an enzyme called reverse transcriptase. After the cDNA is made, regular PCR can be used to amplify it.

Gel electrophoresis

Gel electrophoresis is a technique used to separate DNA fragments of different sizes. Usually the gel is made of a chemical called agarose or polyacylamide depending on the sample being used. The DNA has a net negative charge and moves from the negative electrode toward the positive electrode. The electric current is applied for sufficient time to let the DNA separate according to size; the smallest fragments will be farthest from the well (where the DNA was loaded), and the heavier molecular weight fragments will be closest to the well. Once the DNA is separated, the gel is stained with a DNA-specific dye for viewing it.

Hybridization, southern blotting, and northern blotting

Different types of electrophoresis can be used to look at various changes at the level of the DNA (genome), RNA (transcriptome), or protein (proteome). In all cases, a sample (DNA, RNA, protein) is run on a gel (electrophoresis) and is then examined using a probe specific to the sample.

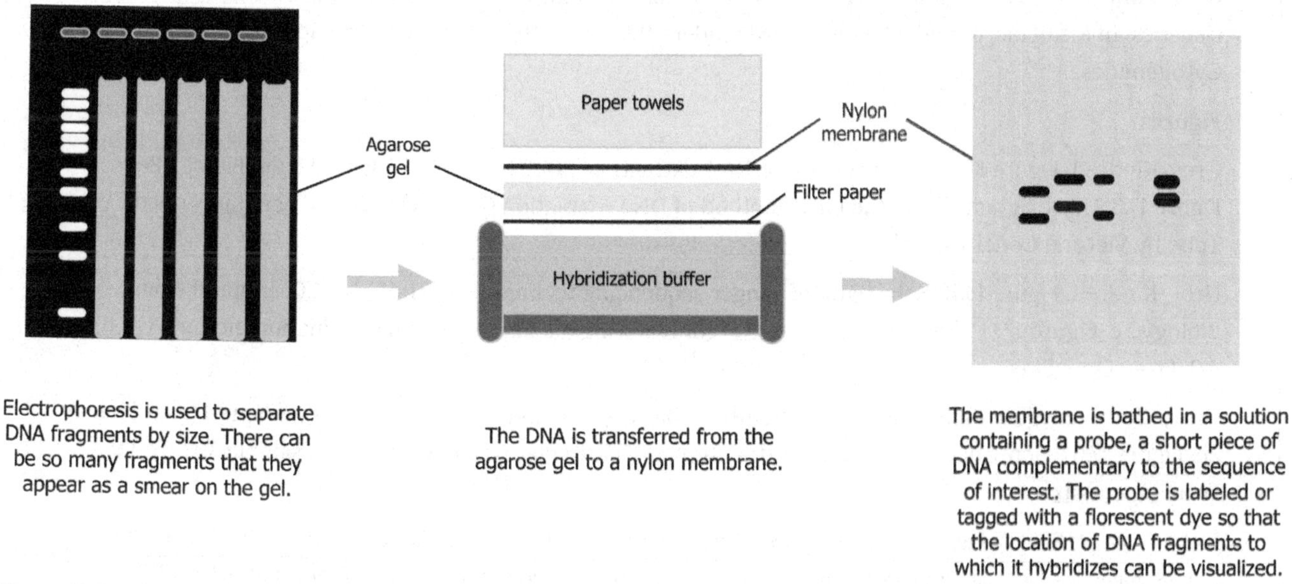

Figure 13.12: Schematic of southern blotting technique.

Southern blots are designed to examine changes in DNA. DNA, typically genomic DNA, is probed with a DNA probe complementary to the region of interest in the genome (figure 13.12).

Northern blots are designed to examine changes in RNA. RNA is probed with a DNA probe complementary to the transcript of interest. This will detect changes in gene expression.

Western blots are designed to examine changes in protein size and amount. Cell lysates or protein isolates are probed with an antibody specific to the protein of interest. This will detect changes in protein expression.

13.2 References and resources

Text

Clark, M. A. *Biology*, 2nd ed. Houston, TX: OpenStax College, Rice University, 2018, Chapter 10: Cell Reproduction, Chapter 11: Meiosis and Sexual Reproduction, Chapter 13: Modern Understandings of Inheritance, Chapter 17: Biotechnology and Genomics.

Le, T., and V. Bhushan. *First Aid for the USMLE Step* 1, 29th ed. New York: McGraw Hill Education, 2018, 52–55.

LeClair, R. J., and R. G. Best. "Chromosome Mechanics." *eLS* (2016): 1–11. https://onlinelibrary.wiley.com/doi/....a0001441.pub3.

Nussbaum, R. L., R. R. McInnes, H. F. Willard, A. Hamosh, and M. W. Thompson. *Thompson & Thompson Genetics in Medicine*, 8th ed. Philadelphia: Saunders/Elsevier, 2016, Chapter 5: Principles of Clinical Cytogenetics.

Figures

Grey, Kindred, Figure 13.8 Basic process for DNA extraction. 2021. CC BY 4.0. Adapted from Biology 2e. Figure 17.3 This diagram shows the basic method of DNA extraction.CC BY 4.0. From OpenStax. Added Test Tube by Victoria Codes from the Noun Project.

Grey, Kindred, Figure 13.10 Schematic of Sanger sequencing technique. 2021. CC BY 4.0. Adapted from Biology 2e. Figure 17.14 This figure illustrates Frederick Sanger's dideoxy chain termination method. CC BY 4.0. From OpenStax.

Grey, Kindred, Figure 13.12 Schematic of Southern Blotting technique. 2021. CC BY 4.0. Adapted from Biology 2e. Figure 17.6 Scientists use Southern blotting to find a particular sequence in a DNA sample. CC BY 4.0. From OpenStax.

Lieberman M, Peet A. Figure 13.11 Overview of polymerase chain reaction. Adapted under Fair Use from Marks' Basic Medical Biochemistry. 5th Ed. pp 329. Figure 17.10 Polymerase chain reaction (PCR). 2017.

National Cancer Institute. Figure 13.9 Male karyotype with G-banding patterns. Karyotype (normal). Public domain. From Wikimedia Commons.

14. Linkage Studies, Pedigrees, and Population Genetics

Learning Objectives

Linkage studies and pedigrees

- Interpret a pedigree for type of inheritance.
- Describe how Mendelian disease genes are identified by linkage mapping.

Population genetics

- Perform simple Hardy-Weinberg calculations for autosomal recessive disease.
- Recognize populations that are not in Hardy-Weinberg equilibrium.
- Understand the following terms related to genetic variation: polymorphism, SNP, haplotype, HapMap.

About this Chapter

Single gene inheritance is also referred to as Mendelian inheritance and follows transmission patterns he observed in his research on peas. These are the most basic patterns of inheritance, and within each category, there can be nuances of disease presentation. The frequency of these disorders in populations can be determined using Hardy-Weinberg calculations.

It is important to remember that these inheritance patterns are not characteristic of all genetic traits, and there are many factors that influence an individual's phenotype.

14.1 Mendelian Inheritance

There are four basic types of Mendelian inheritance patterns: autosomal dominant, autosomal recessive, X-linked recessive, and X-linked dominant. Autosomal inheritance patterns suggest that the gene responsible for the phenotype is located on one of the twenty-two pairs of autosomes (non-sex determining chromosomes). This is in contrast to X-linked traits where the gene that encodes for the trait is located on the X chromosome.

Traits can be either dominant or recessive in nature such that in the case of dominant traits conditions manifest in heterozygotes (individuals with just one copy of the mutant allele).

Recessive traits

- Recessive conditions are expressed in individuals who have two copies of the mutant allele. Keep in mind, the two recessive alleles may have two different mutations to produce a recessive individual (heteroallelic).
- When just one copy of the mutant allele is present, an individual is a carrier of the mutation but does not develop the condition.
- Females and males are affected equally by traits transmitted by autosomal recessive inheritance.
- A heterozygous carrier for a recessive mutation has a 50 percent probability of transmitting this mutation to a child (figure 14.1).
- If both partners are heterozygous carriers for the same autosomal recessive disease, the risk for transmission to offspring is as follows:
  - 25 percent of the offspring of the couple will be homozygous (or compound heterozygous) for the disease-causing allele and thus be affected by the disorder.
  - 50 percent of the offspring will be healthy heterozygous carriers just as their parents.
  - 25 percent will be homozygous for the wild-type allele.

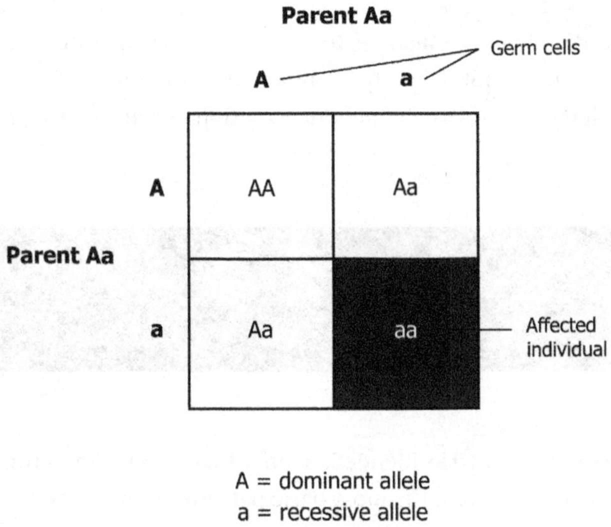

Figure 14.1: Punnett square illustrating allelic distribution of recessive traits.

When speaking of the children of carrier parents, two-thirds of the healthy siblings of an affected child are heterozygous carriers.

If an individual with an autosomal recessive disorder has children, a disease-causing mutation will be transmitted to all of them (either of the two mutant alleles). The consequences for the child depends on this individual's partner. If the partner is homozygous for the normal allele of the respective gene (as in the majority of cases), all offspring will be nonaffected heterozygous carriers. If the partner, however, is a carrier (the likelihood is approximately 0.5 to 1 percent for the more frequent recessive disorders), statistically, half of the offspring will be affected (homozygous or compound heterozygous), and the other half will be carriers. If both partners should have the same recessive disorder (caused by mutations in the same gene), all offspring will be homozygous/compound heterozygous and affected.

Dominant traits

- Dominant conditions are expressed in individuals who have just one copy of the mutant allele.
- Females and males are affected equally by traits transmitted in an autosomal dominant fashion.
- Affected individuals have one normal copy of the gene and one mutant copy of the gene; thus each offspring has a 50 percent chance on inheriting the mutant allele (figure 14.2).

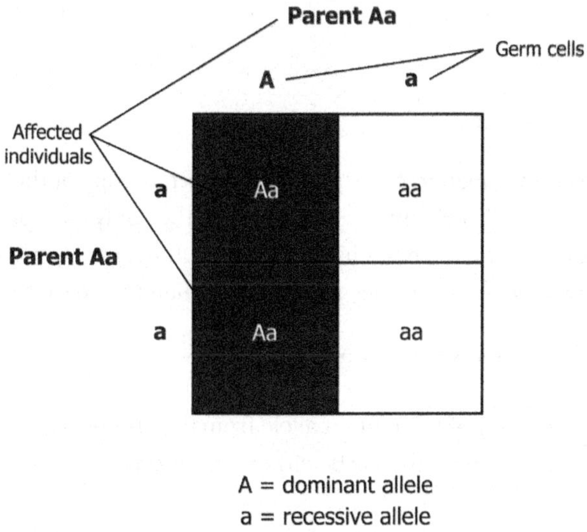

Figure 14.2: Allelic distributions in dominant traits.

Semidominance or incomplete dominance

For most disorders inherited as dominant traits, homozygosity for a disease-causing mutation results in a much more severe clinical phenotype than heterozygosity. An example is familial hypercholesterolemia, a genetic disorder resulting from mutations of the low-density lipoprotein (LDL) receptor gene. Individuals with a heterozygous loss-of-function mutation show elevated LDL cholesterol levels (greater than 7 to 10 mmol/ L) and typically suffer their first myocardial infarction in midlife. Homozygous individuals have a much higher LDL cholesterol level (10 to 30 mmol/ L), with the onset of symptoms in early childhood and coronary heart disease as early as school age.

In these examples, the phenotype of heterozygotes (Aa) is somewhere in between the phenotypes of wild-type and mutant homozygotes (AA and aa). The inheritance pattern is called semidominant or incompletely dominant, in contrast to complete dominance that is found in very few conditions, such as Huntington's disease, in which the phenotype of the heterozygous and homozygous mutation carriers is more or less identical. It is worth thinking about reasons why a condition may show complete penetrance. For practical purposes, both types of conditions may be called dominant because the definition rests on the clinical phenotype in the heterozygote, irrespective of what is observed in the homozygote.

Codominance

There are a few cases in which two alleles of the same gene code for proteins with different specific functions, both of which may be found simultaneously in (compound) heterozygous individuals. Such alleles are said to be codominant to each other. The classic example is the ABO blood group system, in which individuals with genotype AB show phenotypic characteristics of allele A as well as allele B, and there is also a null allele that causes complete loss of protein function.

Sex-linked traits

X-linked recessive traits do not typically manifest when there is a normal copy of the gene (e.g., in females). In contrast nearly all X-linked recessive traits are fully evident in males because they only have one copy of the X chromosome, and thus do not have a normal copy of the gene to compensate for the mutant copy. For that same reason, women are rarely affected by X-linked recessive diseases, however, they are affected when they have two copies of the mutant allele.

If a man is affected with an X-linked recessive condition:

- All his daughters will inherit one copy of the mutant allele from him; there is no male-to-male transmission.
- All daughters are obligate heterozygotes and may be either asymptomatic carriers or have variable (less severe) symptoms of the disorder.
- On average, 25 percent of the daughters' children (50 percent of her sons) will be affected with the disorder of their grandfather, 25 percent of children (50 percent of her daughters) will be heterozygous females, while 50 percent of the children will inherit the normal allele from their mother.
- All sons of an affected male will have inherited the Y chromosome of their father and, therefore, will not be affected and will not transmit the disorder to their children.

X-linked dominant disorders clinically manifest when only one copy of the mutant allele is present. There is no transmission from father to son, but there can be transmission from father to daughter (all daughters of an affected male will be affected since the father has only one X chromosome to transmit). Children of an affected woman have a 50 percent chance of inheriting the X chromosome with the mutant allele. Phenotypic presentation of X-linked traits can be influenced by lyonization or X-inactivation. As one X chromosome is randomly expressed in all female cells, the differential patterns of X-inactivation can alter phenotype in female carriers of X-linked recessive disorders and X-linked dominant disorders.

Calculation of risk

One of the most important considerations of genetic counseling is calculating risk. Mathematics is only the first step; equally important is communicating the probability that the event will occur. There are a number of ways to say that an event will not occur with absolute certainty. Studies have shown that these terms are understood and evaluated differently by different individuals. Another factor that varies between patients is that events are evaluated according to whether the result will be considered positive or negative and by which consequences they will have. For example, the probability that, beginning at age forty-five, mothers have a 5 percent risk of giving birth to a child with a chromosomal disorder is generally considered a high risk. In cancer, on the other hand, a survival chance of 5 percent is considered low.

Hardy-Weinberg equations

The Hardy-Weinberg law rests on the assumption that there are two different alleles at a certain locus; these alleles are named "p" and "q" (i.e., a normal allele [traditionally p] and a variant allele [traditionally q]). Since there are only these two alleles, $p + q = 1$.

In humans, if the respective gene occurs in two copies on only one autosome, the frequency of the three possible genotypes is calculated from the binominal distribution, which is often represented as:

$p^2 + 2pq + q^2 = 1$

p is the frequency of the 'A' allele

q is the frequency of the 'a' allele

p^2 = the frequency of the AA genotype

q^2 = the frequency of the aa genotype

$2pq$ = the frequency of the Aa genotype

The Hardy-Weinberg law only applies to an "ideal population" that meets the following criteria:

- Mating within the population occurs randomly, with equal probability and equal success for the various genotypes.
- The population is large enough to prevent random events (gene drift) from affecting the allele frequency.
- There is no selection advantage or disadvantage for carriers of certain genotypes.
- There are no new mutations.
- There are no migration events that might alter the allele frequency.

The one factor that has practical implications among this group of criteria is random mating, since the Hardy-Weinberg law cannot be applied if there is frequent intermarriage. In such cases, rare recessive disorders occur with much greater frequency than would be expected from the frequency of heterozygosity. The other criteria are more relevant to whether or not the allele or genotype frequencies remain constant or whether the incidence of a disorder changes.

Example

Cystic fibrosis is a recessive condition that affects 1/2,500 births in the Caucasian population:

Frequency of the recessive allele:

$q^2 = 1/2{,}500 = 0.0004$

$q = 0.02$

Frequency of the dominant allele:

$1 - 0.02 = 0.98 = p$

14.1 References and resources

Text

Clark, M. A. *Biology*, 2nd ed. Houston, TX: OpenStax College, Rice University, 2018, Chapter 10: Cell Reproduction, Chapter 12: Mendel's Experiments and Heridity, Chapter 13: Modern Understandings of Inheritance.

Le, T., and V. Bhushan. *First Aid for the USMLE Step 1*, 29th ed. New York: McGraw Hill Education, 2018, 55–59.

Nussbaum, R. L., R. R. McInnes, H. F. Willard, A. Hamosh, and M. W. Thompson. *Thompson & Thompson Genetics in Medicine*, 8th ed. Philadelphia: Saunders/Elsevier, 2016, Chapter 7: Patterns of Single Gene Inheritance, Chapter 9: Genetic Variations in Populations, Chapter 10: Identifying the Genetic Basis for Human Disease.

Figures

Grey, Kindred, Figure 14.1 Punnett square illustrating allelic distribution of recessive traits. 2021. https://archive.org/details/14.1_20210926. CC BY 4.0.

Grey, Kindred, Figure 14.2 Allelic distributions in dominant traits. 2021. https://archive.org/details/14.2_20210926. CC BY 4.0.

Additional resources

- Hardy-Weinberg problems: https://www.k-state.edu/parasitology…/hardwein.html
- Practice pedigrees: https://ocw.mit.edu/courses/biology/…ntals-of-biology-fall-2011/genetics/pedigrees/MIT7_01SCF11_3.3sol1.pdf
- Practice pedigrees: https://www.khanacademy.org/science/high-school-biology/hs-classical-genetics/hs-pedigrees/a/hs-pedigrees-review

14.2 Non-Mendelian Inheritance

The majority of genetic disorders are not inherited in a Mendelian fashion. Even in cases where Mendelian genetics can predict genotype, the disease phenotype may not be displayed or may be variable due to external influences. This section describes some additional factors that influence presentation and inheritance patterns.

Penetrance refers to the display of any signs or symptoms if you have the genetic abnormality; this does not describe the variety of phenotype. As illustrated in figure 14.3, this refers to the number of "affected (purple)" versus "unaffected (white)" cells in an individual. Individuals with a greater number of purple cells may have a more pronounced phenotype than individuals with greater numbers of white cells.

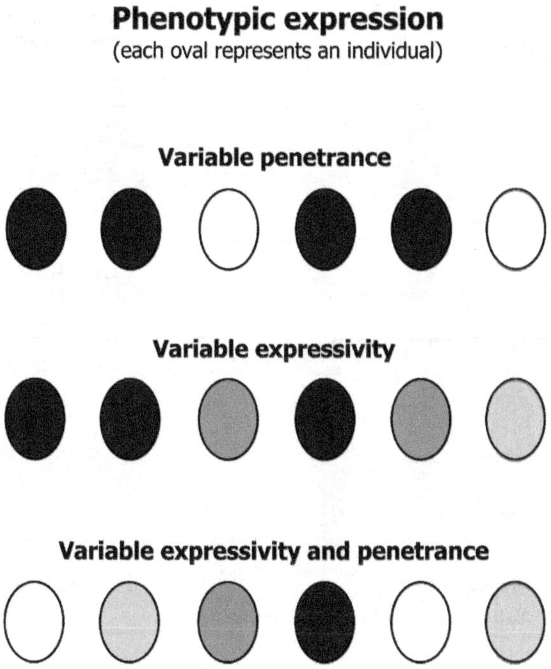

Figure 14.3: Graphic representation of penetrance and expressivity.

Variable phenotypes can present due to changes in expressivity or pleiotropy. These terms refer to the variety of presentations from a single genetic disorder (variable expression). As illustrated in figure 14.3, expressivity can be a range of "purplish" colors, which may give rise to a variable phenotype. In other more complicated genetic cases, both penetrance and expressivity must be considered when making a diagnosis. Pleiotropy of a disorder is best described as a single gene disorder having implications on several different organ systems.

Extranuclear inheritance

Mitochondria are unique in that they have multiple copies of a circular chromosome. This DNA is independent of nuclear DNA and inherited from the mother.

Therefore in this inheritance modality, the females can transmit the trait to all offspring (figure 14.4), however, only female offspring will continue to transmit the disorder. Disease phenotype in mitochondrial disease is extremely variable due to mitochondrial heteroplasmy.

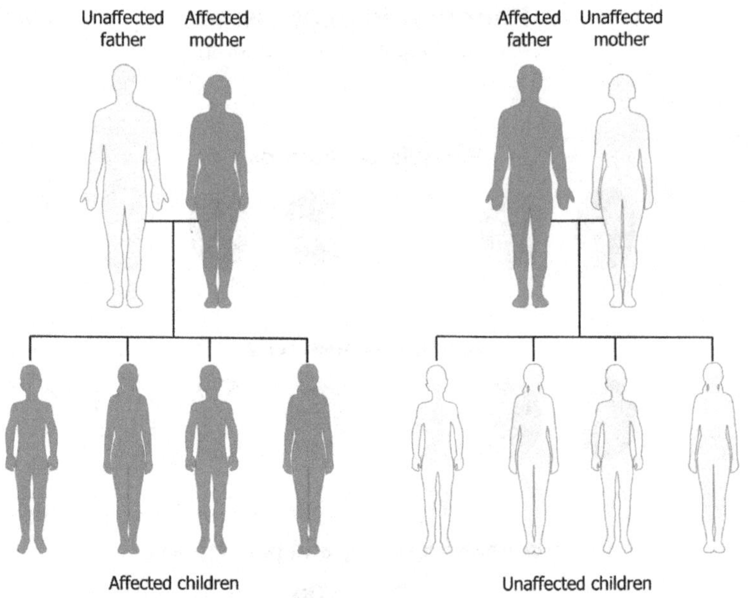

Figure 14.4: Mitochondrial inheritance pattern.

Heteroplasmy is a term referring to the diversity of the mitochondrial genome within each cell. During cell division, mitochondria are divided randomly between the two daughter cells, and therefore the percentage of affected mitochondrial DNA (mtDNA) will also be variable within the offspring. The mitochondria generate energy for the rest of the cell, therefore disease transmitted through mitochondrial inheritance affects high-energy organs (this is a good example of pleiotropy).

Genomic imprinting

Genetic information is not just stored in the actual code (e.g., ATCG), but also for many genes hereditary information is transmitted with a parental-specific imprint based on whether the gene was transmitted from the father or from the mother. This imprint can be thought of as the font of the genome (e.g., ATCG vs. ATCG vs. ATCG). For these imprinted genes, even though the nucleotide sequence in the maternal and paternal copies is identical, the expression differs depending on the parental imprint. Genomic imprinting is the most well-characterized epigenetic transmission of gene regulation. Often in cases, the imprinting of one allele is essential for a normal phenotype, and loss of imprinting or uniparental disomy (inheritance of both loci from a single parental source) can cause inappropriate expression patterns.

Differential methylation of genomic DNA is a central mechanism in the regulation of the expression of genes. Of special importance is the methylation of cytosine in CpG (cytosine-phosphorus-guanine) dinucleotides. Many genes have numerous "CpG islands" with a large number of CpG dinucleotides located upstream of the transcriptional start. Hypermethylation in this region results in transcriptional silencing, meaning the gene can no longer be read. The methylation pattern of DNA and, consequently, the activity pattern of the genes are generally transmitted as a stable trait in mitosis; however, for imprinted or epigenetically sensitive genes, this "trait" is reset in meiosis.

Trinucleotide repeat disorders

Disorders in this category are caused by expansion of tandem trinucleotide repeats (figure 14.5). These repetitive regions can be within upstream regulatory elements or within the coding region themselves; typically these repeated regions are of low copy number. In each generation there is the potential for these repetitive sequences to expand, and the expansion will change gene expression.

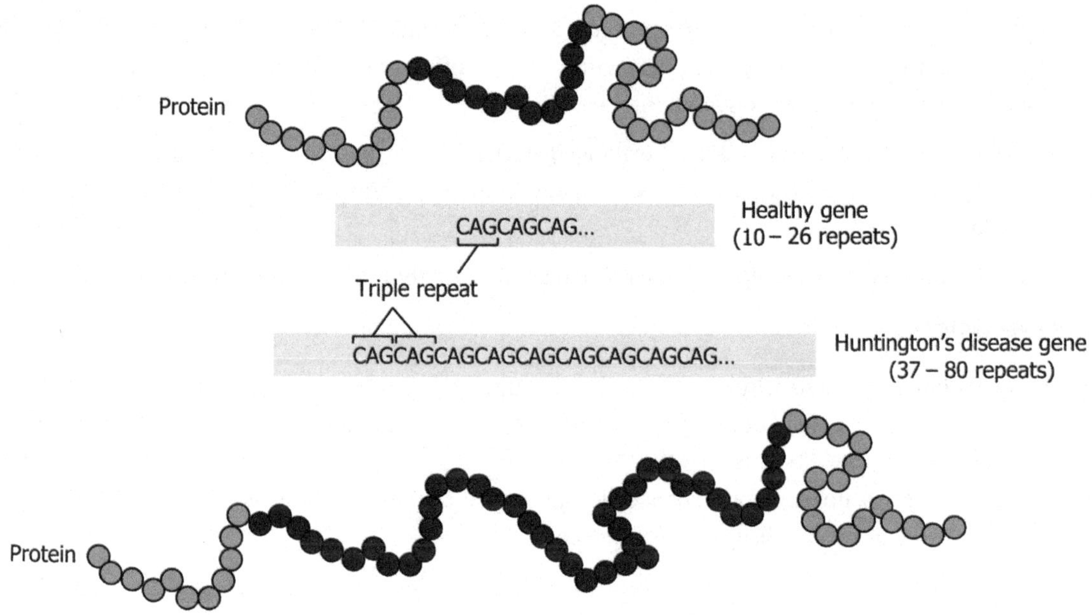

Figure 14.5: Trinucleotide repeat expansion characteristic of Huntington's disease.

Triplicate repeat disorders are also characteristic of anticipation where the affected phenotype of individuals becomes progressively worse with each generation. Classic repeat disorders include Fragile X and Huntington's disease. In the case of Fragile X, the repeated region becomes hypermethylated and the methylation pattern expands into the promoter region for the gene. This will lead to silencing of the transcript. The gene itself, FMR1, is involved in mRNA splicing, and the loss of this gene product has a pleiotropic effect.

14.2 References and resources

Text

Clark, M. A. *Biology*, 2nd ed. Houston, TX: OpenStax College, Rice University, 2018, Chapter 10: Cell Reproduction, Chapter 12: Mendel's Experiments and Heridity, Chapter 13: Modern Understandings of Inheritance.

Le, T., and V. Bhushan. *First Aid for the USMLE Step 1*, 29th ed. New York: McGraw Hill Education, 2018, 55–59.

Nussbaum, R. L., R. R. McInnes, H. F. Willard, A. Hamosh, and M. W. Thompson. *Thompson & Thompson Genetics in Medicine*, 8th ed. Philadelphia: Saunders/Elsevier, 2016, Chapter 7: Patterns of Single Gene Inheritance, Chapter 9: Genetic Variations in Populations, Chapter 10: Identifying the Genetic Basis for Human Disease.

Figures

Grey, Kindred, Figure 14.3 Graphic representation of penetrance and expressivity. 2021. CC BY4.0. Adapted from Introduction to Genetic Analysis 7th Ed. Figure 4.33 The effects of penetrance and expressivity through a hypothetical character "pigment intensity. From NCBI.

Grey, Kindred, Figure 14.4 Mitochondrial inheritance pattern. 2021. https://archive.org/details/14.4_20210926. CC BY-SA 4.0. Added Mitochondrial inheritance by Domaina, Angelito7 and SUM1. CC BY-SA 4.0. From Wikimedia Commons.

Grey, Kindred, Figure 14.5: Trinucleotide repeat expansion characteristic of Huntington's disease. 2021.

Additional resources

- Hardy-Weinberg problems: https://www.k-state.edu/parasitology.../hardwein.html
- Practice pedigrees: https://ocw.mit.edu/courses/biology/...ntals-of-biology-fall-2011/genetics/pedigrees/MIT7_01SCF11_3.3sol1.pdf
- Practice pedigrees: https://www.khanacademy.org/science/high-school-biology/hs-classical-genetics/hs-pedigrees/a/hs-pedigrees-review

14.3 Linkage Analysis and Genome-Wide Association Studies (GWAS)

There is tremendous interest in finding specific genes that predispose individuals to common disease traits, most of which follow complex inheritance patterns rather than Mendelian (single gene) patterns. Physicians will find frequent references in the medical literature related to the search for genes with high predictive value in common disorders.

While we know the DNA sequence of the vast majority of the coding regions of the genome, we still do not understand the full function of the majority of genes or how they are involved in human health conditions. There are two major approaches to identifying genetic loci, which contribute to disease presentation: linkage analysis and genome-wide association studies.

Linkage analysis

Linkage analysis relies on the fact that disease-causing mutations are inherited jointly (linked) with genetic markers located in their immediate vicinity. In order for a gene and a genetic marker to be linked, they must be syntenic, meaning they must be located on the same chromosome. Most genes or markers within the human genome are inherited independently of one another, and therefore are transmitted together 50 percent of the time.

Linkage between two genes means that they tend to be inherited together more often than expected by chance.

For linkage to occur, two conditions must be met:

- First, the genes must be syntenic.
- Second, they need to reside relatively close to one another.

Syntenic genes may become detached from one another through crossing over (or recombination). For large chromosomes, crossing over is so common that genes at opposite ends of the chromosome are inherited together no more often than if they resided on entirely different chromosomes.

When markers are close enough together on the same chromosome, crossing over fails to separate them frequently enough for them to be inherited independently of one another. This is evidenced by coinheritance of greater than 50 percent.

The unit of measure in linkage studies is "centimorgans." This concept can be confusing because we refer to the "distance" between two traits, but what is measured experimentally is the frequency of coinheritance, not physical distance.

A very small linkage distance means the traits are rarely separated during meiosis. A distance of 0 cM means two traits always stay together, implying that they are extremely close to one another on the same chromosome. If the two traits separate from one another 1 percent of the time during meiosis, they are described as being 1 cM apart; if the two traits separate from one another 5 percent of the time during meiosis, they are described as being 5 cM apart (figure 14.6).

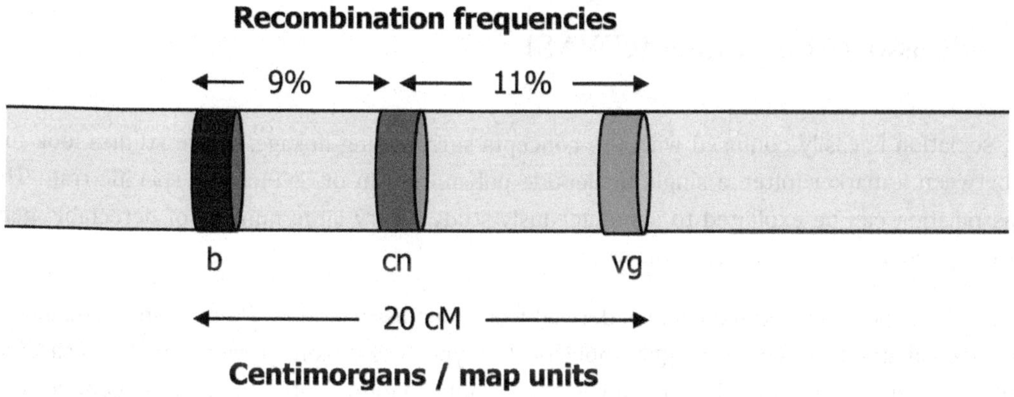

Figure 14.6: Relationship between centimorgans and recombination frequency.

The further apart two genes or markers are on the same chromosome increases the probability of a crossover occurring in between the two markers. Studies to determine linkage require the careful study of large numbers of parents and their offspring. Careful study of the family relationships across three generations allows linkage phases to be determined. In this case, the grandparents' information is required to determine how the genes are initially linked in the parents, and the grandchildren are studied to determine recombination events (crossing over) that separate the genes or markers during meiosis in the parents.

Distance can be expressed in cM as described previously, or in terms of theta (θ), which are proportions. Remember, both are measures of probability, not physical distance. Linkage determinations are based on the fundamental rules of probability and binomial mathematics. Like any probability issue, a ratio greater than one reflects odds in favor (of linkage), and less than one reflects odds against.

For linkage studies, each family represents an independent estimate of the odds in favor of (or against) linkage. The property within standard probability laws is the concept of joint probability. To determine joint probability, meaning the chance that BOTH of two events will happen, we use what is often called the "AND rule." The AND rule applies whenever the probabilities under study are independent of one another.

Multiplying the results of many families is challenging, and was particularly so before computer resources became readily available. It is simpler mathematically to add numbers. We can move from multiplication to addition if we simply use the log of the probability instead of the probability number itself. Remember that the log of a number that is less than one is a negative number, and for a number greater than one, it is a positive number. Using a log conversion makes it simple to see if the ratio of the odds is favorable (positive) or unfavorable. The term "LOD score" refers to the log (base 10) of the odds of linkage, looking across a series of independent families.

There really are just two things to remember about LOD scores:

- First, it is a convenient system for combining the observations across a large number of families to describe the odds of linkage.
- Second, the values of LOD scores define "proof" that two genes or markers are linked or not linked.
- When the odds reach an LOD score of 3, the two markers are considered to be proven to be linked.
- When odds reach a level of -2, this is taken as conclusive evidence that the two genes or markers are not linked. LOD scores appear in a great deal of medical literature where the identification or location of disease-related genes is being considered.

Genome-wide association studies (GWAS)

Population association is easily confused with the concepts surrounding linkage. These studies look for a statistical association between a marker (often a single nucleotide polymorphism or SNP) and a specific trait. The concept of population association can be exploited to simultaneously study a very large number of detectable genetic markers (SNPs) in patient populations with common disorders.

Much of the power of personalized medicine is derived from such associations. There is an abundance of GWAS that appear in the medical literature. This is a highly sophisticated type of case-control study for which careful study design is required to avoid spurious findings. These studies provide information related to common genetic traits but do not help address genetic manifestations of rare traits in a population (figure 14.7).

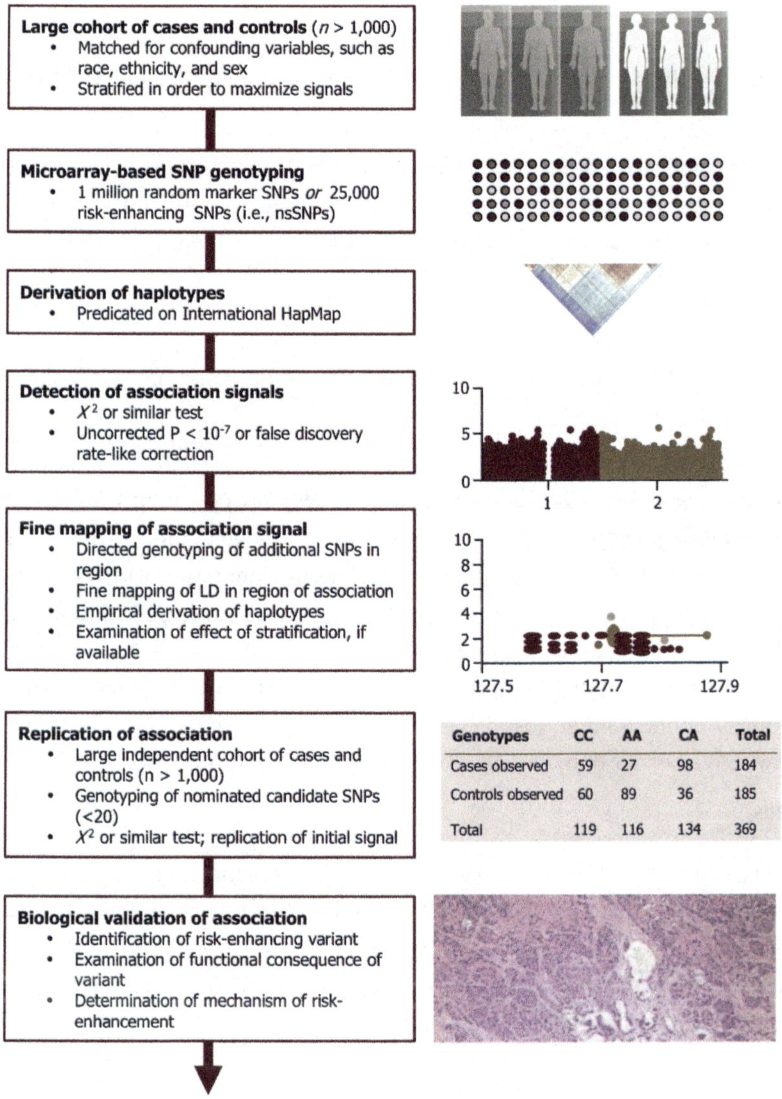

Genotypes	CC	AA	CA	Total
Cases observed	59	27	98	184
Controls observed	60	89	36	185
Total	119	116	134	369

Figure 14.7: Schematic of GWAS.

For more information on these types of studies, please see: https://www.genome.gov/20019523/geno...ies-factsheet/.

14.3 References and resources

Text

Clark, M. A. *Biology*, 2nd ed. Houston, TX: OpenStax College, Rice University, 2018, Chapter 10: Cell Reproduction, Chapter 12: Mendel's Experiments and Heridity, Chapter 13: Modern Understandings of Inheritance.

Le, T., and V. Bhushan. *First Aid for the* USMLE *Step* 1, 29th ed. New York: McGraw Hill Education, 2018, 55–59.

Nussbaum, R. L., R. R. McInnes, H. F. Willard, A. Hamosh, and M. W. Thompson. *Thompson & Thompson Genetics in Medicine*, 8th ed. Philadelphia: Saunders/Elsevier, 2016, Chapter 7: Patterns of Single Gene Inheritance, Chapter 9: Genetic Variations in Populations, Chapter 10: Identifying the Genetic Basis for Human Disease.

Figures

Grey, Kindred, Figure 14.6 Relationship between centimorgans and recombination frequency. 2021. https://archive.org/details/14.6_20210926. CC BY 4.0.

Tam, V., Patel, N., Turcotte, M. et al. Figure 14.7 Schematic of GWAS study. Adapted under Fair Use from Benefits and limitations of genome-wide association studies. Nat Rev Genet 20, 467–484 (2019). https://pubmed.ncbi.nlm.nih.gov/31068683/. Fig. 1: GWAS study design. Added Mitochondrial inheritance by Domaina, Angelito7 and SUM1. CC BY-SA 4.0. From Wikimedia Commons. Added Genetic similarities between 51 worldwide human populations (Euclidean genetic distance using 289,160 SNPs) by Tiago R. Magalhães, Jillian P. Casey, Judith Conroy, Regina Regan, Darren J. Fitzpatrick, Naisha Shah, João Sobral, Sean Ennis. CC BY 2.5. From Wikimedia Commons. Added Histopathology of adenosquamous carcinoma of the pancreas by Yeung, Vincent; Palmer, Joshua D.; Williams, Noelle; Weinstein, Jonathan C.; Fortuna, Danielle; Sama, Ashwin; Winter, Jordan; Bar-Ad, Voichita. CC BY 4.0. From Wikimedia Commons.

Additional resources

- Hardy-Weinberg problems: https://www.k-state.edu/parasitology.../hardwein.html
- Practice pedigrees: https://ocw.mit.edu/courses/biology/...ntals-of-biology-fall-2011/genetics/pedigrees/MIT7_01SCF11_3.3sol1.pdf
- Practice pedigrees: https://www.khanacademy.org/science/high-school-biology/hs-classical-genetics/hs-pedigrees/a/hs-pedigrees-review

15. Cellular Signaling

Learning Objectives

- Outline the general characteristics of signal transduction systems.
- Describe the mechanism by which G protein coupled receptors produce secondary messengers.
- Describe the points at which cascades can be regulated by phosphatases and inhibitors.
- Describe phosphatidylinositol-derived second messengers and the functions of Ca_2^{+} as a second messenger and the downstream effectors that both activate.
- Describe the characteristics of the receptor tyrosine kinase signaling pathway.
- Describe the signal transduction principles used in regulating glucose levels (pathways initiated by glucagon, epinephrine, and insulin).
- Describe the general processes of cellular apoptosis
- Describe the physiological role of membrane potential in signal transduction.

15.1 Cell Communication

Cell communication is a fundamental homeostatic process.

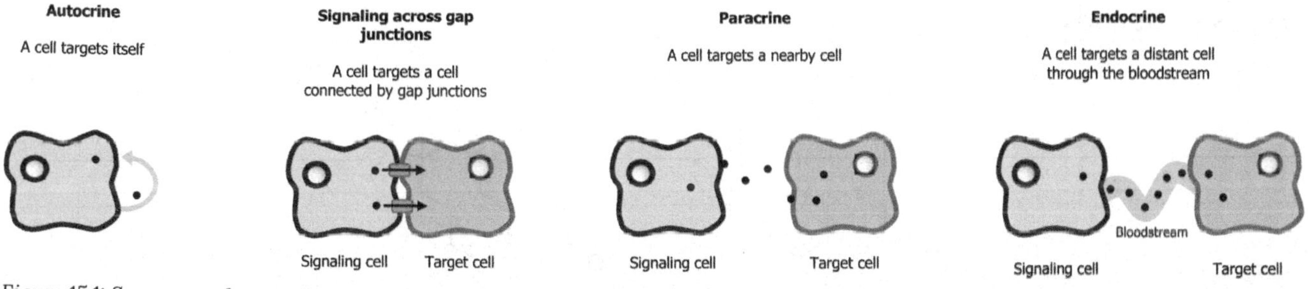

Figure 15.1: Summary of types of cell signaling.

Generally speaking, it uses various communication modalities to sense and respond to neighboring cells and environmental cues, which can be categorized into the following types of communication (figure 15.1):

- Autocrine: These signals act on the cell from which it is secreted or on nearby cells that are the same type of cell as the secreting cell. Most autocrine cells are also paracrine cells.
- Juxtocrine or signaling through gap junctions: These types of signals require physical contact between cells in order for a signal to be transduced. These are two different types of signaling that both involve cell contact.

- Paracrine: The paracrine substance is secreted from cells that are not normally thought of as endocrine cells. Actions are performed on nearby cells and very low amounts are too dilute to affect distance cells. The location of the cell plays a role in the specificity of the response.
- Endocrine: Endocrine cells secrete the hormone into the blood and exerts its action on specific target cells that can be very far away (for example: insulin, glucagon, and cortisol).

General characteristics:

- Cellular signaling begins with the release of a chemical messenger, which will either diffuse or is transported in the blood/extracellular fluids to its location of action.

Once at the intended location it will bind to its receptor, which can be intracellular or extracellular, to elicit a response.

This could be in the form of:

- A conformational change
- Activation of a second messenger
- Protein recruitment
- Cleavage of a receptor

Finally, the signal can be terminated by:

- Degradation of the receptor or ligand.

The outcome of a signaling cascade is diverse. For example, elevated insulin may signal for increased uptake and storage of glucose (see section 15.3) or a signal may initiate apoptosis (see section 15.2).

Types of ligands

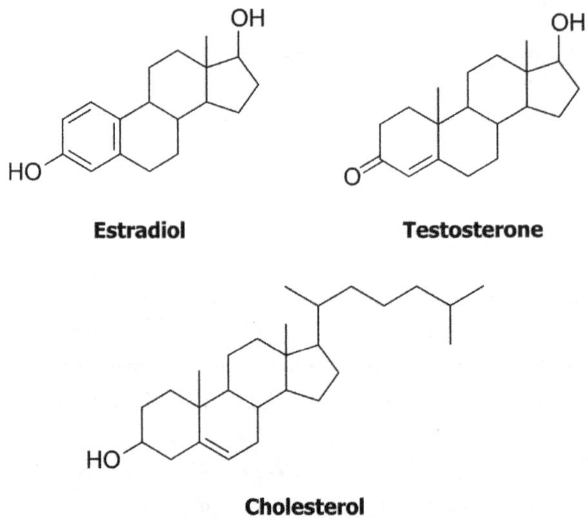

Figure 15.2: Examples of steroid hormones.

- Steroid hormones: These are often cholesterol-derived and can diffuse through membranes to bind intracellular receptors (figure 15.2).
- Amino acid metabolites: These types of hormones are often neurotransmitters and contain nitrogenous groups.
- Gases: Both NO and CO are common gases that elicit unique signaling cascades.
- Proteins: These can be small polypeptides (e.g., insulin) or larger membrane-bound proteins that elicit a cellular response.
- Lipids: Eicosanoids and other phospholipids can function as cell signals either in a membrane bound or free form.

General G-protein-coupled receptor cascade

G-protein-coupled receptors (GPCR) can come in several different classes: $G\alpha_s$, $G\alpha_i$, and $G\alpha_q$. Activation of a $G\alpha_s$ (activated by glucagon) will increase the second messenger cAMP, while both $G\alpha_i$ or $G\alpha_t$ cascades function to reduce cAMP, either through inhibition of adenylyl cyclase (also known as adenylate cyclase) or through activation of phosphodiesterase, respectively.

The classic cascade starts with hormone binding, to an extracellular domain of a seven-helix receptor (GPCR), which causes a conformational change in the receptor that is transmitted to a G protein on the cytosolic side of the membrane (figure 15.3).

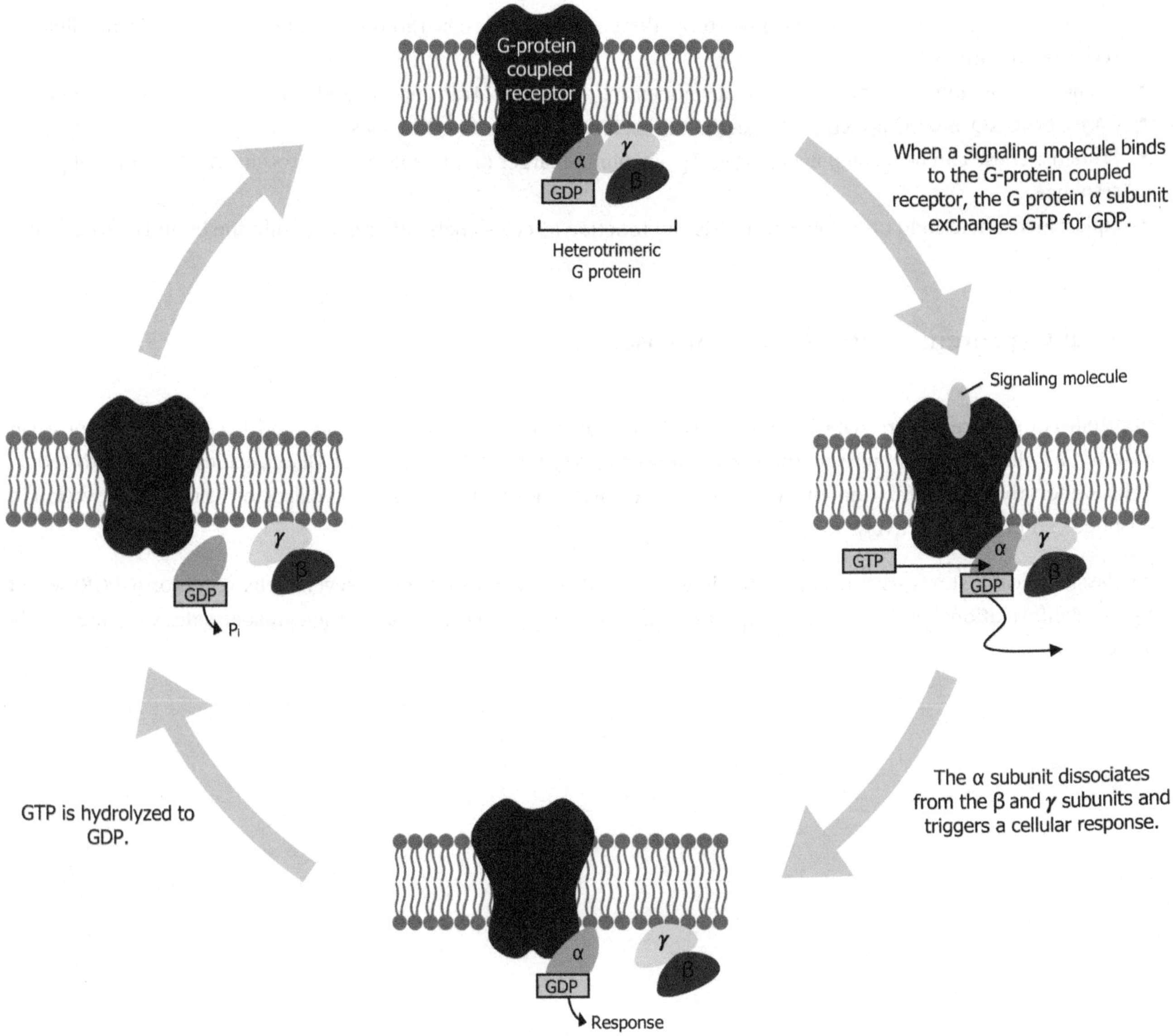

Figure 15.3: Common G-protein-coupled receptor signaling cascade.

- The nucleotide-binding site on $G\alpha_S$ becomes more accessible to the cytosol, where [GTP] is usually higher than [GDP]. Gα releases GDP and binds GTP (GDP–GTP exchange). Substitution of GTP for GDP causes another conformational change in Gα.
- Gα-GTP dissociates from the inhibitory subunit complex and activates adenylyl cyclase.
- Adenylyl cyclase catalyzes synthesis of cAMP (second messenger), and in turn cAMP activates protein kinase A (cAMP-dependent protein kinase).
- The cascade can be terminated by the action of phosphodiesterase, which can degrade cAMP and terminate signal.

Phosphatidylinositol-derived second messengers

Phosphatidylinositols are membrane-bound compounds that can be phosphorylated or cleaved to function as second messengers in a signaling cascade (figure 15.4).

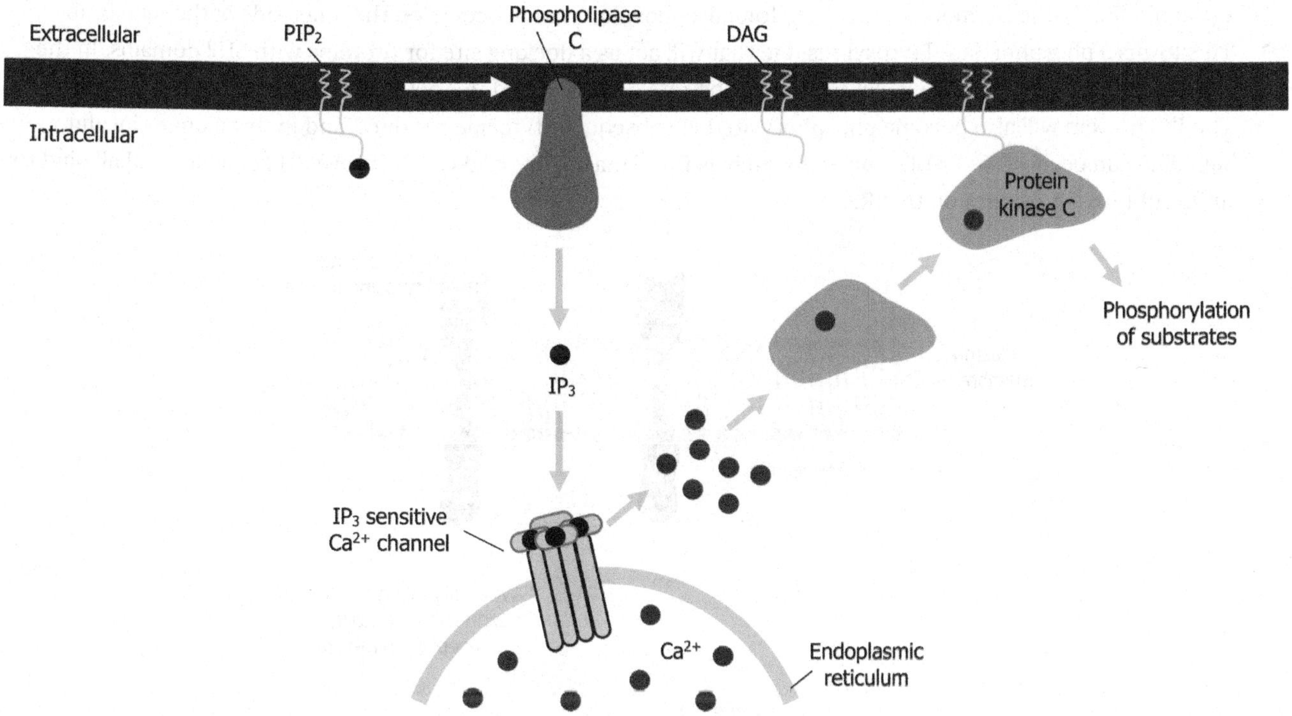

Figure 15.4: Signaling cascade initiated by DAG and IP3.

The common membrane component, phosphatidylinositol (PI), can be phosphorylated (by any number of kinases) to form PI 4,5-bisphosphate. This molecule can undergo two different fates.

1. First it could be phosphorylated by a kinase, such as P-I3kinase, downstream of insulin; this produces phosphatidylinositol 3′,4′,5′-trisphosphate (PI-3,4,5-trisP), which can serve as a plasma-membrane docking site for signal transduction proteins with pleckstrin homology domains (PH).
2. Alternatively, PI 4,5-bisphosphate can be cleaved into two second messengers: inositol-1,4,5-trisphosphate (IP_3) and diacylglycerol (DAG) by activation of phospholipase C (PLC). Phospholipase C is downstream of a Gαq cascade.

This cascade will become important for calcium signaling, which is modulated through interactions of IP_3 with the mitochondria.

1. DAG recruits protein kinase C.
2. IP_3 initiates release of CA^{2+} from the smooth ER.

Changes in intracellular calcium can alter membrane permeability through calcium-induced calcium release.

Receptor Tyrosine Kinase (RTK)

RTKs are in the cell membrane and typically function as a dimer.

- Upon binding of the hormone to the receptor, autophosphorylation occurs on the inner side of the membrane. This forms a phosphorylated tyrosyl residue that will act as a docking site for proteins with SH2 domains. In the case of insulin signaling, the insulin receptor substrate (IRS) will bind this activated receptor (figure 15.5).
- The IRS protein will also become phosphorylated at subsequent tyrosine residues, and in this manner insulin signaling can be amplified. Other proteins such as PI 3-kinase, PLC, and Grb2 all have SH2 domains and all bind to different tyrosyl residues on the IRS.

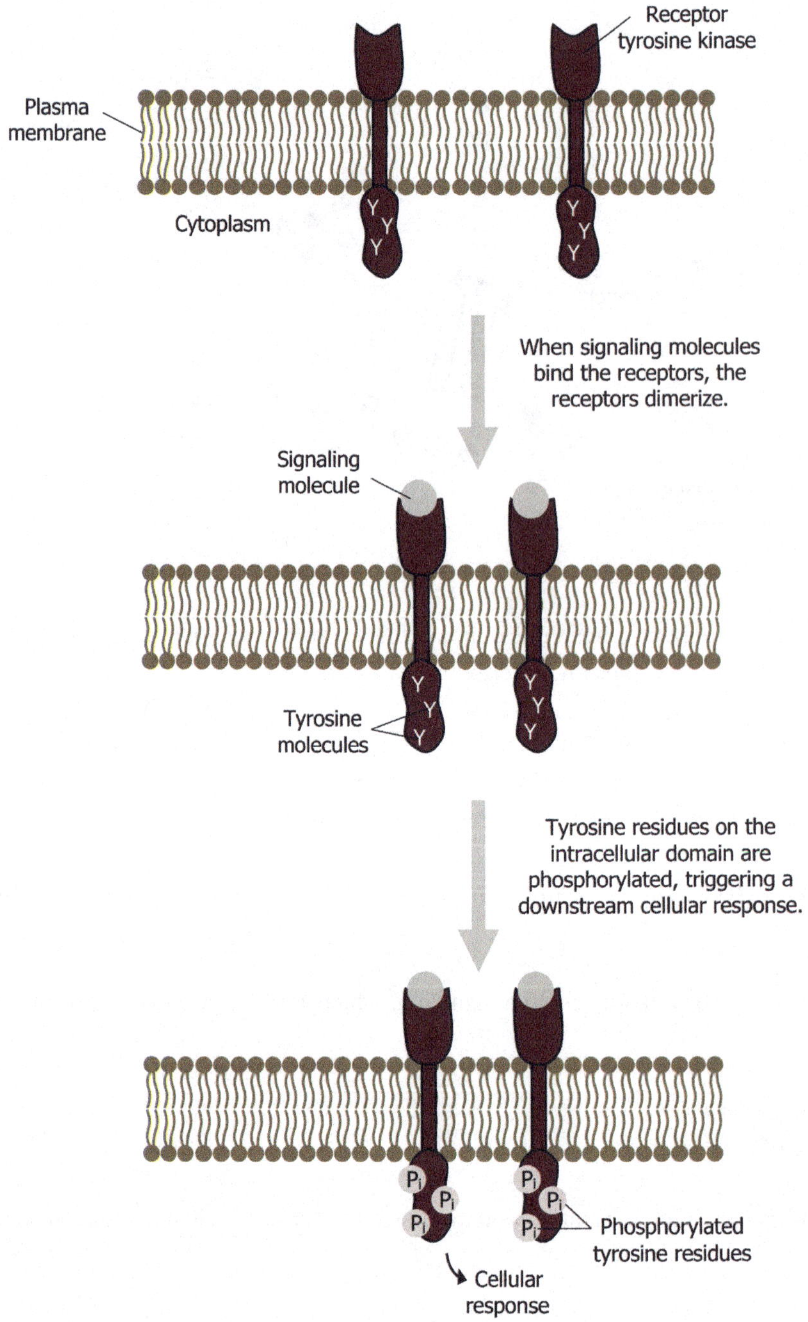

Figure 15.5: Receptor tyrosine kinase signaling.

Two major cascades are activated downstream of insulin and other growth hormones:

- Ras-dependent signaling: The activated Grb2 binds a SOS-Ras complex leading to a conformational change exchanging GDP for GTP. Ras-GTP binds Raf, and activated Raf is the first step in a MAP-kinase cascade that can lead to a change in gene transcription.
- Ras-independent signaling: This involves activation of phosphoinositol 3-kinase and is discussed under phosphatidylinositol-derived second messengers.

Jak-STAT and serine threonine kinases

Jak-STATs are also types of tyrosine kinases. The difference here is that these receptors lack autocatalytic abilities and require an intracellular kinase (Jak) to phosphorylate the transcription factor STAT. Jak-STAT signaling is most commonly associated with immune cell signaling.

Serine threonine kinase

This receptor family encompasses many of the growth factors for the body (EGF, VEGF, and TGF-β). These receptors usually form heterodimers, and the Type II receptor will autophosphorylate the Type I receptor upon ligand binding. These receptors have an autocatalytic domain that will phosphorylate and typically activate a transcription factor.

Intracellular receptors

Intracellular receptors bind hydrophobic chemical messengers such as steroid hormones. Binding of the intracellular receptor (which could be cytosolic or nuclear) usually elicits a transcriptional response. Cortisol is an example of a hormone that binds an intracellular receptor. It is released from the adrenal cortex and diffuses into the bloodstream attached to serum albumin and steroid hormone-binding globulin. After diffusing through the plasma membrane, it binds to the cortisol receptor (intracellular receptor) in the cytosol and forms a homodimer exposing a nuclear localization signal (NLS). Exposure of the NLS targets the complex to the nucleus.

Intracellular receptors commonly have three domains:

- Transactivation domain,
- DNA-binding domain, and
- Ligand-binding domain.

Intracellular receptors will function as a transcriptional activator by binding specific DNA elements, altering transcription of downstream genes. The signal is terminated by the lowering of the concentration of the hormone.

NO as a messenger

Nitric oxide NO is a gas that also acts as a ligand. It is able to diffuse directly across the plasma membrane, and one of its roles is to interact with receptors in smooth muscle and induce relaxation of the tissue.

NO has a very short half-life and, therefore, only functions over short distances. It activates guanylyl cyclase to synthesize cGMP. This in turn results in smooth muscle relaxation.

Nitroglycerin, a treatment for heart disease, acts by triggering the release of NO, which causes blood vessels to dilate (expand), thus restoring blood flow to the heart. NO has become better known recently because the pathway that it affects is targeted by prescription medications for erectile dysfunction, such as Viagra (erection involves dilated blood vessels).

15.1 References and resources

Text

Clark, M. A. *Biology*, 2nd ed. Houston, TX: OpenStax College, Rice University, 2018, Chapter 9: Cell Communication, Chapter 10: Cell Reproduction.

Karp, G., and J. G. Patton. *Cell and Molecular Biology: Concepts and Experiments*, 7th ed. Hoboken, NJ: John Wiley, 2013, Chapter 15: Cell Signaling and Signal Transduction.

Le, T., and V. Bhushan. *First Aid for the USMLE Step 1*, 29th ed. New York: McGraw Hill Education, 2018, 85, 208, 238.

Figures

Grey, Kindred, Figure 15.1 Summary of types of cell signaling. 2021. https://archive.org/details/15.1_20210926. CC BY 4.0.

Grey, Kindred, Figure 15.2 Examples of steroid hormones. 2021. Chemical structure by Henry Jakubowski. https://archive.org/details/15.2_20210926. CC BY 4.0.

Grey, Kindred, Figure 15.3 Common G-protein coupled receptor signaling cascade. 2021. CC BY 4.0. Added ion channel by Léa Lortal from the Noun Project.

Grey, Kindred, Figure 15.4 Signaling cascade initiated by DAG and IP3. 2021. https://archive.org/details/15.4_20210926. CC BY 4.0.

Grey, Kindred, Figure 15.5 Receptor Tyrosine kinase signaling. 2021. CC BY 4.0. Added ion channel by Léa Lortal from the Noun Project.

15.2 Apoptosis

Both cell proliferation and apoptosis (controlled/programed cell death) are decisive processes within a cell. Keep in mind, apoptosis is distinct from cell necrosis, in which cell death is usually attributable to physical or chemical damage and rapidly spontaneous; think explosion.

Apoptosis is genetically programmed cell death, which leads to "tidy" breakdown and disposal of cells. Morphologically, apoptosis is characterized by shrinking of the cell, changes in the cell membrane (with the formation of small blebs known as "apoptotic bodies"), shrinking of the nucleus, chromatin condensation, and fragmentation of DNA. Macrophages and other phagocytic cells recognize this signal and remove apoptotic cells by phagocytosis without inflammatory phenomena developing. Apoptosis regulates the growth of normal tissues and removes unwanted cells in a controlled manner.

Caspases are a family of enzymes that control this process. These are cysteine proteases that cleave proteins next to aspartate residues when they become activated. When a cell receives an apoptotic signal, the procaspases become active and begin the process of protein degradation starting with the cleavage of laminins in the nuclear envelope, protein kinases, transcription factors, snRP proteins, and inhibitors of special DNAses, which are able to fragment the nuclear DNA (figure 15.6).

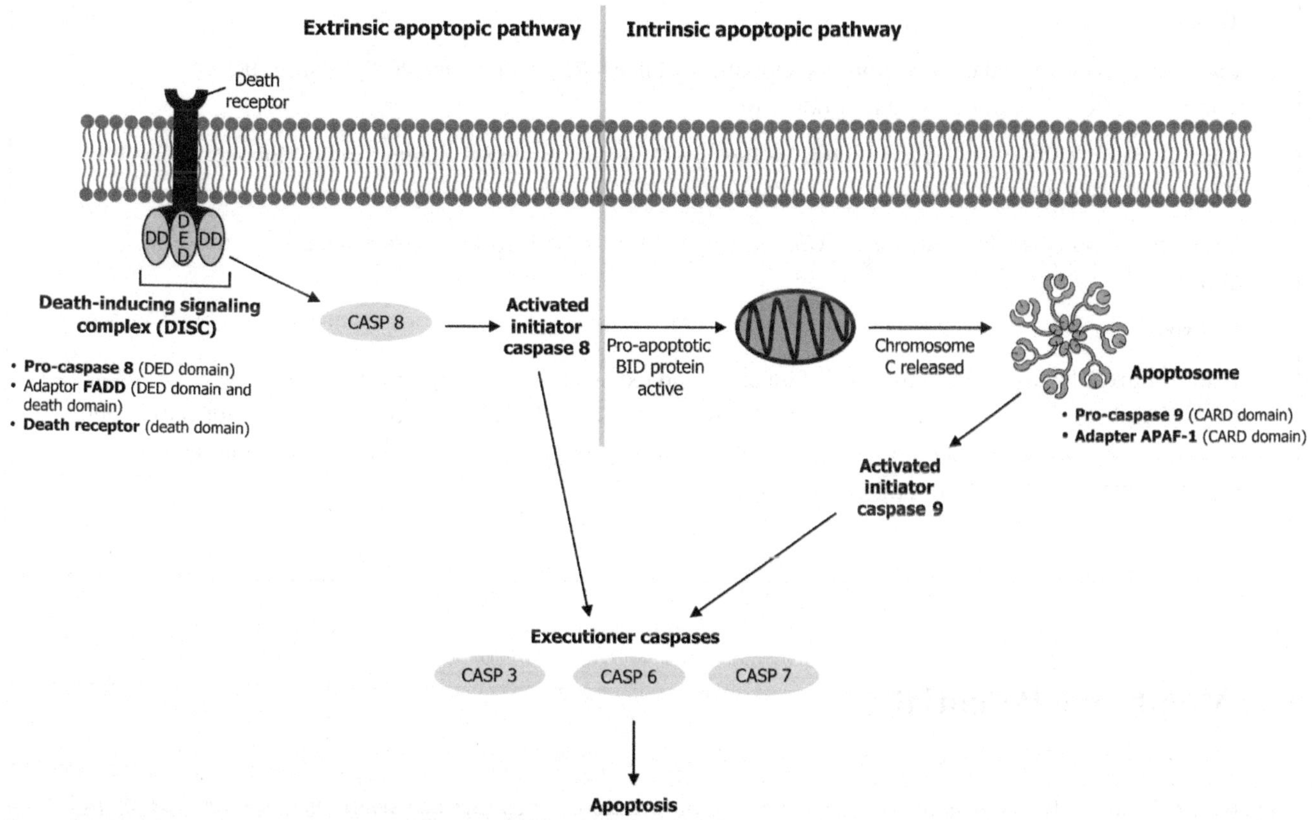

Figure 15.6: Comparison of intrinsic and extrinsic apoptosis pathways.

The extrinsic pathway for apoptosis is triggered on the cell surface by ligands that bind to receptors of the tumor necrosis factor family (TNFR, "death receptors"). These include Fas receptors, which are present on the plasma membrane of most cells in the body. When Fas ligands bind to a cell's Fas receptors, trimerization of the receptors takes place via the adapter protein FADD ("Fas-associated death domain"), which activates the initiator caspases 8 and 10 inside the cell, setting in motion the apoptotic process.

The intrinsic, mitochondrial pathway is triggered by genotoxic (DNA damage) or oxidative stress. Aided by Bcl proteins, chemical stress makes the outer mitochondrial membrane leaky. As a result, mitochondrial proteins reach the cytoplasm. Cytochrome c in particular then triggers the caspase cascade by binding to the adapter protein Apaf1 and promoting formation of an apoptosome, a wheel-shaped heptamer that recruits initiator procaspase 9 and activates it to caspase 9.

The Bcl protein family not only includes proapoptotic proteins (Bax, Bak, and Bim) but also proteins that inhibit apoptosis (including Bcl2). Extracellular growth factors ensure inactivation of Bad or replication of Bcl 2, thus preventing apoptosis.

15.2 References and resources

Text

Clark, M. A. *Biology*, 2nd ed. Houston, TX: OpenStax College, Rice University, 2018, Chapter 9: Cell Communication, Chapter 10: Cell Reproduction.

Karp, G., and J. G. Patton. *Cell and Molecular Biology: Concepts and Experiments*, 7th ed. Hoboken, NJ: John Wiley, 2013, Chapter 15: Cell Signaling and Signal Transduction.

Le, T., and V. Bhushan. *First Aid for the USMLE Step 1*, 29th ed. New York: McGraw Hill Education, 2018, 85, 208, 238.

Figures

Grey, Kindred, Figure 15.6 Comparison of intrinsic and extrinsic apoptosis pathways. 2021. https://archive.org/details/15.6_20210926. CC BY-SA 3.0. Added Model № 2 of apoptosome formation and activation of caspase-9 and caspase-3 (hy) by Brat Ural. CC BY-SA 3.0. From Wikimedia Commons. Added ion channel by Léa Lortal from the Noun Project.

15.3 Membrane Potential

The electrical state of the cell membrane can have several variations. These are all variations in the membrane potential. A potential is a distribution of charge across the cell membrane, measured in millivolts (mV). The standard is to compare the inside of the cell relative to the outside, so the membrane potential is a value representing the charge on the intracellular side of the membrane based on the outside being zero, relatively speaking. Neurons harvest this membrane potential to generate or propagate a nerve impulse (figure 15.7).

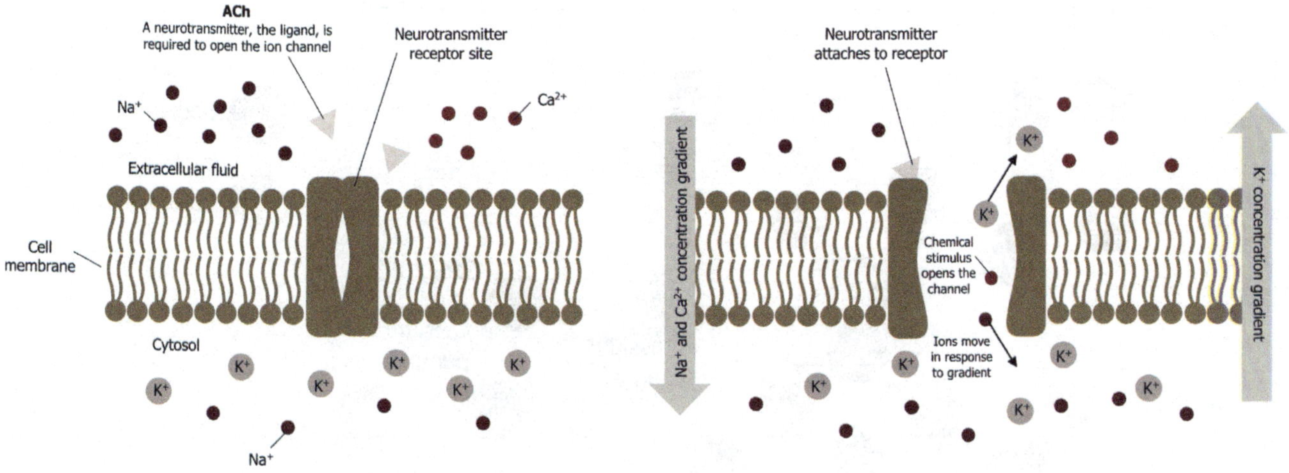

Figure 15.7: Neurotransmission by acetylcholine.

The action potential

Resting membrane potential describes the steady state of the cell, which is a dynamic process that is balanced by ion leakage and ion pumping. Without any outside influence, it will not change. To get an electrical signal started, the membrane potential has to change (summary in figures 15.8 and 15.9).

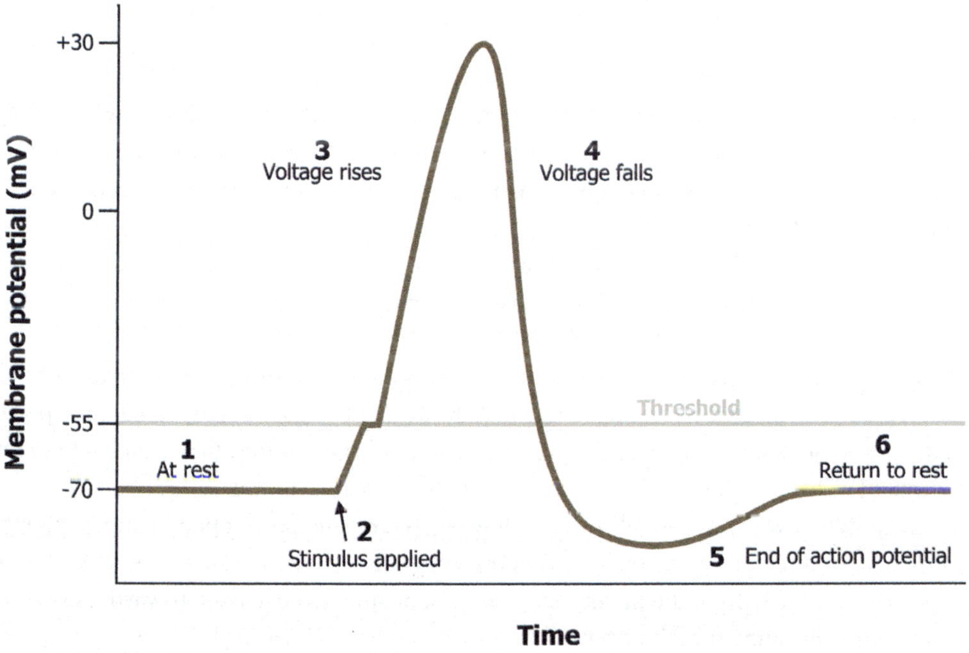

Figure 15.8: Summary of the action potential to membrane potential.

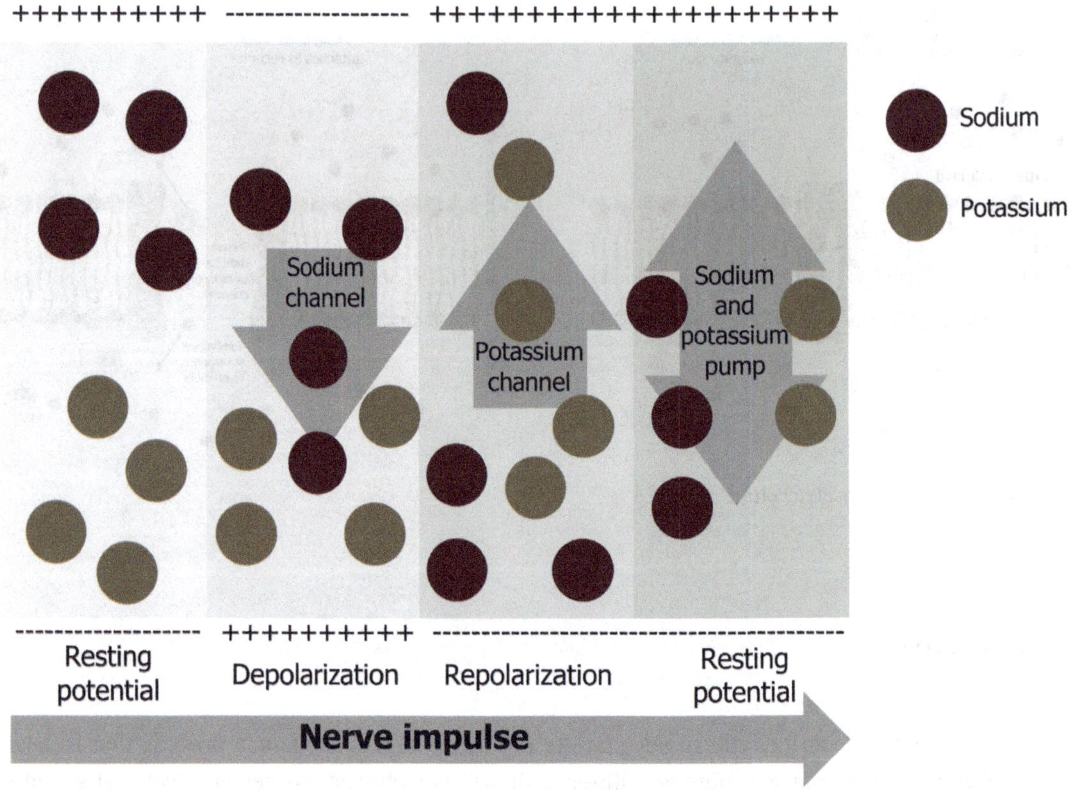

Figure 15.9: Summary of the action potential as it relates to change in ion concentration across the membrane.

- This starts with a channel opening for Na^+ in the membrane. Because the concentration of Na^+ is higher outside the cell than inside the cell by a factor of 10, ions will rush into the cell that are driven largely by the concentration gradient. Because sodium is a positively charged ion, it will change the relative voltage immediately inside the cell relative to immediately outside.
- The resting potential is the state of the membrane at a voltage of −70 mV, so the sodium cation entering the cell will cause it to become less negative. This is known as depolarization, meaning the membrane potential moves toward zero.
- The concentration gradient for Na^+ is so strong that it will continue to enter the cell even after the membrane potential has become zero, so that the voltage immediately around the pore begins to become positive. The electrical gradient also plays a role, as negative proteins below the membrane attract the sodium ion. The membrane potential will reach +30 mV by the time sodium has entered the cell.
- As the membrane potential reaches +30 mV, other voltage-gated channels are opening in the membrane. These channels are specific for the potassium ion. A concentration gradient acts on K^+ as well. As K^+ starts to leave the cell, taking a positive charge with it, the membrane potential begins to move back toward its resting voltage. This is called repolarization, meaning that the membrane voltage moves back toward the −70 mV value of the resting membrane potential.
- Repolarization returns the membrane potential to the −70 mV value that indicates the resting potential, but it actually overshoots that value. Potassium ions reach equilibrium when the membrane voltage is below −70 mV, so a period of hyperpolarization occurs while the K^+ channels are open. Those K^+ channels are slightly delayed in closing, accounting for this short overshoot.

15.3 References and resources

Text

Clark, M. A. *Biology*, 2nd ed. Houston, TX: OpenStax College, Rice University, 2018, Chapter 9: Cell Communication, Chapter 10: Cell Reproduction.

Karp, G., and J. G. Patton. *Cell and Molecular Biology: Concepts and Experiments*, 7th ed. Hoboken, NJ: John Wiley, 2013, Chapter 15: Cell Signaling and Signal Transduction.

Le, T., and V. Bhushan. *First Aid for the USMLE Step 1*, 29th ed. New York: McGraw Hill Education, 2018, 85, 208, 238.

Figures

Grey, Kindred, Figure 15.7 Neurotransmission by acetylcholine. 2021. https://archive.org/details/15.7_20210926. CC BY 4.0. Added ion channel by Léa Lortal from the Noun Project.

Grey, Kindred, Figure 15.9 Summary of the action potential as it relates to change in ion concentration across the membrane. 2021. https://archive.org/details/15.9_20210926. CC BY 4.0.

Lieberman M, Peet A. Figure 15.8 Summary of the action potential to membrane potential. Adapted under Fair Use from Marks' Basic Medical Biochemistry. 5th Ed. pp 199. Figure 11.11 Signal transduction by tyrosine receptors. 2017.

16. Plasma Membrane

Learning Objectives

- Describe the structure and functions of cellular membranes.
- Describe the chemical components of cell membranes and review their chemical properties.
- Explain carbohydrate involvement in membrane structure, and their possible functions and location.
- Describe the types of proteins found in membranes and the roles they play in membrane function.
- Stress the importance of membrane fluidity to living cells and the mechanisms by which cells maintain an appropriate level of fluidity.
- Describe biological membrane asymmetry and the dynamic nature of membrane structure and function.
- Describe the different mechanisms employed by cells to transport materials across membranes: simple and facilitated diffusion, channel proteins, and active transport.

About this Chapter

Plasma membranes must allow certain substances to enter and leave a cell, and prevent some harmful materials from entering and some essential materials from leaving. In other words, plasma membranes are selectively permeable — they allow some substances to pass through, but not others. If they were to lose this selectivity, the cell would no longer be able to sustain itself, and it would be destroyed. There are four major types of transport across the cell membrane:

1. Diffusion,
2. Diffusion through a channel,
3. Facilitated diffusion (selective binding), and
4. Active transport (requires ATP).

16.1 Components and Structure

A cell's plasma membrane defines the cell, outlines its borders, and determines the nature of its interaction with its environment. Cells exclude some substances, take in others, and excrete still others, all in controlled quantities. The plasma membrane has many significant functions:

- It must be very flexible to allow certain cells, such as red and white blood cells, to change shape as they pass through narrow capillaries.
- It carries markers that allow cells to recognize one another, which is vital for tissue and organ formation during early development, and which later plays a role in the immune response's "self" versus "nonself" distinction.
- It functions as a medium for complex, integral proteins, and receptors to transmit signals. These proteins act both as extracellular input receivers and as intracellular processing activators.
- It imparts selective permeability essential for maintaining a resting membrane potential and osmoregulation.

Fluid mosaic model

The fluid mosaic model describes the plasma membrane structure as a mosaic of components – including phospholipids, cholesterol, proteins, and carbohydrates – that gives the membrane a fluid character. Plasma membranes range from 5 to 10 nm in thickness (figure 16.1). The protein, lipid, and carbohydrate proportions in the plasma membrane vary with cell type.

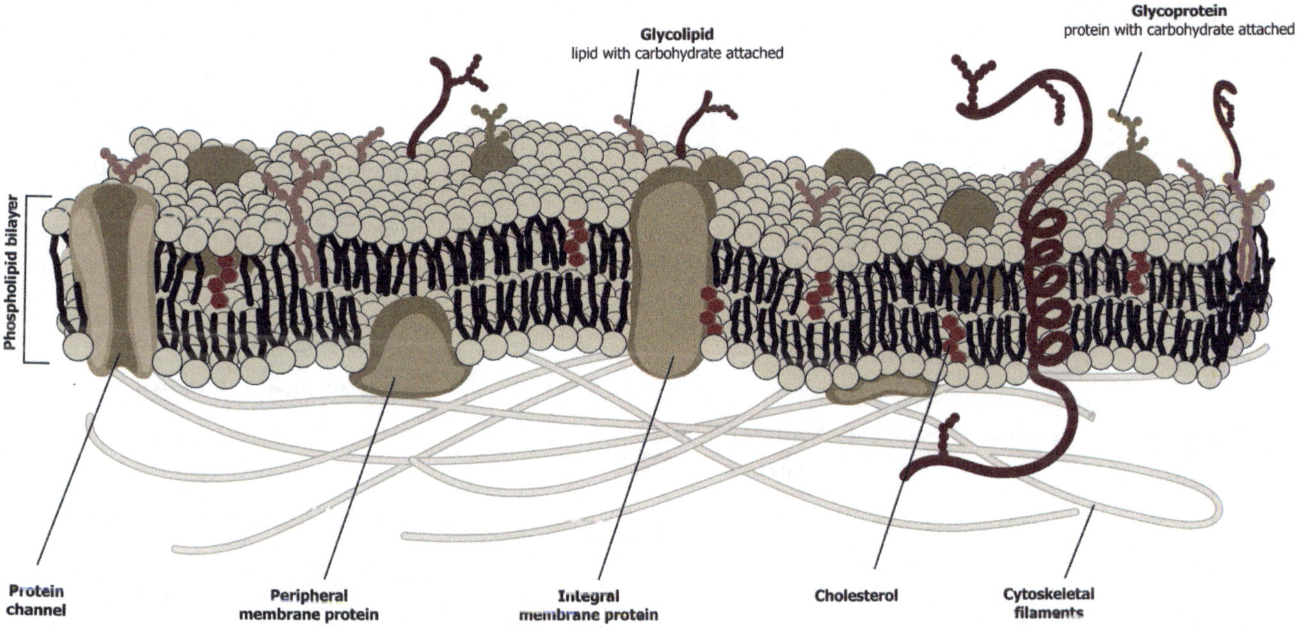

Figure 16.1: Schematic of the cell membrane. Plasma membranes range from 5 to 10 nm in thickness.

Lipids

The membrane's main fabric comprises amphiphilic, phospholipid molecules. The hydrophilic or "water-loving" areas of these molecules (figure 16.2) are in contact with the aqueous fluid both inside and outside the cell. Hydrophobic or "water-hating" molecules tend to be nonpolar. They interact with other nonpolar molecules in chemical reactions, but generally do not interact with polar molecules. A phospholipid molecule consists of a three-carbon glycerol backbone with two fatty acid molecules attached. This arrangement gives the overall molecule a head area (the phosphatecontaining group), which has a polar character or negative charge, and a tail area (the fatty acids), which has no charge. The head can form hydrogen bonds, but the tail cannot (figure 16.2).

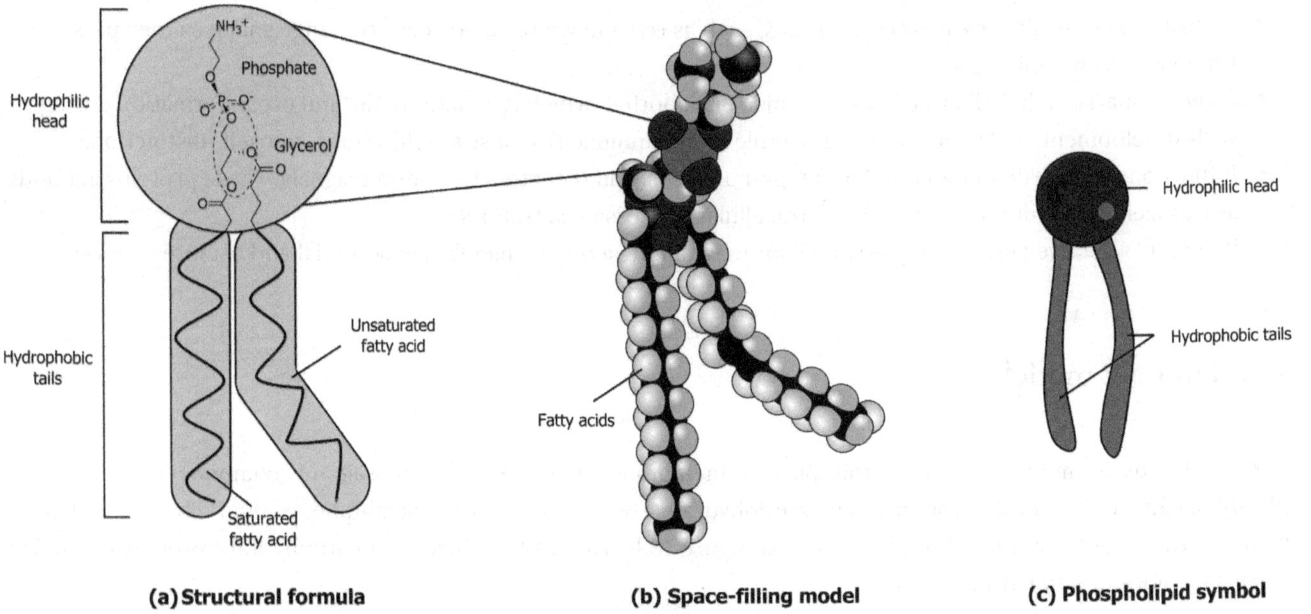

Figure 16.2: Structure of a phospholipid.

Cholesterol, another lipid comprised of four fused carbon rings, is situated alongside the phospholipids in the membrane's core (figure 16.2).

Specific phospholipids play key roles in the membrane; phosphatidylcholine, serine, inositol, and ethanolamine (figure 16.3) play various roles in the membrane.

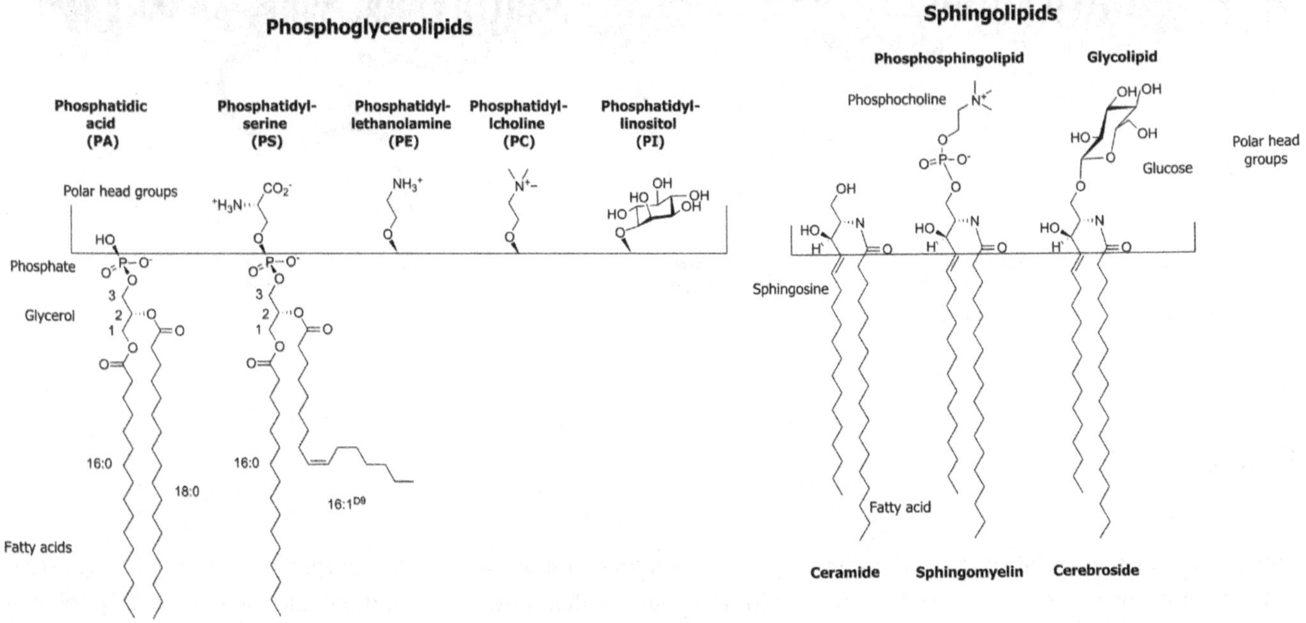

Figure 16.3: Important membrane lipids.

- Phoshatidylcholine is primarily found on the outer leaflet, while phosphatidylserine, inositol, and ethanolamine are all located predominately on the inner leaflet.

- Both phosphatidylserine and inositol are negatively charged at physiological pH allowing for binding of positively charged molecules.
- Sphingolipids and glycolipids are less abundant and play key roles in nervous tissue membranes. Disorders of sphingolipid or glycolipid metabolism are often severe (e.g., Tay-Sachs or Neimann-Pick disease).

Proteins

Proteins comprise the plasma membrane's second major component. Integral proteins, or integrins, as their name suggests, integrate completely into the membrane structure, and their hydrophobic membranespanning regions interact with the phospholipid bilayer's hydrophobic region.

Peripheral proteins are on the membrane's exterior and interior surfaces, attached either to integral proteins or to phospholipids. Peripheral proteins, along with integral proteins, may serve as enzymes, as structural attachments for the cytoskeleton's fibers, or as part of the cell's recognition sites. Scientists sometimes refer to these as "cell-specific" proteins. The body recognizes its own proteins and attacks foreign proteins associated with invasive pathogens. Additional proteins can be lipid anchored on the exterior of the membrane.

Carbohydrates

Carbohydrates are the third major plasma membrane component. They are always on the cell's exterior surface and are bound either to proteins (forming glycoproteins) or to lipids (forming glycolipids). These carbohydrate chains may consist of two to sixty monosaccharide units and can be either straight or branched. Along with peripheral proteins, carbohydrates form specialized sites on the cell surface that allow cells to recognize each other. We collectively refer to these carbohydrates on the cell's exterior surface – the carbohydrate components of both glycoproteins and glycolipids – as the glycocalyx (meaning "sugar coating"). The glycocalyx is highly hydrophilic and attracts large amounts of water to the cell's surface. This aids in the cell's interaction with its watery environment and in the cell's ability to obtain substances dissolved in the water.

Membrane fluidity

The integral proteins and lipids exist in the membrane as separate but loosely attached molecules. The membrane's mosaic characteristics explain some but not all of its fluidity. There are two other factors that help maintain this fluid characteristic.

One factor is the nature of the phospholipids themselves. In their saturated form, the fatty acids in phospholipid tails are saturated with bound hydrogen atoms. There are no double bonds between adjacent carbon atoms. This results in tails that are relatively straight. In contrast, unsaturated fatty acids do not contain a maximal number of hydrogen atoms, but they do contain some double bonds between adjacent carbon atoms.

Temperature can also influence membrane rigidity. Decreasing temperatures compress saturated fatty acids with their straight tails, and they press in on each other, making a dense and fairly rigid membrane. If unsaturated fatty acids are compressed, the "kinks" in their tails elbow adjacent phospholipid molecules away, maintaining some space between the phospholipid molecules. This "elbow room" helps maintain fluidity in the membrane at temperatures at which membranes with saturated fatty acid tails in their phospholipids would "freeze" or solidify.

16.1 References and resources

Text

Clark, M. A. *Biology*, 2nd ed. Houston, TX: OpenStax College, Rice University, 2018, Chapter 4: Cell Structure, Chapter 5: Structure and Function of the Plasma Membranes.

Karp, G., and J. G. Patton. *Cell and Molecular Biology: Concepts and Experiments*, 7th ed. Hoboken, NJ: John Wiley, 2013, Chapter 4: The Structure and Function of the Plasma Membrane.

Le, T., and V. Bhushan. *First Aid for the USMLE Step 1*, 29th ed. New York: McGraw Hill Education, 2018, 49.

Figures

Grey, Kindred, Figure 16.1 Schematic of the cell membrane. Plasma membranes range from 5 to 10 nm in thickness. 2021. https://archive.org/details/16.1_20210926. CC BY 4.0. Added Cell membrane detailed diagram blank by LadyofHats. Public domain. From Wikimedia Commons.

Grey, Kindred, Figure 16.2 Structure of a phospholipid. 2021. Chemical structure by Henry Jakubowski. https://archive.org/details/16.2_20210926. CC BY-SA 4.0. Added Cell membrane detailed diagram 4 vi by P.T.Đ. CC BY-SA 4.0. From Wikimedia Commons.

Grey, Kindred, Figure 16.3 Important membrane lipids. 2021. Chemical structure by Henry Jakubowski. https://archive.org/details/16.3_20210926. CC BY 4.0.

16.2 Passive Transport

Plasma membranes must allow certain substances to enter and leave a cell, and prevent some harmful materials from entering and some essential materials from leaving. In other words, plasma membranes are selectively permeable; they allow some substances to pass through, but not others. If they were to lose this selectivity, the cell would no longer be able to sustain itself, and it would be destroyed. There are four major types of transport across the cell membrane:

1. Diffusion,
2. Diffusion through a channel,
3. Facilitated diffusion (selective binding), and
4. Active transport (requires ATP).

Recall that plasma membranes are amphiphilic: they have hydrophilic and hydrophobic regions. This characteristic helps move some materials through the membrane and hinders the movement of others.

Nonpolar and lipid-soluble material with a low molecular weight can easily slip through the membrane's hydrophobic lipid core. Substances such as the fat-soluble vitamins A, D, E, and K readily pass through the plasma membranes in the digestive tract and other tissues. Fat-soluble drugs and hormones also gain easy entry into cells and readily transport themselves into the body's tissues and organs. Oxygen and carbon dioxide molecules have no charge and pass through membranes by simple diffusion.

Polar substances present problems for the membrane. While some polar molecules connect easily with the cell's outside, they cannot readily pass through the plasma membrane's lipid core.

Additionally, while small ions could easily slip through the spaces in the membrane's mosaic, their charge prevents them from doing so. Ions such as sodium, potassium, calcium, and chloride must have special means of penetrating plasma membranes. Simple sugars and amino acids also need the help of various transmembrane proteins (channels) to transport themselves across plasma membranes.

Diffusion

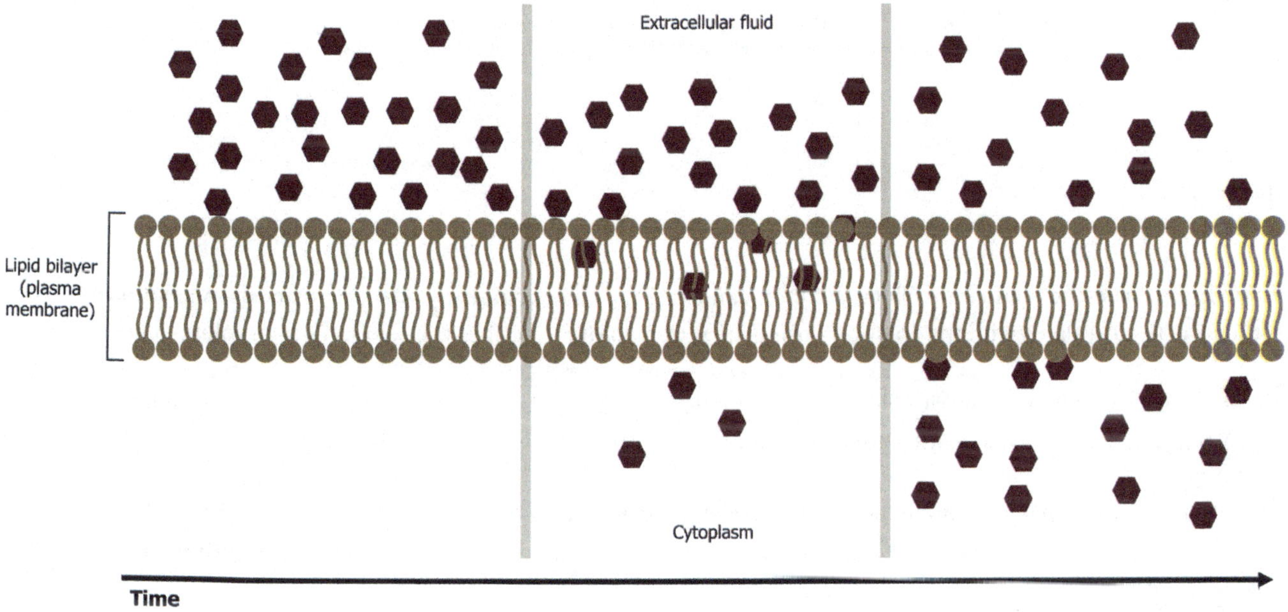

Figure 16.4: Diffusion across the plasma membrane.

Diffusion is a passive process of transport. A single substance moves from a high concentration to a low concentration area until the concentration is equal across a space (figure 16.4). Materials move within the cell's cytosol by diffusion, and certain materials move through the plasma membrane by diffusion such as lipids and fat-soluble vitamins. Diffusion expends no energy. On the contrary, concentration gradients are a form of potential energy, which dissipates as the gradient is eliminated.

Osmosis

Osmosis is the movement of water through a semipermeable membrane according to the water's concentration gradient across the membrane, which is inversely proportional to the solute's concentration. While diffusion transports material across membranes and within cells, osmosis transports only water across a membrane, and the membrane limits the solute's diffusion in the water (figure 16.5). Not surprisingly, the aquaporins that facilitate water movement play a large role in osmosis, most prominently in red blood cells and the membranes of kidney tubules. In osmosis, water always moves from an area of higher water concentration to one of lower concentration.

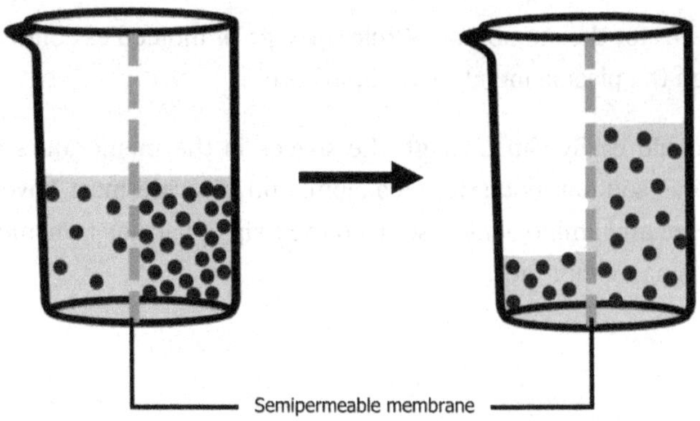

Figure 16.5: Illustration of osmosis. In the diagram, the solute cannot pass through the selectively permeable membrane, but the water can.

Tonicity

Tonicity describes how an extracellular solution can change a cell's volume by affecting osmosis. A solution's tonicity often directly correlates with the solution's osmolarity. Osmolarity describes the solution's total solute concentration.

- A solution with low osmolarity has a greater number of water molecules relative to the number of solute particles.
- A solution with high osmolarity has fewer water molecules with respect to solute particles.

In a situation in which a membrane, permeable to water though not to the solute, separates two different osmolarities, water will move from the membrane's side with lower osmolarity (and more water) to the side with higher osmolarity (and less water).

Hypotonic solutions

In a hypotonic situation, the extracellular fluid has lower osmolarity than the fluid inside the cell, and water enters the cell. It also means that the extracellular fluid has a higher water concentration in the solution than does the cell. In this situation, water will follow its concentration gradient and enter the cell.

Hypertonic solutions

As for a hypertonic solution, the prefix "hyper" refers to the extracellular fluid having a higher osmolarity than the cell's cytoplasm; therefore, the fluid contains less water than the cell does. Because the cell has a relatively higher water concentration, water will leave the cell.

Isotonic solutions

In an isotonic solution, the extracellular fluid has the same osmolarity as the cell. If the cell's osmolarity matches that of the extracellular fluid, there will be no net movement of water into or out of the cell, although water will still move in and out. Osmotic pressure changes red blood cells' shape in hypertonic, isotonic, and hypotonic solutions (figure 16.6).

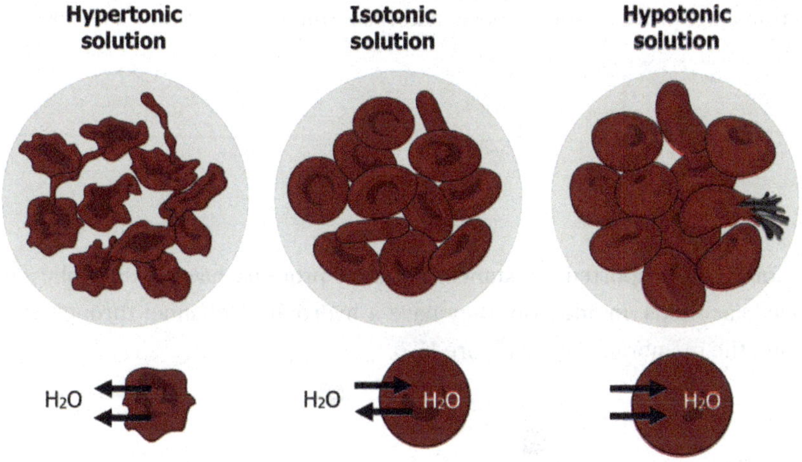

Figure 16.6: Comparison of red blood cell morphology in isotonic, hypertonic, and hypotonic solutions.

Factors that affect diffusion

Molecules move constantly in a random manner, at a rate that depends on their mass, their environment, and the amount of thermal energy they possess, which in turn is a function of temperature. While diffusion will go forward in the presence of a substance's concentration gradient, several factors affect the diffusion rate:

- Extent of the concentration gradient: The greater the difference in concentration, the more rapid the diffusion. The closer the distribution of the material gets to equilibrium, the slower the diffusion rate.
- Mass of the molecules diffusing: Heavier molecules move more slowly; therefore, they diffuse more slowly. The reverse is true for lighter molecules.
- Temperature: Higher temperatures increase the energy and therefore the molecules' movement, increasing the diffusion rate. Lower temperatures decrease the molecules' energy, thus decreasing the diffusion rate.
- Solvent density: As the density of a solvent increases, the diffusion rate decreases. The molecules slow down because they have a more difficult time passing through the denser medium.
- Solubility: Nonpolar or lipid-soluble materials pass through plasma membranes more easily than polar materials, allowing for a faster diffusion rate.
- Surface area and plasma membrane thickness: Increased surface area increases the diffusion rate, whereas a thicker membrane reduces it.
- Distance traveled: The greater the distance that a substance must travel, the slower the diffusion rate.

Facilitated transport (diffusion)

In facilitated transport, or facilitated diffusion, materials diffuse across the plasma membrane with the help of membrane proteins. A concentration gradient exists that would allow these materials to diffuse into the cell without expending cellular energy. However, these materials are polar molecules or ions that the cell membrane's hydrophobic parts repel. Facilitated transport proteins shield these materials from the membrane's repulsive force, allowing them to diffuse into the cell.

Ion channels

Channels are specific for the transported substance. Channel proteins have hydrophilic domains exposed to the intracellular and extracellular fluids. In addition, they have a hydrophilic channel through their core that provides a hydrated opening through the membrane layers (figure 16.7).

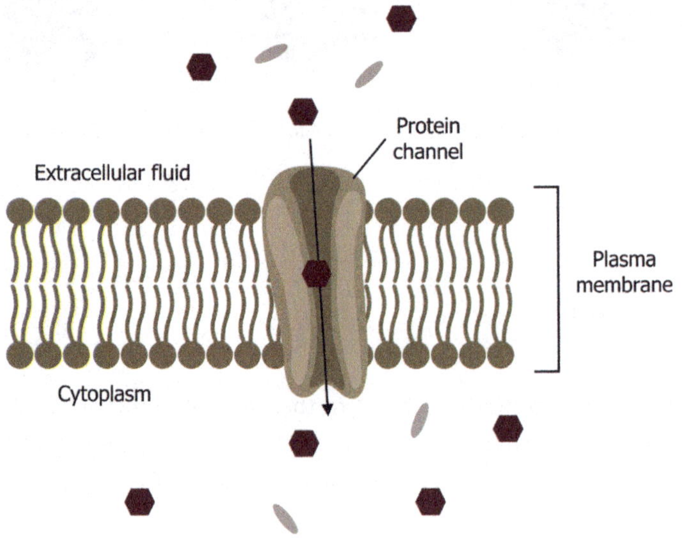

Figure 16.7: Protein channel.

Channel proteins are either open at all times or they are "gated," which controls the channel's opening. The gating can be controlled by volatage, ligand (such as ATP), or mechanical stimulus. When a particular ion attaches to the channel protein, it may control the opening, or other mechanisms or substances may be involved.

In some tissues, sodium and chloride ions pass freely through open channels, whereas in other tissues a gate must open to allow passage. Cells involved in transmitting electrical impulses, such as nerve and muscle cells, have gated channels for sodium, potassium, and calcium in their membranes. Opening and closing these channels changes the relative concentrations on opposing sides of the membrane of these ions, resulting in facilitating electrical transmission along membranes (in the case of nerve cells) or in muscle contraction (in the case of muscle cells).

Carrier proteins

Another type of protein embedded in the plasma membrane is a carrier protein. This aptly named protein binds a substance and, thus triggers a change of its own shape, moving the bound molecule from the cell's outside to its interior (figure 16.8).

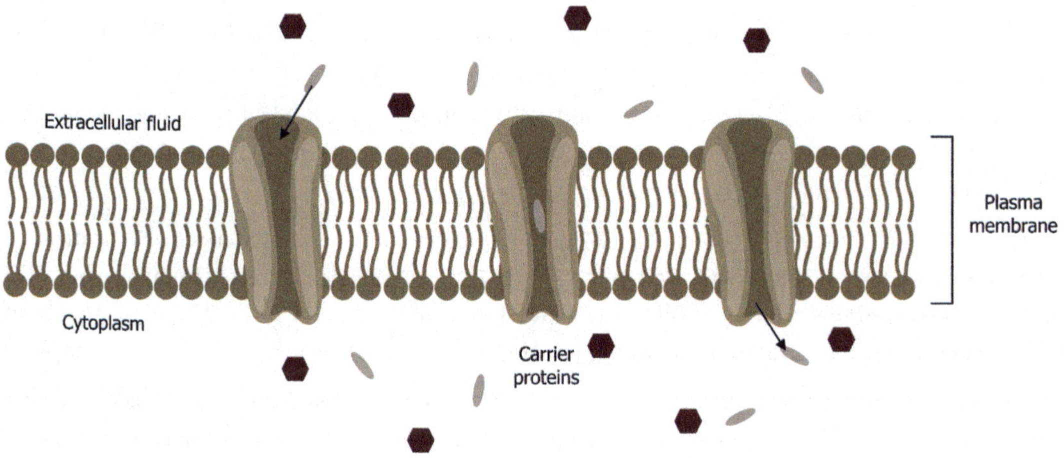

Figure 16.8: Carrier proteins. This aptly named protein binds a substance and thus triggers a change of its own shape, moving the bound molecule from the cell's outside to its interior.

Depending on the gradient, the material may move in the opposite direction. Carrier proteins are typically specific for a single substance. This selectivity adds to the plasma membrane's overall selectivity. One group of carrier proteins, glucose transport proteins, or GLUTs, are involved in transporting glucose and other hexose sugars through plasma membranes within the body.

Channel and carrier proteins transport material at different rates. Channel proteins transport much more quickly than carrier proteins. Channel proteins facilitate diffusion at a rate of tens of millions of molecules per second, whereas carrier proteins work at a rate of a thousand to a million molecules per second.

16.2 References and resources

Text

Clark, M. A. *Biology*, 2nd ed. Houston, TX: OpenStax College, Rice University, 2018, Chapter 4: Cell Structure, Chapter 5: Structure and Function of the Plasma Membranes.

Karp, G., and J. G. Patton. *Cell and Molecular Biology: Concepts and Experiments*, 7th ed. Hoboken, NJ: John Wiley, 2013, Chapter 4: The Structure and Function of the Plasma Membrane.

Le, T., and V. Bhushan. *First Aid for the USMLE Step 1*, 29th ed. New York: McGraw Hill Education, 2018, 49.

Figures

Grey, Kindred, Figure 16.4 Diffusion across the plasma membrane. 2021. https://archive.org/details/16.4_20210926. CC BY 4.0. Added ion channel by Léa Lortal from the Noun Project.

Grey, Kindred, Figure 16.5 Illustration of osmosis. In the diagram, the solute cannot pass through the selectively permeable membrane, but the water can. 2021. https://archive.org/details/16.5_20210926. CC BY 4.0.

Grey, Kindred, Figure 16.6 Comparison of red blood cell morphology in isotonic, hypertonic and hypotonic solutions. 2021. https://archive.org/details/16.6_20210926. CC BY 4.0. Added Osmotic pressure on blood cells diagram by LadyofHats. Public domain. From Wikimedia Commons.

Lieberman M, Peet A. Figure 16.7 Protein channel. Adapted under Fair Use from Marks' Basic Medical Biochemistry. 5th Ed. pp 175 Figure 10.7 Common types of transport mechanisms for human cells. 2017. Added Cell membrane detailed diagram blank by LadyofHats. Public domain. From Wikimedia Commons. Added ion channel by Léa Lortal from theNoun Project.

Lieberman M, Peet A. Figure 16.8 Carrier proteins… Adapted under Fair Use from Marks' Basic Medical Biochemistry. 5th Ed. pp 175 Figure 10.7 Common types of transport mechanisms for human cells. 2017. Added Cell membrane detailed diagram blank by LadyofHats. Public domain. From Wikimedia Commons. Added ion channel by Léa Lortal from the Noun Project.

16.3 Active Transport

Active transport mechanisms require the cell's energy, usually in the form of adenosine triphosphate (ATP). If a substance must move into the cell against its concentration gradient — that is, if the substance's concentration inside the cell is greater than its concentration in the extracellular fluid (and vice versa) — the cell must use energy to move the substance.

Electrochemical gradient

We have discussed simple concentration gradients — a substance's differential concentrations across a space or a membrane — but in living systems, gradients are more complex. Because ions move into and out of cells and because cells contain proteins that do not move across the membrane and are mostly negatively charged, there is also an electrical gradient, a difference of charge, across the plasma membrane.

The interior of living cells is electrically negative with respect to the extracellular fluid in which they are bathed, and at the same time, cells have higher concentrations of potassium (K^+) and lower concentrations of sodium (Na^+) than the extracellular fluid. Thus in a living cell, the concentration gradient of Na^+ tends to drive it into the cell, and its electrical gradient (a positive ion) also drives it inward to the negatively charged interior. However, the situation is more complex for other elements such as potassium. The electrical gradient of K^+, a positive ion, also drives it into the cell, but the concentration gradient of K^+ drives K^+ out of the cell (figure 16.9). We call the combined concentration gradient and electrical charge that affects an ion its electrochemical gradient.

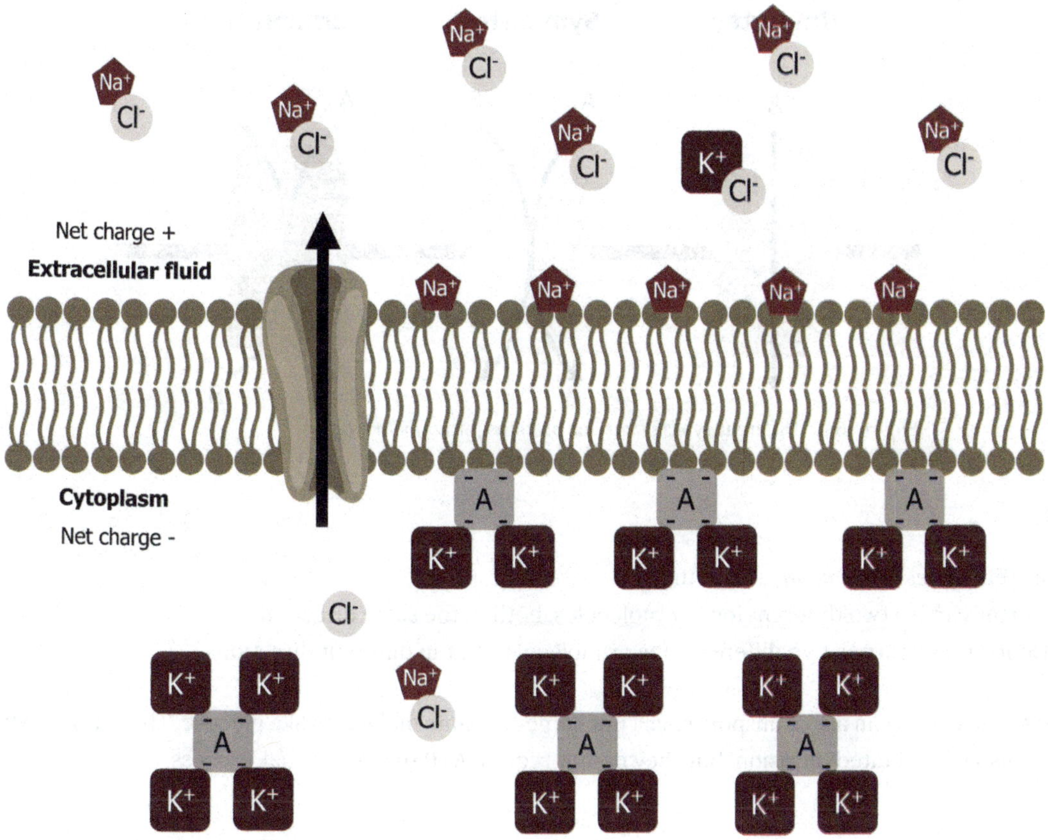

Figure 16.9: Electrochemical gradients.

Moving against a gradient

Two mechanisms exist for transporting small molecular weight material and small molecules:

1. Primary active transport moves ions across a membrane and creates a difference in charge across that membrane, which is directly dependent on ATP.
2. Secondary active transport does not directly require ATP; instead, it is the movement of material due to the electrochemical gradient established by primary active transport.

Carrier proteins for active transport

An important membrane adaptation for active transport is the presence of specific carrier proteins or pumps to facilitate movement. There are three protein types or transporters (figure 16.10).

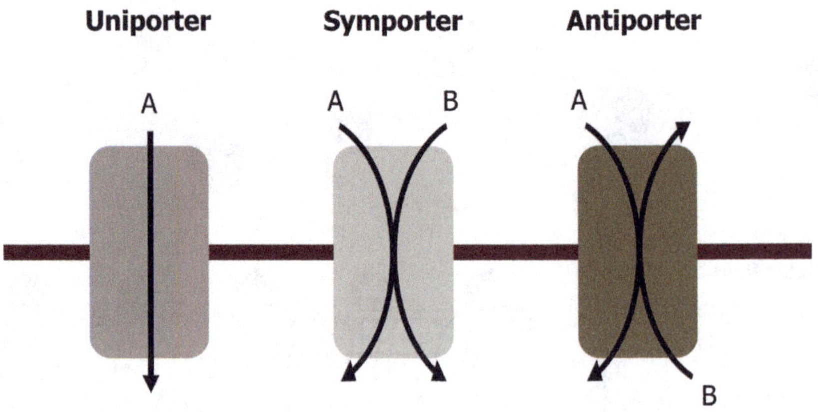

Figure 16.10: Different types of carrier proteins for active transport.

- A uniporter carries one specific ion or molecule.
- A symporter carries two different ions or molecules, both in the same direction.
- An antiporter also carries two different ions or molecules, but in different directions.

All of these transporters can also transport small, uncharged organic molecules like glucose. These three types of carrier proteins are also in facilitated diffusion, but they do not require ATP to work in that process.

Primary active transport

The primary active transport that functions with the active transport of sodium and potassium allows secondary active transport to occur. The second transport method is still active because it depends on using energy as does primary transport (figure 16.11).

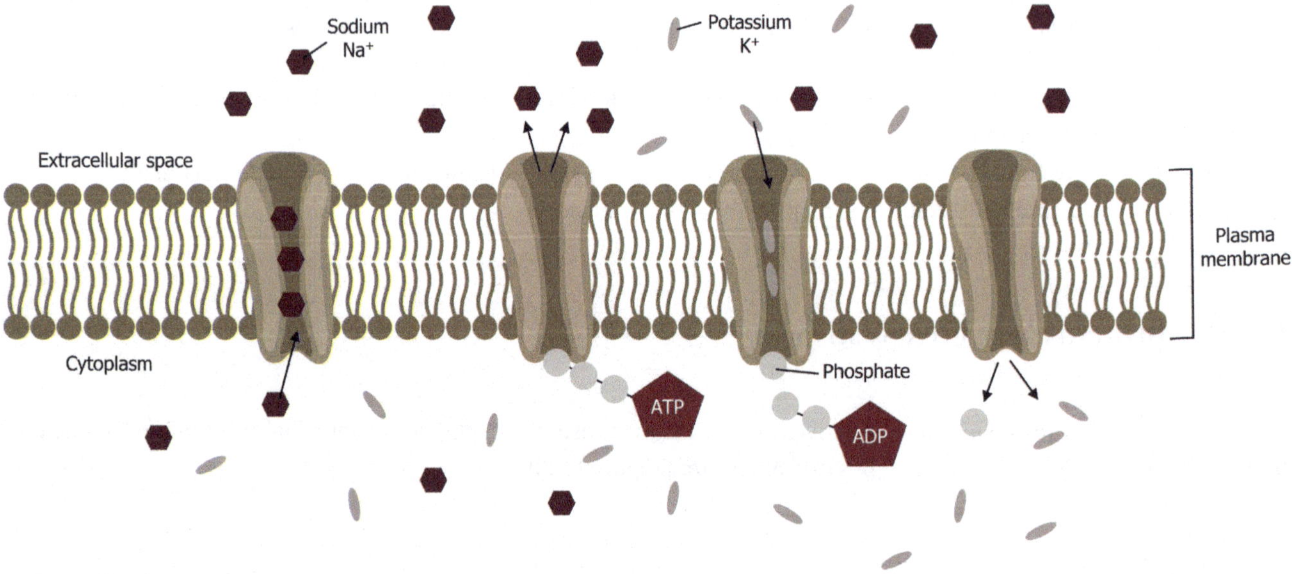

Figure 16.11: Primary active transport.

One of the most important pumps in animal cells is the sodium-potassium pump (Na^+-K^+ ATPase), which maintains the electrochemical gradient (and the correct concentrations of Na^+ and K^+) in living cells. The sodium-potassium pump moves K^+ into the cell while moving Na^+ out at the same time, at a ratio of three Na^+ for every two K^+ ions moved in. The Na^+-K^+ ATPase exists in two forms, depending on its orientation to the cell's interior or exterior and its affinity for either sodium or potassium ions. The process consists of the following six steps.

1. With the protein oriented toward the cell's interior, the carrier has a high affinity for sodium ions. Three ions bind to the protein.
2. The protein carrier hydrolyzes ATP, and a low-energy phosphate group attaches to it.
3. As a result, the carrier changes shape and reorients itself toward the membrane's exterior. The protein's affinity for sodium decreases, and the three sodium ions leave the carrier.
4. The shape change increases the carrier's affinity for potassium ions, and two such ions attach to the protein.
5. With the phosphate group removed and potassium ions attached, the carrier protein repositions itself toward the cell's interior.
6. The carrier protein, in its new configuration, has a decreased affinity for potassium, and the two ions move into the cytoplasm. The protein now has a higher affinity for sodium ions, and the process starts again.

Secondary active transport (cotransport)

Secondary active transport brings sodium ions, and possibly other compounds, into the cell. As sodium ion concentrations build up outside of the plasma membrane because of the primary active transport process, this creates an electrochemical gradient. If a channel protein exists and is open, the sodium ions will pull through the membrane. This movement transports other substances that can attach themselves to the transport protein through the membrane. Many amino acids, as well as glucose, enter a cell this way.

16.3 References and resources

Text

Clark, M. A. *Biology*, 2nd ed. Houston, TX: OpenStax College, Rice University, 2018, Chapter 4: Cell Structure, Chapter 5: Structure and Function of the Plasma Membranes.

Karp, G., and J. G. Patton. *Cell and Molecular Biology: Concepts and Experiments*, 7th ed. Hoboken, NJ: John Wiley, 2013, Chapter 4: The Structure and Function of the Plasma Membrane.

Le, T., and V. Bhushan. *First Aid for the USMLE Step 1*, 29th ed. New York: McGraw Hill Education, 2018, 49.

Figures

Grey, Kindred, Figure 16.9 Electrochemical gradients. 2021. https://archive.org/details/16.9_20210926. CC BY 4.0. Added Cell membrane detailed diagram blank by LadyofHats. Public domain. From Wikimedia Commons. Added ion channel by Léa Lortal from the Noun Project.

Grey, Kindred, Figure 16.10 Different types of carrier proteins for active transport. 2021. https://archive.org/details/16.10. CC BY 4.0.

Lieberman M, Peet A. Figure 16.11 Primary active transport. Adapted under Fair Use from Marks' Basic Medical Biochemistry. 5th Ed. pp 175 Figure 10.10 Active transport by Na+,K+-ATPase. 2017. Added Cell membrane detailed diagram blank by LadyofHats. Public domain. From Wikimedia Commons. Added ion channel by Léa Lortal from the Noun Project.

17. Cytoplasmic Membranes

Learning Objectives

- Emphasize the dynamic nature of the endomembrane system within the cell.
- Elucidate the structure and function of the rough and smooth endoplasmic reticulum.
- Describe the basic synthetic pathways for secretory and integral membrane proteins.
- Describe the role and sites of glycosylation in the processing of secretory and integral membrane proteins.
- Elucidate the structure, function, and polarization of the Golgi complex.
- Explain the signals used to target proteins to their appropriate cellular location.
- Describe lysosomal structure and function and the diseases caused by lysosome malfunction.
- Distinguish between phagocytosis, bulk phase endocytosis, and receptor-mediated endocytosis.

17.1 Cellular Organelles and the Endomembrane System

Organization of the nucleus

Like most other cellular organelles, the nucleus is surrounded by a membrane called the nuclear envelope. This membranous covering consists of two adjacent lipid bilayers with a thin fluid space in between them. Spanning these two bilayers are nuclear pores. A nuclear pore is a tiny passageway for the passage of proteins, RNA, and solutes between the nucleus and the cytoplasm.

Proteins called pore complexes lining the nuclear pores regulate the passage of materials into and out of the nucleus.

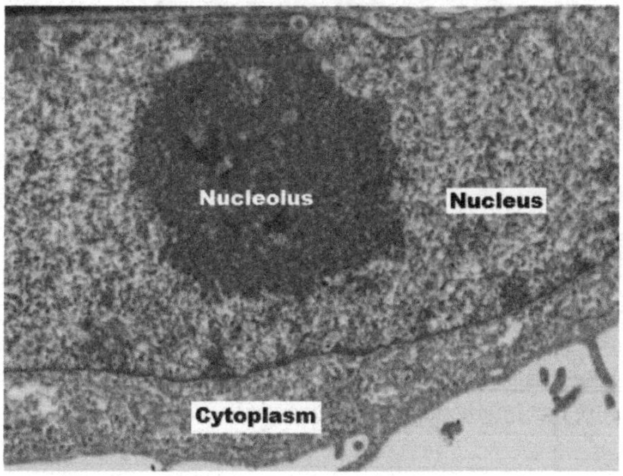

Figure 17.1: EM of the nucleus and nucleolus.

Inside the nuclear envelope is a gel-like nucleoplasm with solutes that include the building blocks of nucleic acids. There also can be a dark-staining mass often visible under a simple light microscope, called a nucleolus (plural = nucleoli). The nucleolus is a region of the nucleus that is responsible for manufacturing the RNA necessary for construction of ribosomes. Once synthesized, newly made ribosomal subunits exit the cell's nucleus through the nuclear pores (figure 17.1). Proteins entering the nucleus require nuclear localization signals, while proteins exiting require nuclear export signals.

Endomembrane system

The endomembrane system (endo = "within") is a group of membranes and organelles (figure 17.2) in eukaryotic cells that work together to modify, package, and transport lipids and proteins. It includes the nuclear envelope as well as:

- Endoplasmic reticulum,
- Golgi apparatus,
- Endosomes,
- Lysosomes,
- Vacuoles, and
- Peroxisomes.

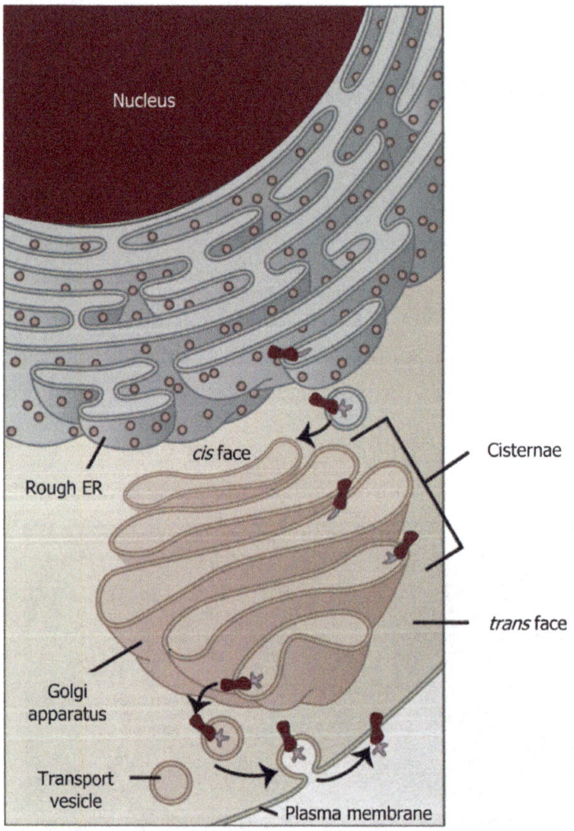

Figure 17.2: Interaction of the endomembrane systems.

Although not technically within the cell the plasma membrane is included in the endomembrane system because, it interacts with the other endomembranous organelles. The endomembrane system does not include the mitochondria. The system of intracellular membranes is designed to move proteins through both the secretory pathway (constitutive or regulated) and the endocytic pathways.

The endoplasmic reticulum (ER)

The endoplasmic reticulum (ER) (figure 17.2) is a series of interconnected membranous sacs and tubules that collectively modify proteins and synthesize lipids. However, these two functions take place in separate areas of the ER: the rough ER and the smooth ER, respectively.

Smooth ER

The smooth endoplasmic reticulum (SER) is continuous with the rough ER (RER) but has few or no ribosomes on its cytoplasmic surface. SER functions include synthesis of carbohydrates, lipids, and steroid hormones; detoxification of medications and poisons; and storing calcium ions. In muscle cells, a specialized SER, the sarcoplasmic reticulum, is responsible for storing calcium ions that are needed to trigger the muscle cells' coordinated contractions.

Rough ER

Scientists have named the rough endoplasmic reticulum (RER) as such because the ribosomes attached to its cytoplasmic surface give it a studded appearance when viewing it through an electron microscope.

Ribosomes transfer their newly synthesized proteins into the RER's lumen where they undergo structural modifications, such as folding or acquiring side chains. These modified proteins incorporate into cellular membranes, the ER, or other organelles' membranes. The proteins can also be secreted from the cell (such as protein hormones and enzymes). The RER also makes phospholipids for cellular membranes.

If the phospholipids or modified proteins are not destined to stay in the RER, they will reach their destinations via transport vesicles that bud from the RER's membrane.

Glycosylation

Nearly all RER-synthesized proteins are glycosylated with short-branched oligosaccharides. This occurs in an N-linked fashion on asparagine residues.

Protein degradation

If proteins aren't folded properly, this can contribute to a host of disease processes related to misfolding events.

Typically, folding is facilitated in the ER using chaperones (BiP), but if the protein is altered (due to mutation), this can lead to aggregation. Accumulation of BiP can initiate the unfolded protein response (UPR) (figure 17.3).

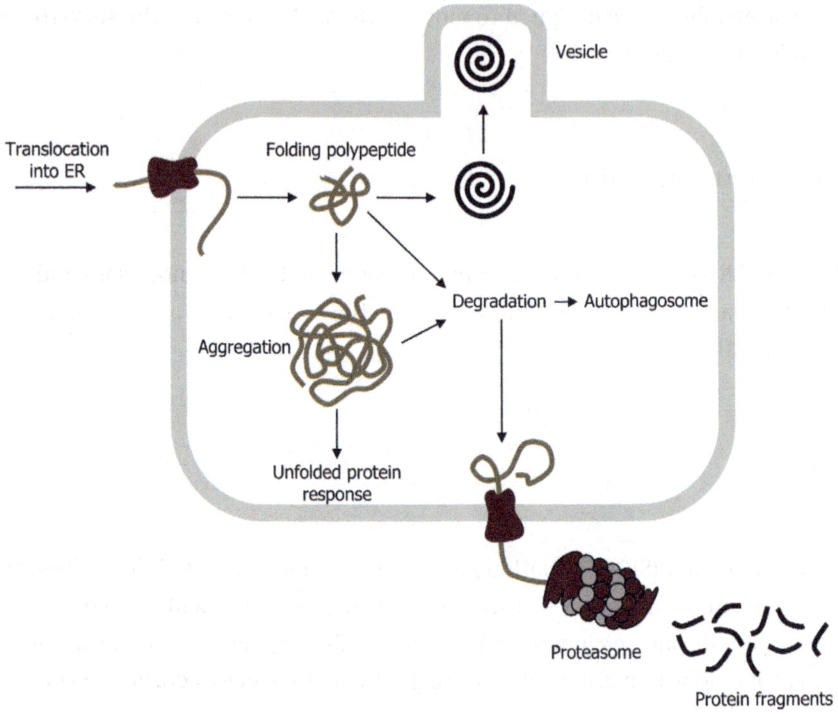

Figure 17.3: Unfolded protein response in the RER.

E3 ubiquitin ligase is often responsible for tagging aggregates with ubiquitin, which targets the protein to the proteasome. The proteasome consists of two subunits (19S and 20S) to make a functional 26S proteasome. Inside the proteasome, the polypeptide chains are cleaved back to their native amino acids and can be reused in other translational events. However, if the aggregates accumulate, in some instances they can contribute to any number of neurodegenerative disorders.

Golgi

When proteins exit the RER they are trafficked to the Golgi where they will incur further post-translational modifications and will translocate to their final destination. These modifications will include "pruning" of large oligosaccharides that were attached in the RER, glycosylation, sulfation, and phosphorylation. Additionally, some proteins require Golgi-associated cleavage to produce a mature protein ready for trafficking.

The Golgi is divided into trans and cis networks.

- Cis Golgi is close to the ER and sorts proteins back to the ER.
- Trans Golgi sorts proteins into vesicles bound for the plasma membrane and intracellular vesicles.

In the Golgi, O-linked glycosylation happens, and most mannose residues are removed. This is done by a large family of enzymes known as glycosyltranferases.

Protein localization

Protein translation can take place on both free ribosomes and the RER. Free ribosomes translate proteins bound for the mitochondria, nucleus, and peroxisomes.

The RER translates proteins for secretion, membrane-bound proteins, or soluble proteins.

Proteins translated on the RER are folded and processed into mature proteins in the lumen of the ER. Transcripts for protein products to be translated on the RER are characteristic of a signal sequence that is recognized by a signal recognition peptide. The signal sequence on the nascent polypeptide will be used to later target the protein to its correct location. The signal recognition peptide facilitates the docking of the ribosome complex on the ER, and the peptide is translated into the lumen of the ER. Inside the ER, the peptide is often associated with chaperones to assist in correct protein folding.

Localization using coat proteins (COP)

Once translated in the RER, proteins are trafficked in the cell using vesicle transport systems. The direction of the transport, ER to Golgi or Golgi to ER, is determined by the coat proteins on the vesicles.

- Retrograde transport: The coat protein COPI is used for retrograde transport, from the cis-Golgi to the ER.
- Anterograde transport: The coat protein COPII is used for anterograde transport from the ER to the cis-Golgi.
- Additional transport mechanisms: Clathrin is used for trans-Golgi transport to lysosomes. It is also used in endocytosis in transporting proteins from the plasma membrane to the endosomes.

The vesicles are targeted to the intended membrane by transport over microtubules in the cytosol. The fusion itself requires surface proteins, Snares, which facilitate the formation of a docking complex stabilizing the interaction between the vesicle and the intended membrane. GTP is required for fusion of the two membranes.

Lysosomes and peroxisomes

Lysosomes are organelles formed by the fusion of a late endosome and a lysosomal-enzyme-filled vesicle secreted from the Golgi. Proteins are targeted to lysosomes by the presence of mannose 6-phosphate (acquired in the RER), and the presence of these tags are essential for trafficking to the lysosome.

The major function for these organelles is to break down macromolecules through enzymatic degradation. Both processes of autophagy and exocytosis can be facilitated. Lysosomal storage diseases are inherited metabolic diseases characterized by an abnormal buildup of various metabolic intermediates. Collectively, there are approximately fifty of these disorders, and they may affect different parts of the body. Clinical correlates include: Gaucher disease, Fabry disease, glycogen storage disease, mucopolisacaridosis, and sphingolipidoses.

This is in contrast to peroxisomes, which are formed by budding from the ER. They primarily perform hydrogen peroxide-mediated degradation of lipids (i.e., very long-chain fatty acids) and some amino acids. Zellweger syndrome is one of the heritable disorders of peroxisome biogenesis and results in infant death before six months.

17.1 References and resources

Text

Clark, M. A. *Biology*, 2nd ed. Houston, TX: OpenStax College, Rice University, 2018, Chapter 4: Cell Structure, Chapter 5: Structure and Function of the Plasma Membranes.

Karp, G., and J. G. Patton. *Cell and Molecular Biology: Concepts and Experiments*, 7th ed. Hoboken, NJ: John Wiley, 2013, Chapter 8: Cytoplasmic Membrane Systems: Structure, Function, and Membrane Trafficking.

Le, T., and V. Bhushan. *First Aid for the USMLE Step 1*, 29th ed. New York: McGraw Hill Education, 2018, 46–47.

Figures

Grey, Kindred, Figure 17.2 Interaction of the endomembrane systems. 2021. https://archive.org/details/17.2_20210926. CC BY 4.0. Adapted from Figure 4.18. CC BY 4.0. From OpenStax.

Grey, Kindred, Figure 17.3: Unfolded protein response in the RER. 2021. CC BY 4.0. Adapted from ProteinQS en by Vojtěch Dostál. Public domain. From Wikimedia Commons.

Orlov I, Schertel A, Zuber G, et al. Figure 17.1 EM of the nucleus and nucleolus. CC BY-SA 4.0. From Wikimedia Commons.

Additional resources

- Some helpful animations related to this content
  - Translocation into ER: https://youtu.be/pxG8-BWbpnU
  - Proteasome: https://youtu.be/Gp8lhKghckY
  - Clathrin: https://youtu.be/o_EUHu4OJus

17.2 Endocytosis

Endocytosis

Endocytosis is a type of active transport that moves particles, such as large molecules, parts of cells, and even whole cells, into a cell. There are different endocytosis variations, but all share common characteristics:

1. The cell's plasma membrane invaginates, forming a pocket around thc target particle.
2. The pocket pinches off.
3. This results in the particle containing itself in a newly created intracellular vesicle formed from the plasma membrane.

Phagocytosis

Phagocytosis (the condition of "cell eating") is the process by which a cell takes in large particles, such as other cells or relatively large particles. For example, when microorganisms invade the human body, a type of white blood cell, a neutrophil, will remove the invaders through this process, surrounding and engulfing the microorganism, which the neutrophil then destroys (figure 17.4).

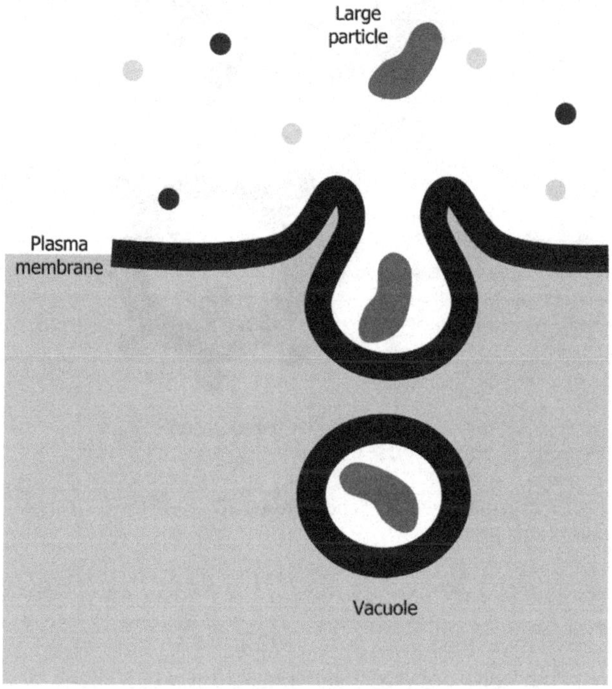

Figure 17.4: General process of phagocytosis. In phagocytosis, the cell membrane surrounds the particle and engulfs it.

In preparation for phagocytosis, a portion of the plasma membrane's inward-facing surface becomes coated with the protein clathrin, which stabilizes this membrane's section. The membrane's coated portion then extends from the cell's body and surrounds the particle, eventually enclosing it. Once the vesicle containing the particle is enclosed within the cell, the clathrin disengages from the membrane ,and the vesicle merges with a lysosome for breaking down the material in the newly formed compartment (endosome). When accessible nutrients from the vesicular contents' degradation have been extracted, the newly formed endosome merges with the plasma membrane and releases its contents into the extracellular fluid. The endosomal membrane again becomes part of the plasma membrane.

Receptor-mediated endocytosis

A targeted variation of endocytosis employs receptor proteins in the plasma membrane that have a specific binding affinity for certain substances (figure 17.5).

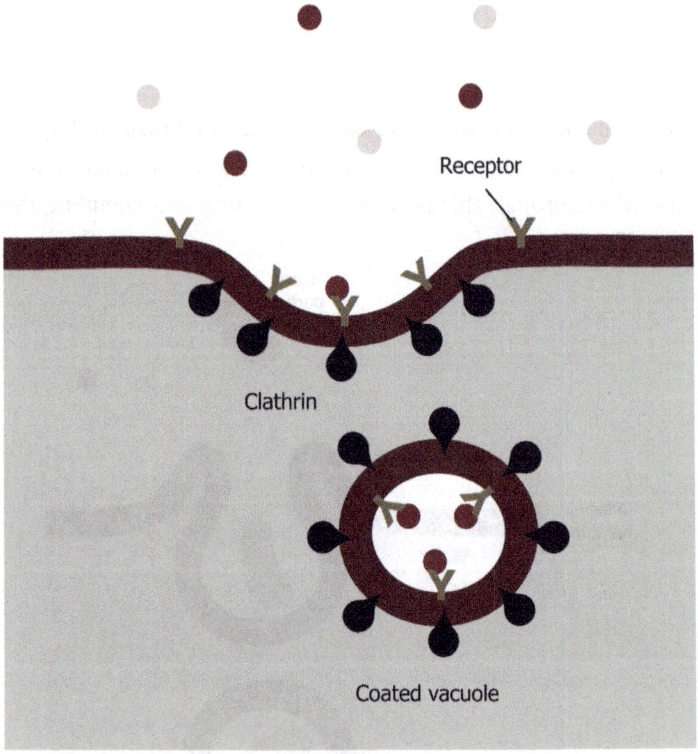

Figure 17.5: Receptor-mediated endocytosis; LDL receptor is a classic example of this process.

In receptor-mediated endocytosis, the cell's uptake of substances targets a single type of substance that binds to the receptor on the cell membrane's external surface.

Clathrin attaches to the plasma membrane's cytoplasmic side. If a compound's uptake is dependent on receptor-mediated endocytosis and the process is ineffective, the material will not be removed from the tissue fluids or blood. Instead, it will stay in those fluids and increase in concentration. The failure of receptor-mediated endocytosis causes some human diseases.

For example, receptor-mediated endocytosis removes low-density lipoprotein or LDL from the blood. In the human genetic disease familial hypercholesterolemia, the LDL receptors are defective or missing entirely. People with this condition have life-threatening levels of cholesterol in their blood because their cells cannot clear LDL particles. See chapter 6.

Exocytosis

Exocytosis is the opposite of the processes we discussed above in that its purpose is to expel material from the cell into the extracellular fluid. Waste material is enveloped in a membrane and fuses with the plasma membrane's interior. This fusion opens the membranous envelope on the cell's exterior, and the waste material expels into the extracellular space. Other examples of cells releasing molecules via exocytosis include extracellular matrix protein secretion and neurotransmitter secretion into the synaptic cleft by synaptic vesicles (figure 17.6).

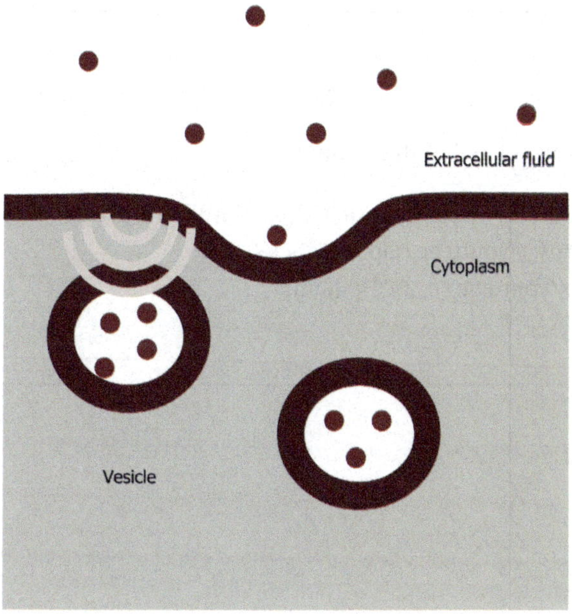

Figure 17.6: Exocytosis: vesicles containing substances fuse with the plasma membrane. The contents then release to the cell's exterior.

17.2 References and resources

Text

Clark, M. A. *Biology*, 2nd ed. Houston, TX: OpenStax College, Rice University, 2018, Chapter 4: Cell Structure, Chapter 5: Structure and Function of the Plasma Membranes.

Karp, G., and J. G. Patton. *Cell and Molecular Biology: Concepts and Experiments*, 7th ed. Hoboken, NJ: John Wiley, 2013, Chapter 8: Cytoplasmic Membrane Systems: Structure, Function, and Membrane Trafficking.

Le, T., and V. Bhushan. *First Aid for the USMLE Step 1*, 29th ed. New York: McGraw Hill Education, 2018, 46–47

Figures

Alberts B, Johnson A, Lewis J, et al. Figure 17.4 General process of phagocytosis… Adapted under Fair Use from Cell and Molecular Biology. 6th Ed. pp 308. Figure 8.46 A summary of phagocytic pathway. 2014.

Alberts B, Johnson A, Lewis J, et al. Figure 17.5 Receptor mediated endocytosis, LDL-receptor is a classic example of this process. Adapted under Fair Use from Cell and Molecular Biology. 6th Ed. pp 306. Figure 8.42 The endocytic pathway. 2014.

Alberts B, Johnson A, Lewis J, et al. Figure 17.6 Exocytosis: vesicles containing substances fuse with the plasma membrane… Adapted under Fair Use from Cell and Molecular Biology. 6th Ed. pp 299. Figure 35 A summary of the autophagic pathway. 2014.

Additional resources

- Some helpful animations related to this content
    - Translocation into ER: https://youtu.be/pxG8-BWbpnU
    - Proteasome: https://youtu.be/Gp8lhKghckY
    - Clathrin: https://youtu.be/o_EUHu4OJus

18. Cytoskeleton

Learning Objectives

- Describe the traits and functions of the various cytoskeletal elements (microtubules, microfilaments, and intermediate filaments).
- Elucidate the general mechanism by which molecular motors move along cytoskeletal elements.
- Identify the molecular motors (dyneins, kinesins, and myosins) that partner with various cytoskeletal elements.
- Describe microtubule organizing centers, and their structures and functions.
- Explain the dynamic properties of cytoskeletal elements and how this relates to their construction and functioning.
- Elucidate the structure and function of cilia and flagella, and their differences and similarities.
- Elucidate the existence and importance of nonmuscle motility.

Key Takeaways

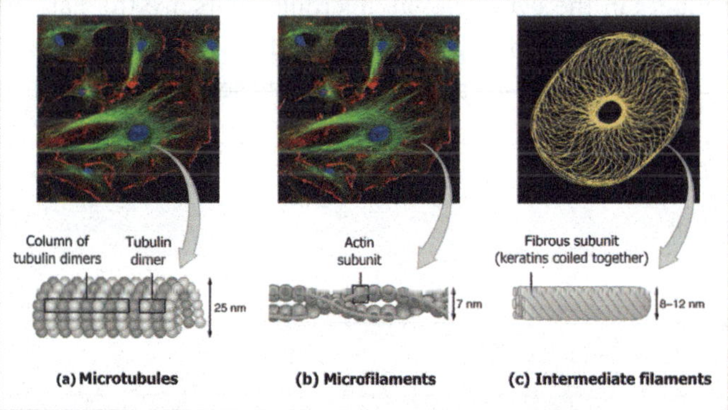

Figure 18.1: Summary of the three major types of structural filaments.

If you were to remove all the organelles from a cell, would the plasma membrane and the cytoplasm be the only components left? No. Within the cytoplasm, there would still be ions and organic molecules, plus a network of protein fibers that help maintain the cell's shape, secure some organelles in specific positions, allow cytoplasm and vesicles to move within the cell, and enable cells within multicellular organisms to move. Collectively, scientists call this network of protein fibers the cytoskeleton.

18.1 The Cytoskeleton

There are three types of fibers within the cytoskeleton:

- Microfilaments,
- Intermediate filaments, and
- Microtubules.

The collection of these fibers plays key roles in structure and support, intracellular transport, contractility and motility, as well as spacial organization (figure 18.2).

Microfilaments thicken the cortex around the cell's inner edge. Like rubber bands, they resist tension. There are microtubules in the cell's interior where they maintain their shape by resisting compressive forces. There are intermediate filaments throughout the cell that hold organelles in place.

Microfilaments

Of the three types of protein fibers in the cytoskeleton, microfilaments are the narrowest. They function in cellular movement, have a diameter of about 7 to 8 nm, and are comprised of two globular protein intertwined strands, which we call actin (figure 18.3). For this reason, we also call microfilaments actin filaments.

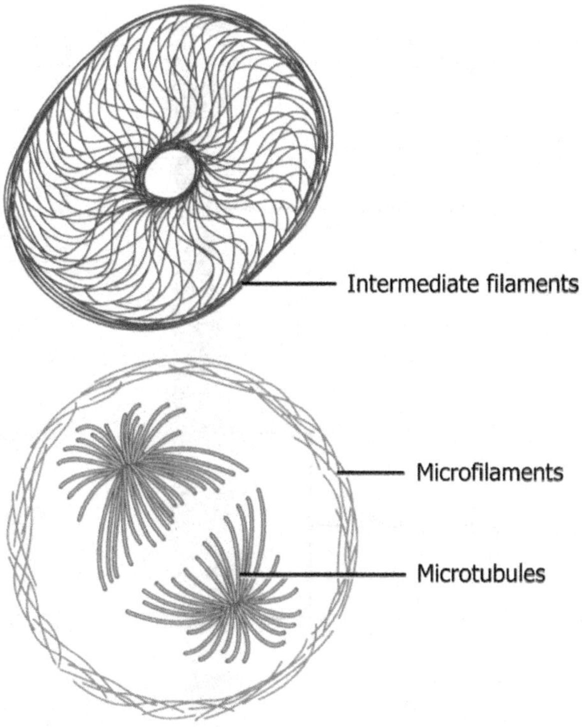

Figure 18.2: Spatial organization of the three types of fibers. Microfilaments thicken the cortex around the cell's inner edge. Intermediate filaments have no role in cell movement. Their function is purely structural. They help the cell resist compression, provide a track along which vesicles move through the cell, and pull replicated chromosomes to opposite ends of a dividing cell.

ATP powers actin to assemble its filamentous form, which serves as a track for the movement of a motor protein we call myosin. This enables actin to engage in cellular events requiring motion, such as cell division in eukaryotic cells. Actin and myosin are plentiful in muscle cells.

Microfilaments also provide some rigidity and shape to the cell. They can depolymerize (disassemble) and reform quickly, thus enabling a cell to change its shape and move.

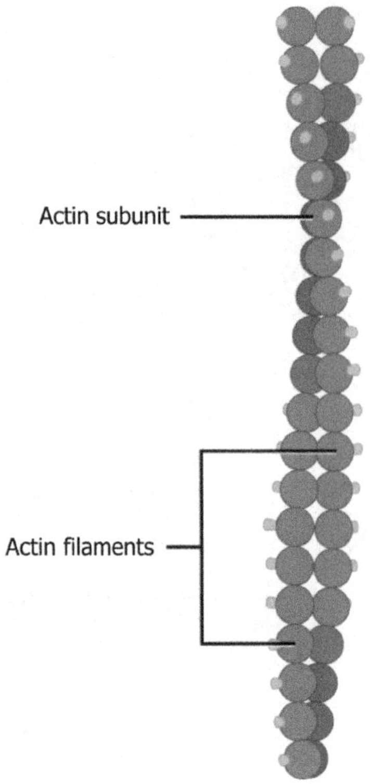

Figure 18.3: Microfilaments are comprised of two globular protein intertwined strands, which we call actin. For this reason, we also call microfilaments actin filaments.

Intermediate filaments

Several strands of fibrous proteins that are wound together comprise intermediate filaments (figure 18.4). These cytoskeleton elements get their name from the fact that their diameter, 10 to 12 nm, is between those of microfilaments and microtubules.

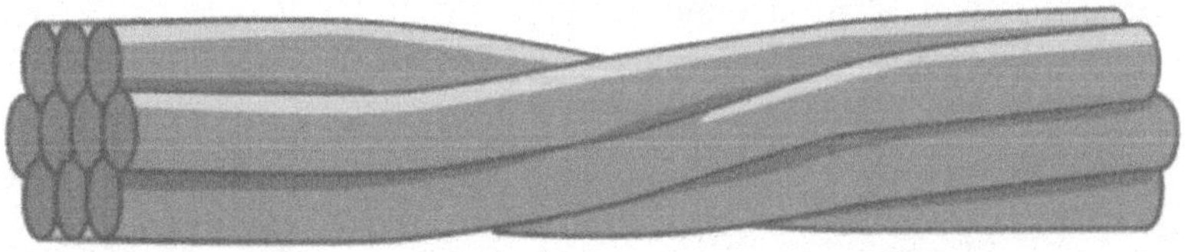

Figure 18.4: Several strands of fibrous proteins that are wound together comprise intermediate filaments.

Intermediate filaments have no role in cell movement. Their function is purely structural. They bear tension, thus maintaining the cell's shape, and anchor the nucleus and other organelles in place (figure 18.1).

The intermediate filaments are the most diverse group of cytoskeletal elements. They are unbranched and rope-like with long fibrous subunits. There is no polarity associated with their assembly. Intermediate filaments are classified by their location and function. The table below summarizes various types of intermediate filaments.

Class	Protein type	Location	Function
1 & 2	Keratins	Epithelial cells	Structural support, stretching
3	Vimentin	Fibroblasts/Epithelial cells	Cage-like structure around the nucleus
	Desmin	Muscle cells	Links myofibrils together
	Glial fibrillary protein (GFAP)	Glial cells	Structural support
4	Neurofilaments	Neurons	Support for axon and dendrites
5	Lamins	Nucleus	Support for inner surface of the nuclear membrane

Table 18.1: Proteins and their functions.

Microtubules

As their name implies, microtubules are small hollow tubes. With a diameter of about 25 nm, microtubules are cytoskeletons' widest components. They help the cell resist compression, provide a track along which vesicles move through the cell, and pull replicated chromosomes to opposite ends of a dividing cell (figure 18.5).

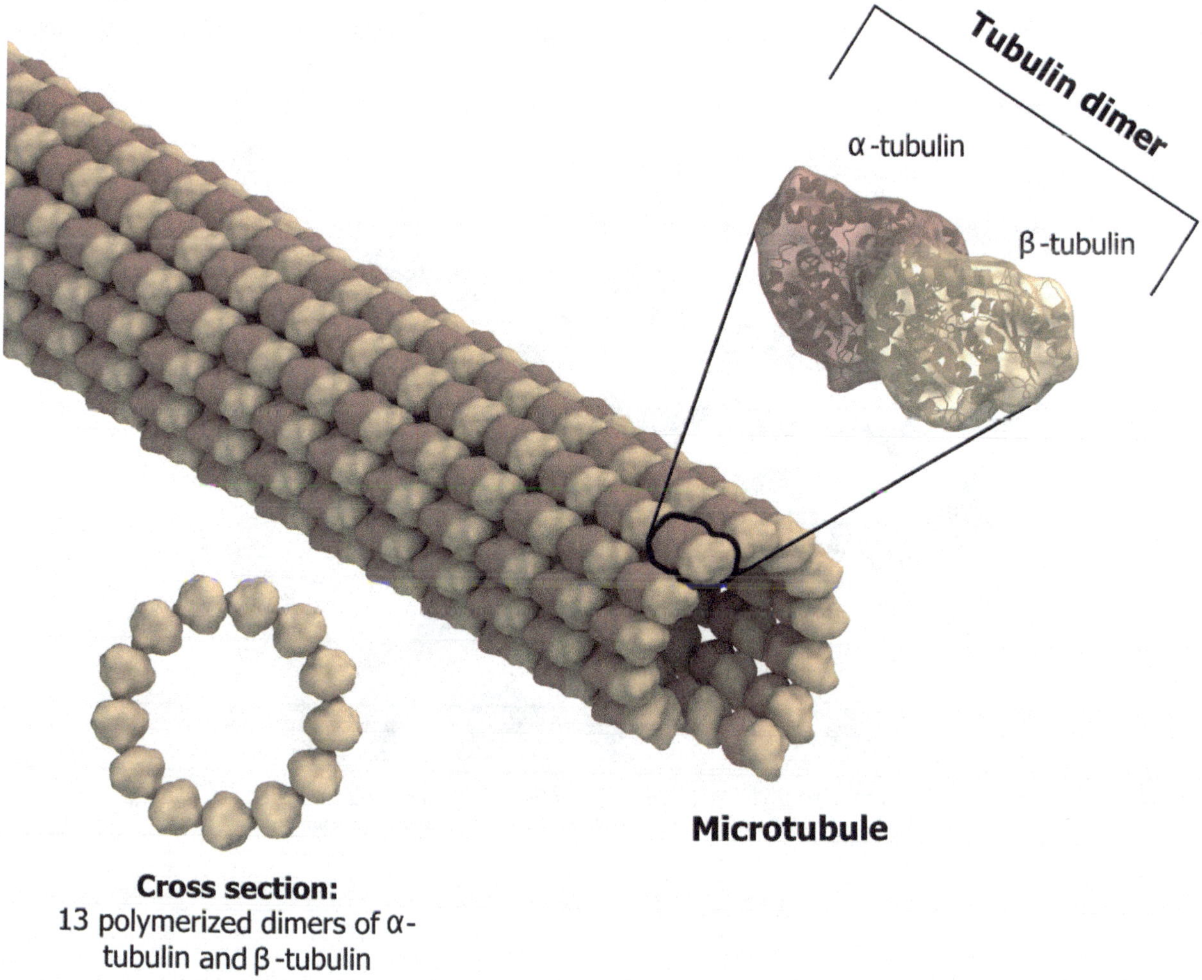

Figure 18.5: Microtubules are hollow. Their walls consist of thirteen polymerized dimers of α-tubulin and β-tubulin. The left image shows the tube's molecular structure.

Like microfilaments, microtubules can disassemble and reform quickly using GTP. The tube is formed from polymerized dimers of α-tubulin and β-tubulin, two globular proteins. These proteins form long chains that comprise the microtubule's walls. The assembly is slow and occurs from the plus end, which is designated by a row of β-tubulin. Disassembly can occur rapidly at the plus end. (Note the minus end has a row of α-tubulin.)

Microtubules are also the structural elements of flagella, cilia, and centrioles (the latter are the centrosome's two perpendicular bodies). In animal cells, the centrosome is the microtubule-organizing center.

Flagella and cilia

The flagella (singular = flagellum) are long, hair-like structures that extend from the plasma membrane and enable an entire cell to move. When present, the cell has just one flagellum or a few flagella.

However, when cilia (singular = cilium) are present, many of them extend along the plasma membrane's entire surface. They are short, hair-like structures that move entire cells (such as paramecia) or substances along the cell's outer surface (for example, the cilia of cells lining the Fallopian tubes that move the ovum toward the uterus, or cilia lining the cells of the respiratory tract that trap particulate matter and move it toward your nostrils).

Despite their differences in length and number, flagella and cilia share a common structural arrangement of microtubules called a "9 + 2 array." This is an appropriate name because a single flagellum or cilium is made of a ring of nine microtubule doublets, surrounding a single microtubule doublet (axoneme) in the center (figure 18.6).

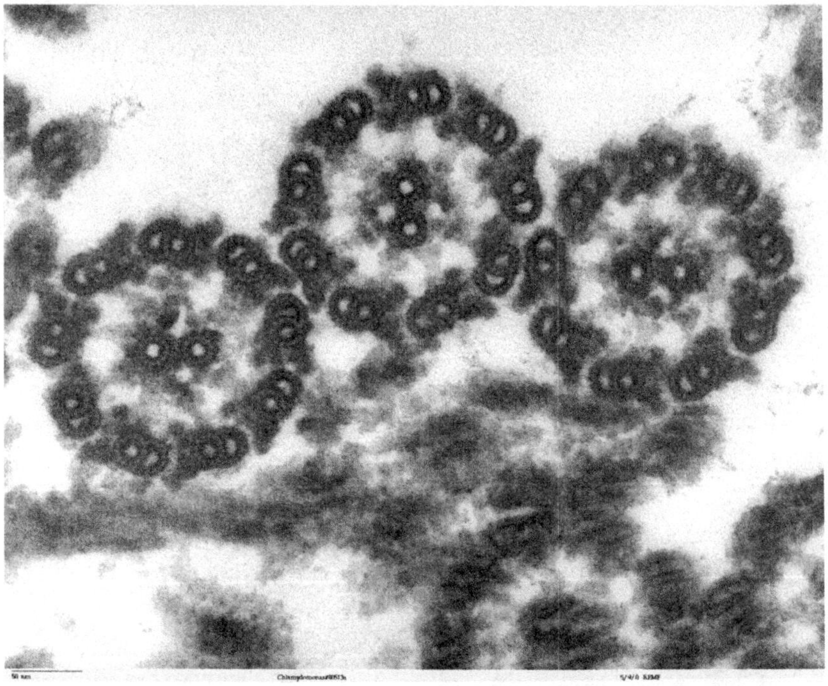

Figure 18.6: This transmission electron micrograph of two flagella shows the microtubules' 9 + 2 array: nine microtubule doublets surround a single microtubule doublet.

18.1 References and resources

Text

Clark, M. A. *Biology*, 2nd ed. Houston, TX: OpenStax College, Rice University, 2018, Chapter 4: Cell Structure, Chapter 5: Structure and Function of the Plasma Membranes.

Karp, G., and J. G. Patton. *Cell and Molecular Biology: Concepts and Experiments*, 7th ed. Hoboken, NJ: John Wiley, 2013, Chapter 9: The Cytoskeleton and Cell Mobility.

Le, T., and V. Bhushan. *First Aid for the* USMLE *Step* 1, 29th ed. New York: McGraw Hill Education, 2018, 48–49.

Figures

Dartmouth Electron Microscope Facility, Dartmouth College. Figure 18.6 This transmission electron micrograph of two flagella shows the microtubules' 9 + 2 array: nine microtubule doublets surround a single microtubule doublet. Scale bar data from Matt Russell. Public domain. From Wikimedia Commons.

Grey, Kindred, Figure 18.1 Summary of the three major types of structural filaments. 2021. https://archive.org/details/18.1_20210926. CC BY 4.0. Adapted from Figure 3.18. CC BY 4.0. From OpenStax.

Grey, Kindred, Figure 18.2 Spatial organization of the three types of fibers... 2021. https://archive.org/details/18.2_20210926. CC BY 4.0. Adapted from Figure 4.22. CC BY 4.0. From OpenStax.

Grey, Kindred, Figure 18.3 Microfilaments are comprised of two globular protein intertwined strands, which we call actin. For this reason, we also call microfilaments actin filaments. 2021. https://archive.org/details/18.3_20210926. CC BY 4.0. Adapted from Figure 4.23. CC BY 4.0. From OpenStax.

Grey, Kindred, Figure 18.4 Several strands of fibrous proteins that are wound together comprise intermediate filaments. 2021. https://archive.org/details/18.4_20210926. CC BY 4.0. Adapted from Figure 4.24. CC BY 4.0. From OpenStax.

Grey, Kindred, Figure 18.5 Microtubules are hollow. Their walls consist of 13 polymerized dimers of \(\alpha\)-tubulin and \(\beta\)-tubulin. The left image shows the tube's molecular structure. 2021. https://archive.org/details/18.5_20210926. CC BY-SA 4.0. Adapted from Microtubule structure csp by Posible2006. CC BY-SA 4.0. From Wikimedia Commons.

18.2 Cell Movement

Motor proteins, such as myosins, dyneins, and kinesins (figure 18.7), move along cytoskeletal filaments via a force-dependent mechanism that is driven by the hydrolysis of ATP molecules. Motor proteins propel themselves along the cytoskeleton using a mechanochemical cycle of filament binding, conformational change, filament release, conformation reversal, and filament rebinding. In most cases, the conformational change(s) on the motor protein prevents subsequent nucleotide binding or hydrolysis until the prior round of hydrolysis and release is complete.

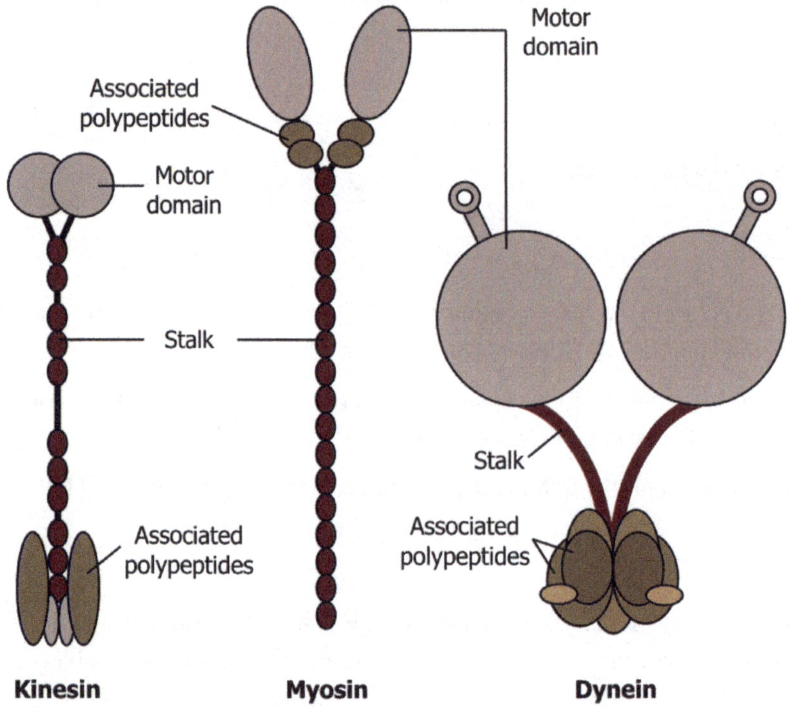

Figure 18.7: Comparison of the three different motor proteins.

Myosin

Myosin can be characterized as conventional or unconventional, with characteristic head groups (that bind ATP) and unique tails. Myosin is essential for muscle contraction, and this occurs in striated muscle (skeletal and cardiac) after specific binding sites on the actin have been exposed in response to the interaction between calcium ions (Ca^{2+}) and proteins (troponin and tropomyosin) that "shield" the actin-binding sites. Ca^{2+} is also required for the contraction of smooth muscle, although its role is different: here Ca^{2+} activates enzymes, which in turn activate myosin heads. All muscles require adenosine triphosphate (ATP) to continue the process of contracting, and they all relax when the Ca^{2+} is removed and the actin-binding sites are re-shielded.

Dynein

Dynein is a large motor protein that typically transports organelles (lysosomes or endosomes). It moves toward the minus end (α-tubulin) of microtubules, which is in the direction of the cell body.

Kinesin

Kinesin is a relatively small motor protein that moves membrane-bound cargo (e.g., vesicles). In contrast to dynein, most move toward the plus end β-tubulin) of the microtubules, which is typically away from the cell body. Figure 18.8 nicely summarizes the location and general role of each of these motor proteins.

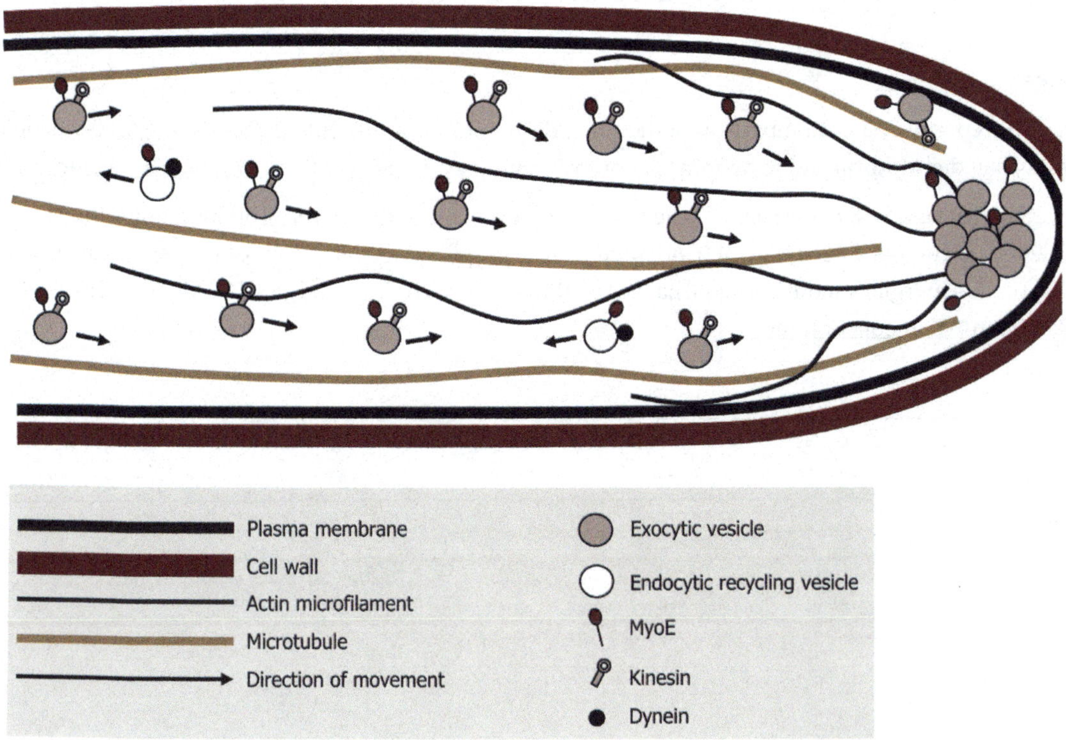

Figure 18.8: Summary of the roles and movement of the motor proteins along various cytoskeletal elements.

- Myosin can be found associated actin filaments, generally moving cargo (exocytic vesicles) away from the cell body. There is also a role in actin polymerization, which is essential for cellular motility.
- Kinesin is associated with microtubules moving cargo away from the cell body.
- In contrast, dynein, is associated with microtubules moving cargo (endocytic vesicles) toward the cell body.

18.2 References and resources

Text

Clark, M. A. *Biology*, 2nd ed. Houston, TX: OpenStax College, Rice University, 2018, Chapter 4: Cell Structure, Chapter 5: Structure and Function of the Plasma Membranes.

Karp, G., and J. G. Patton. *Cell and Molecular Biology: Concepts and Experiments*, 7th ed. Hoboken, NJ: John Wiley, 2013, Chapter 9: The Cytoskeleton and Cell Mobility.

Le, T., and V. Bhushan. *First Aid for the USMLE Step 1*, 29th ed. New York: McGraw Hill Education, 2018, 48–49.

Figures

Grey, Kindred, Figure 18.7 Comparison of the three different motor proteins. 2021. CC BY SA 4.0. Adapted from Aufbau der Motorproteine by keine Autoren genannt. CC BY SA 4.0. From Wikimedia Commons.

Grey, Kindred, Figure 18.8 Summary of the roles and movement of the motor proteins along various cytoskeletal elements. 2021. CC BY 4.0. Adapted from A simplified model for myosin V (MyoE) function at the hyphal tip in Aspergillus nidulans - journal.pone.0031218.g009B by Taheri-Talesh N, Xiong Y, Oakley BR. CC BY 2.5. From Wikimedia Commons.

19. Extracellular Matrix

Learning Objectives

- Define the general structure and function of the glycocalyx and extracellular matrix.
- Describe the function and structure of basement membranes (basal lamina).
- Describe the membrane proteins involved in the adhesion of cells to noncellular surfaces.
- Compare and contrast the structures and functions of the different cell junctions.
- Describe the membrane proteins involved in cell–cell adhesion.

About this Chapter

Most animal cells release materials into the extracellular space. The primary components of these materials are glycoproteins and the protein collagen. Collectively, these materials are called the extracellular matrix. Not only does the extracellular matrix hold the cells together to form a tissue, but it also allows the cells within the tissue to communicate with each other.

19.1 Extracellular Matrix

Extracellular matrix

The extracellular matrix consists of a network of substances secreted by cells (figure 19.1). This dynamic structure has many roles in cellular adhesion, signaling, and overall cellular organization.

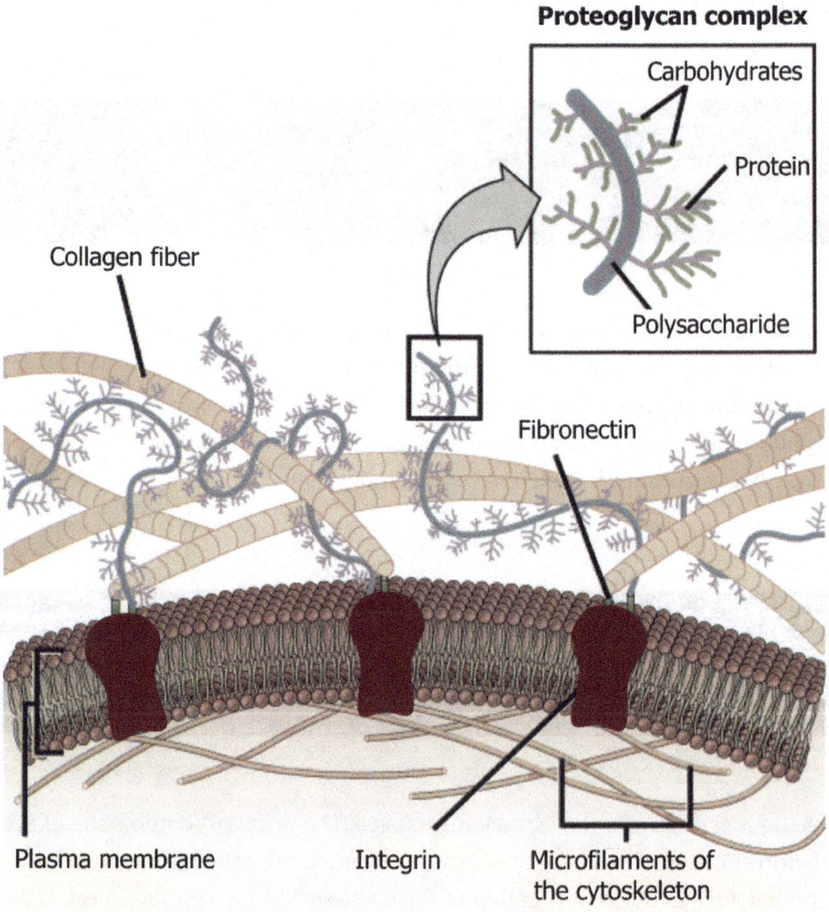

Figure 19.1: Overview of the extracellular matrix.

Glycocalyx

In addition to the many proteins in the matrix, there are some essential carbohydrate components that make up the glycocalyx. This is a carbohydrate "coat" that forms a barrier around the plasma membrane, can bind regulatory factors, and can mediate cell-cell interactions.

Proteins of the matrix

The major components of the extracellular matrix form a fibrous, secreted network.

Fibronectin

Fibronectin is a dimer held together by disulfide bonds. These dimers assemble in structural modules that serve as binding sites for other proteins such as heparin, collagen, and fibrin. These proteins are the "matrix" that allows other proteins to dock, and it has RGD loops that serve as integrin binding sites.

Collagen

Collagen is synthesized by fibroblasts and is the most abundant protein in the body. There are twenty-seven types of collagen, and it is often a triple helix, stabilized by hydrogen bonding. There are additional nonfibrillar forms that can form web-like structures. Synthesis of collagen requires vitamin C for formation of hydroxyproline.

As collagen is a major component to connective tissue, it plays key roles in tendons, cornea, blood vessels, hair, and cartilage. Disorders of collagen synthesis are implicated in osteogenesis imperfecta, dwarfism, and skeletal deformities.

Proteoglycans

Structurally proteoglycans contain both proteins plus glycosaminoglycans (carbohydrates) and take on a bottle-brush structure (figure 19.1). They assemble into larger complexes, bound to a central hyaluronic acid. The overall structure is negatively charged, which attracts water, allowing it to function as a cushion.

Laminin

Laminin consists of three glycoproteins linked through disulfide bonds. They bind cell-surface receptors and are important during development and cell migration.

Integrins

Integrins span the plasma membrane and connect the matrix to the cellular environment (inside-out or outside-in signaling). They are associated with fibronectin (RGD sequences) on the extracellular side and have both active and inactive states (figure 19.2).

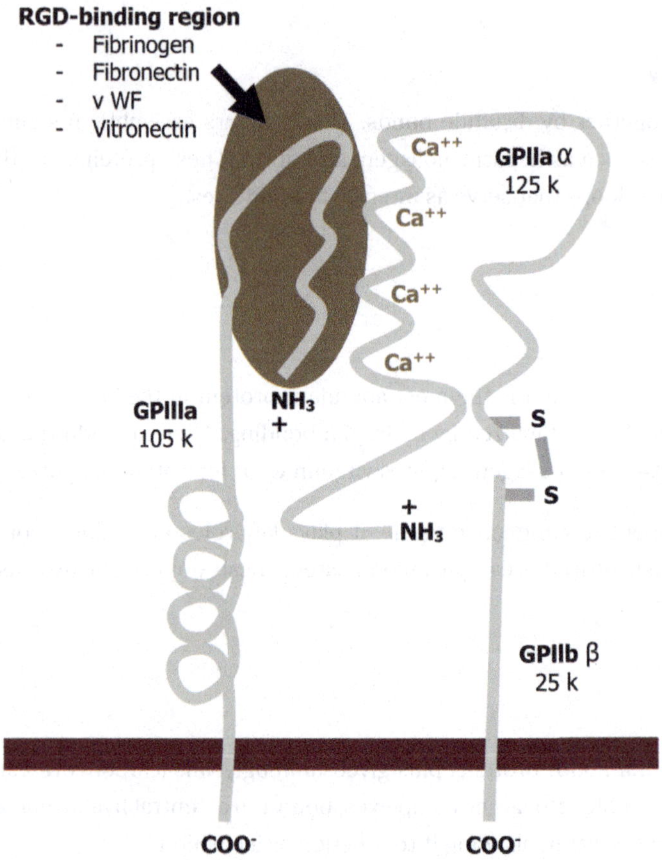

Figure 19.2: Schematic of integrin structure. The protein spans the plasma membrane and is an extracellular domain that can bind other matrix proteins.

Matrix metalloproteinases

The matrix is a dynamic component and is remodeled as a part of normal growth and development. It can also be reorganized as a result of disease or pathology such as arthritis or atherosclerosis.

A family of enzymes, termed matrix metalloproteinases, is responsible for this remodeling, and they require metal for catalysis. Zinc is the typical cofactor, although some enzymes in the family require cobalt.

Cell adhesion to the substratum

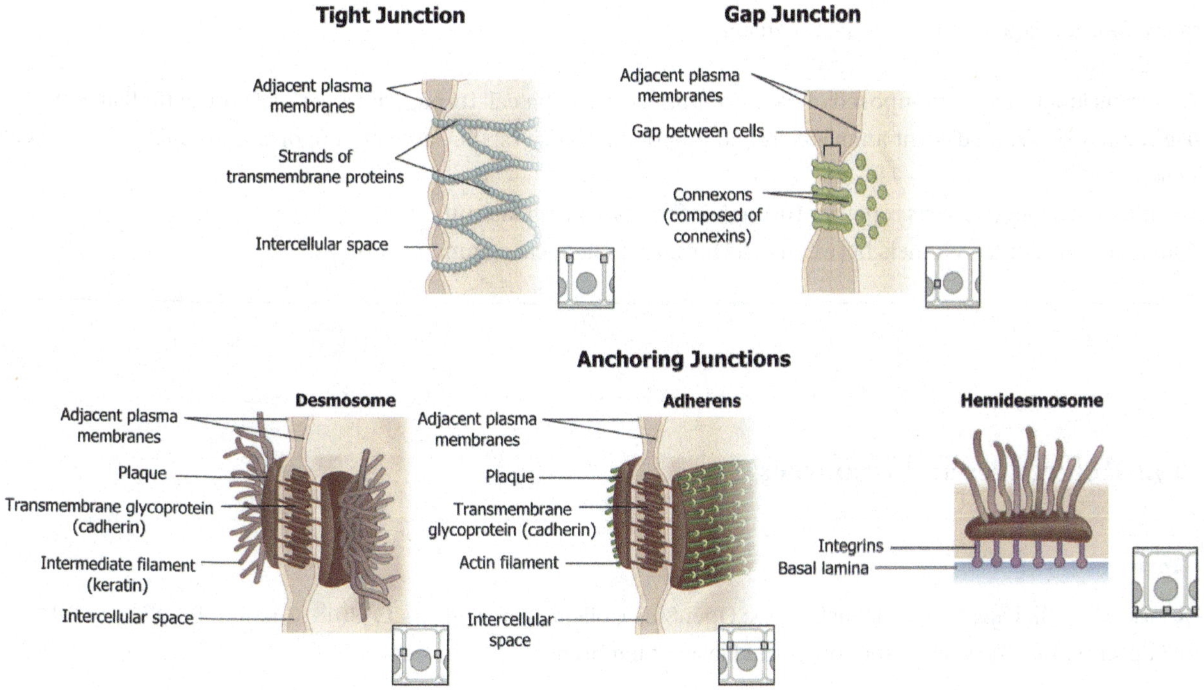

Figure 19.3: Summary of cell adhesion mechanisms.

Focal adhesions and hemidesmosomes (figure 19.3) serve to anchor cells to the substratum.

Focal adhesions are a cluster of rapidly assembling and disassembling proteins that involves a cluster of integrins connected to actin in the cytoskeleton.

Hemidesmosomes are the tightest of all in vivo attachments. They consist of intermediate filaments (keratin) and form an attachment between the basal surface of epithelial cells to the basement membrane.

Cell–cell adhesion

Cells attach to one another through interactions of cell adhesion molecules (CAMs). These interactions can be transient involving one protein on one cell and one on another cell. There are several major classes of CAMs with biological relevance. Their roles are summarized in the table below.

CAM	Characteristics	Role
Selectins (E,L,P)	Membrane glycoproteins	Bind carbohydrate ligands; transient interactions
Ig superfamily	Calcium independent	Modulate interactions with immune cells
Integrins	Interacts with the Ig superfamily	RGD domains for interaction with the matrix
Cadherins	Calcium-dependent glycoproteins	Join similar cells

Table 19.1: Major classes of CAMs with biological relevance.

Cell–cell adhesive junctions

There are four kinds of connections between cells:

1. Adherens junctions are composed of cadherins and anchor the cell through interactions with actin filaments.
2. Tight junctions join adjacent animal cells and function as barriers; they are very important in capillary endothelial cells.
3. Desmosomes join two cells together through interactions with keratin.
4. Gap junctions act as channels between cells for direct chemical communication.

19.1 References and resources

Text

Clark, M. A. *Biology*, 2nd ed. Houston, TX: OpenStax College, Rice University, 2018, Chapter 4: Cell Structure, Chapter 5: Structure and Function of the Plasma Membranes.

Karp, G., and J. G. Patton. *Cell and Molecular Biology: Concepts and Experiments*, 7th ed. Hoboken, NJ: John Wiley, 2013, Chapter 7: Interactions between Cells and Their Environment.

Le, T., and V. Bhushan. *First Aid for the USMLE Step 1*, 29th ed. New York: McGraw Hill Education, 2018, 50–51.

Figures

Grey, Kindred, Figure 19.1 Overview of the extracellular matrix. 2021. https://archive.org/details/19.1_20210926. CC BY 4.0. Adapted from Figure 16. CC BY 4.0. From Open Oregon.

Grey, Kindred, Figure 19.2 Schematic of integrin structure... 2021. CC BY SA 3.0. Adapted from Integrin by Odysseus1479. CC BY SA 3.0. From Wikimedia Commons.

Grey, Kindred, Figure 19.3 Summary of cell adhesion mechanisms. 2021. https://archive.org/details/19.3_20210926. CC BY 3.0. Adapted from 402 Types of Cell Junctions new by OpenStax College. CC BY 3.0. From Wikimedia Commons.

Made in the USA
Monee, IL
02 November 2026

67386641R00155